WQ100

*Recent Advances*

# Obstetrics and Gynaecology 24

35.00

# Recent Advances in Obstetrics and Gynaecology 23
*Edited by John Bonnar and William Dunlop*

*Recent Advances in*

# Obstetrics and Gynaecology 24

*Edited by*

**William Dunlop** PhD FRCSEd FRCOG

Emeritus Professor of Obstetrics and Gynaecology,
Newcastle University,
Newcastle upon Tyne, UK

**William L Ledger** MA DPhil FRCOG

Professor of Obstetrics and Gynaecology,
Head of Department, Academic Unit of Reproductive
and Developmental Medicine,
University of Sheffield,
Sheffield, UK

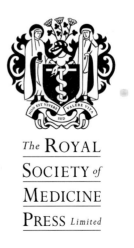

The ROYAL
SOCIETY *of*
MEDICINE
PRESS *Limited*

© 2008 Royal Society of Medicine Press Ltd

Published by the Royal Society of Medicine Press Ltd
1 Wimpole Street, London W1G 0AE, UK
Tel: +44 (0)20 7290 2921
Fax: +44 (0)20 7290 2929
Email: publishing@rsm.ac.uk
Website: www.rsmpress.co.uk

British Library Cataloguing in Publication Data
A catalogue record for this book is available from the British Library
ISBN 978-1-85315-699-1

*Distribution in Europe and Rest of World:*

Marston Book Services Ltd
PO Box 269, Abingdon
Oxon OX14 4YN, UK
Tel: +44 (0)1235 465500
Fax: +44 (0)1235 465555
Email: direct.order@marston.co.uk

*Distribution in the USA and Canada:*

Royal Society of Medicine Press Ltd
c/o BookMasters Inc
30 Amberwood Parkway
Ashland, OH 44805, USA
Tel: +1 800 247 6553/+1 800 266 5564
Fax: +1 419 281 6883
Email: order@bookmasters.com

*Distribution in Australia and New Zealand:*

Elsevier Australia
30–52 Smidmore Street
Marrickville NSW 2204, Australia
Tel: +61 2 9517 8999
Fax: +61 2 9517 2249
Email: service@elsevier.com.au

Editorial services and typesetting by BA & GM Haddock, Ford, Midlothian, UK

Printed in Great Britain by Bell & Bain, Glasgow, UK

# Contents

# Contributors

**Susana Aguilera** MBBS
Specialist in Obstetrics and Gynecology, University of Chile; and Clinical Research Fellow, St Michael's Hospital, University of Bristol, UK

**Gaity Ahmad** MRCOG
Specialist Registrar, Department of Obstetrics and Gynaecology, Stepping Hill Hospital, Stockport, UK

**Saad A.K. Amer** MBChB MSc MD MRCOG
Associate Professor and Consultant Gynaecologist, University of Nottingham, Derby City General Hospital, Derby, UK

**Malathy Appasamy** MRCOG
Clinical Research Fellow, UCL Institute for Women's Health, University College London, London, UK

**Sabaratnam Arulkumaran** PhD FRCOG
Professor, Department of Obstetrics and Gynaecology, St George's Hospital, University of London, London, UK

**Stephen L. Atkin** PhD FRCP
Professor in Diabetes and Enocrinology, The Michael White Centre for Diabetes and Endocrinology, University of Hull, Hull, UK

**Marina Baldi** PhD
GENOMA – Molecular Genetics Laboratories, Rome, Italy

**Chris Brewer** MBBCh
Specialist Registrar in Obstetrics and Gynaecology, Department of Obstetrics and Gynaecology, St James's University Hospital, Leeds, UK

**Stergios K. Doumouchtsis** PhD MRCOG
Senior Specialist Registrar, Department of Obstetrics and Gynaecology, St George's Hospital, University of London, London, UK

**William Dunlop** PhD FRCSEd FRCOG
Emeritus Professor of Obstetrics and Gynaecology, Newcastle University, Newcastle upon Tyne, UK

**Alaa El-Ghobashy** MD MRCOG
Specialist Registrar in Obstetrics and Gynaecology, Department of Obstetrics and Gynaecology, St James's University Hospital, Leeds, UK

**Francesco Fiorentino** PhD
CEO and Lab Director, GENOMA – Molecular Genetics Laboratory, EmbryoGen – Centre for Preimplantation Genetic Diagnosis, Rome, Italy

**Robert Fraser** MD FRCOG
Reader, Reproductive & Developmental Medicine, School of Medicine and Biomedical Sciences, University of Sheffield and Honorary Consultant at Royal Hallamshire Hospital, Sheffield, UK

**WanLye Haw** BMedSci MRCOG
Specialist Registrar in Obstetrics and Gynaecology, Department of Obstetrics and Gynaecology, St James's University Hospital, Leeds, UK

**Tony Hollingworth** MBChB MBA PhD FRCS(Ed) FRCOG
Consultant Obstetrician and Gynaecologist, Whipps Cross University Hospital, Leytonstone, London, UK

**Jane Hook** MBBChir MA(Cantab) MRCP
Specialist Registrar in Medical Oncology, St James' Institute of Oncology, St James' University Hospital, Leeds, UK

**William L. Ledger** MA DPhil FRCOG
Professor of Obstetrics and Gynaecology, Head of Department, Academic Unit of Reproductive and Developmental Medicine, University of Sheffield, Sheffield, UK

**Alastair McKelvey** MRCOG MB MCh BAO
Subspecialty Fellow in Materno-Fetal Medicine, Fetal Medicine Unit, Elizabeth Garrett Anderson Obstetric Hospital, University College London Hospitals NHS Trust, London, UK

**James A. McIntyre** MB ChB FRCOG
Executive Director, Perinatal HIV Research Unit, University of the Witwatersrand, Johannesburg, South Africa

**Deirdre J. Murphy** MD MRCOG
Professor of Obstetrics, University Department of Obstetrics and Gynaecology, Trinity College Dublin & Coombe Women and Infants Hospital, Dublin, Republic of Ireland

**Shanthi Muttukrishna** PhD
Lecturer in Reproductive Science, UCL Institute for Women's Health, University College London, London, UK

**Tom O'Gorman** MBChB BAO DCH MRCOG
Specialist Registrar in Obstetrics and Gynaecology, Whipps Cross University Hospital, Leytonstone, London, UK

**Alka Prakash** MD MRCOG
Sub-specialty Registrar in Reproductive Medicine, Cambridge University Hospitals at Addenbrooke's Hospital, Cambridge, UK

**Norbert Pateisky** MD
Professor of Obstetrics and Gynaecology, Subdepartment of Clinical Risk Management, Department of Obstetrics and Gynecology, University of Vienna, Vienna, Austria

**Lesley Regan** MD FRCOG
Professor and Head, Department of Obstetrics and Gynaecology, Imperial Healthcare NHS Trust at St Mary's Hospital, London, UK

**Charles Rodeck** MBBS BSc DSc(Med) FRCOG FRCPath FMedSci
Emeritus Professor of Obstetrics and Gynaecology, University College London, London, UK

**Thozhukat Sathyapalan** MRCP
Department of Diabetes and Enocrinology, The Michael White Centre for Diabetes and Endocrinology, University of Hull, Hull, UK

**Michael Seckl** MBBS MD FRCP PhD
Professor of Molecular Cancer Medicine and Head of Department of Medical Oncology, Charing Cross Hospital, London, UK

**David Shepherd** MB ChB FRCA
Consultant Obstetric Anaesthetist, Sheffield Teaching Hospitals NHS Foundation Trust, Sheffield, UK

**Peter Soothill** MBBS BSc MD FRCOG
Emeritus Professor of Maternal and Fetal Medicine, University of Bristol, Bristol, UK; and Consultant in Fetal Medicine, St Michael's Hospital, Bristol, UK

**Derek Tuffnell** FRCOG
Honorary Visiting Professor in Obstetrics, Bradford University and Consultant Obstetrician and Gynaecologist, Department of Obstetrics and Gynaecology, Bradford Royal Infirmary, Bradford, UK.

**Jennifer Walsh** MRCOG MRCPI
Specialist Registrar in Obstetrics and Gynaecology, Coombe Women and Infants Hospital, Dublin, Republic of Ireland

**Andrew J.S. Watson** MRCOG
Consultant Obstetrician and Gynaecologist, Tameside General Hospital, Ashton under Lyne, UK

**Sue Zaher** MBChB
Gynaecology Research Fellow, Department of Radiology, Imperial Healthcare NHS Trust at St Mary's Hospital, London, UK

**Ophelia Ziwenga** MBChB(Hons) FRCA FCARCSI
Clinical Research Fellow in Regional Anaesthesia, University of Alberta, Canada

*Alastair McKelvey  Charles Rodeck*

**1**

# Fetal problems associated with recreational drugs

The potential harm that the unborn can suffer as a result of what the pregnant mother takes has been partly understood since ancient times. Aristotle warned against alcohol consumption in pregnancy in the 4th century BC by describing the birth of deformed children to drunken women.[1]

Many of the substances used for pleasure or euphoria diminish the user's capacity to think rationally, and so render the pregnancy vulnerable to further hazards on the part of the disinhibited behaviour of the mother. Some recreational drugs actually change the user's personality. This can result in a solipsistic attitude on the pregnant mother's part, which poses a particular challenge for her carers.

Following this introduction, the three sections of this chapter will look initially at the principles involved, secondly at specific substances and their effects, and finally will conclude with key points for clinical obstetric practice. The effects on the developing fetus of various substances used for pleasure by pregnant women, both legal and illegal are considered. The term 'recreational drugs' is used in its very widest sense to include the major agents, including: drugs of abuse (referred to as narcotics in the US); volatiles, such as glue and aerosol excipients; and the socially wide-spread tobacco, alcoholic and even caffeinated drinks. We consider associated physical anomalies and abnormalities of development and growth which may ensue, as well as the more subtle effects which those substances may have on the formation and function of the central nervous system. We are aware that this will not represent an exhaustive examination of every possible recreational substance

**Alastair McKelvey** MRCOG MB MCH BAO (for correspondence)
Subspecialty Fellow in Materno-Fetal Medicine, Fetal Medicine Unit, Elizabeth Garrett Anderson Obstetric Hospital, University College London Hospitals NHS Trust, Huntley Street, London WC1E 6AU, UK
E-mail: alastairmckelvey@doctors.org.uk

**Charles Rodeck** MB BS BSc DSc(Med) FRCOG FRCPath FMedSci
Emeritus Professor of Obstetrics and Gynaecology, University College London, London, UK

available to the multiplicity of world cultures, but will hopefully provide as basis of understanding mechanisms of harm as well as specific, common examples. Other potential teratogens, such as prescribed drugs, radiation, environmental insults such as temperature imbalance, dietary essential nutrient deficiencies, blood gas composition and stress fall outside the scope of this article.

Long-term effects of fetal exposure, persisting into childhood and adulthood are increasingly recognised as a significant issue. Modifications of fetal programming may play a role in causing deleterious effects on adult physical and mental health. These include increased risks of certain malignant diseases. Although this falls outside our strict remit, the concept must be borne in mind when considering the impact of recreational substance use within pregnancy.

Elucidation of precise associations between recreational drug use and harmful effect is rarely possible, or ethically legitimate, in humans, and so much of the information is derived from the use of animal models. Where human data exist, they are often compromised by factors such as multiple agent usage, poor recall and co-existing medical and social issues. We will look initially at the general principles by which harm can occur, before examining each substance or group of substances and its known, as well as presumed, effects in turn. It is also difficult to draw precise conclusions, even when patterns of use are known. Quantities of active drug vary widely between sources. Even relatively standard production recreational drugs (such as cigarettes) vary in their individual composition from brand to brand. Tobacco also contains multiple compounds each of which may have differing harmful effects on different systems, at different times. We do not all make our coffee to the same strength, alcoholic drinks are of differing strengths and heavy users do not generally monitor the total dosage. Illegal drugs are subject to no quality or dosage control, and so may contain multiple contaminants, each with potential teratogenic activity, as well as massively differing effective doses of the supposed compound. In animal models these dosage and contamination issues can be better controlled, but in human observational studies, they lead to significant problems in data analysis. Thus, while in animals we may be able to determine dosage thresholds above which teratogenic effects are observed and key developmental stages of vulnerability, we cannot necessarily extrapolate those same effective doses or timings to humans.

The incidence of recreational drug use remains elusive. Maternal history-taking is not a reliable way of ascertaining recreational substance usage. Some antenatal units, especially in the US, screen urine and blood samples for illegal drugs and their metabolites. While the ethical basis of this practice is debatable, the practical limits of its usefulness rest on the half-lives of these drugs and the performance of the assays used to test for them. In general, body fluid testing provides only a snapshot of whether the drugs which the testing battery is designed to detect were used in the last few days. The use of more persistent body derivatives, such as hair and nails, has proved useful for analysing drug use over time. These tools have been applied in researching substance abuse and stage of gestation. In one small controlled study, using ELISA analysis, evidence of drug use in the first trimester was found in 10 of 22 women whose babies were affected by gastroschisis, compared to 2 of 25 controls. However, when an apparently more specific assay was used, these data fell to 4 and 0, respectively.[2]

## PRINCIPLES OF RECREATIONAL SUBSTANCE USE IN PREGNANCY

### EMBRYOLOGY

The embryo's susceptibility to teratogens is determined by various factors. These include: (i) the stage(s) of embryonic development at which exposure occurs, the duration and pattern of exposure; and (ii) the pharmacokinetics and pharmacodynamics of the teratogen (including the peak effective dose, the formation of metabolites, their teratogenicity, and half-lives in the fetus and mother). The genotypical susceptibility of the fetus to the teratogen is key. But genetic variations in the ability of both the fetus and mother to metabolise teratogens are also factors in determining the scale of the final insult.

Harmful action upon fetal development and the risk of developing adult disease are influenced by the fetal environment. The development of the pregnancy may be considered in three stages: (i) the fertilisation/implantation stage; (ii) the embryonic stage; and (iii) the fetal stage. Environmental insults in the first stage of development tend to exert an 'all or nothing' effect, namely a catastrophic impact with failure of the pregnancy (miscarriage), or apparently unimpaired survival. The embryonic stage involves the intricate development of organ foundation. The primordial organs and their structural development each have key time periods when exposure to specific agents can induce profound and permanent malformation or agenesis. Examples of these will be discussed below under specific drugs. The third (fetal) stage of development sees the differentiation of tissues, organ growth and maturation. Recreational substances used in the fetogenic period thus have the potential to cause functional defects in organ or organ systems or neurodevelopmental problems. The use of the same substance (*e.g.* tobacco) may thus have different effects depending on the stage of pregnancy at which exposure occurs.

An example of a specific anomaly, which is suspected of being linked with recreational substance use, is gastroschisis. Its aetiology is felt to be vascular, with interruption of blood supply at a key period resulting in the anterior wall defect.[3] The vascular disruptive effects of many recreational substances, notably vasoconstrictors such as cocaine and amphetamines, are well described in animals.[4] It is, therefore, reasonable to consider the possibility that these agents may cause gastroschisis. The rising incidence of gastroschisis has prompted many to consider whether an increase in recreational substance use could account for the increase.[5] However, the increasing rate of teenage pregnancy may also be a significant factor. One small study has suggested that the mothers of affected fetuses are more likely to show evidence of recreational substance use.[2]

The formation of the central nervous system needs to be considered separately. This is partly because of its immense complexity and its uniqueness in developing well beyond the period *in utero* into childhood. This is well illustrated by the simple consideration that the neonatal brain tissue mass is approximately 25% of the mass in the adult, but in the 24-month-old child it is 75% of the final adult mass. This relatively prolonged neurodevelopment is peculiar to our species amongst the animals and renders the use of other species models in assessing the effects of substances on brain and behaviour highly problematic. Another reason why the developing central nervous system is vulnerable to many recreational substances is because of the very reason that the mother takes the psychotrophic substance in the first place, for the perceived pleasurable impact on her central nervous system. Recreational substances are typically lipophilic and so, characteristically, cross the placental barrier and blood–brain barrier well, exerting their desired effect on mood or perception. So those substances, or their active metabolites, which can cross the placenta, will also cross the fetal blood–brain barrier.

The embryonic organogenesis of the brain is followed by two stages. Initially, neurones multiply. This is followed by the proliferation of glial cells. In the second stage, axonal growth with synaptic formation and dendritic branching occurs. The processes of myelination and neurotransmitter system development also occur in this second phase. There is considerable heterogeneity in the rate and timing of the development of neuronal groups, allowing teratogens to cause harm at many different phases of development. Harm can manifest as the depletion in total number of neuronal cells globally or as localised lesions, if sufficient, leading to microcephaly. This damage may be perpetuated during post-natal development by the body's own repair and re-organisation. A permanent reduction in the neuronal population size and density compromises the scope of synaptic connections with other brain areas, leading to intellectual impairment. The effect of damage to the formation of neurotransmitter systems can start a process of secondary injury, affecting subtle functions such as behaviour and thought processes.

Fetal brain development involves the organisation and differentiation of neurones and connections. This process is most marked at the cerebral cortex.

## MANAGING SUBSTANCE ABUSE IN PREGNANCY

Women using illicit drugs pose a significant challenge to obstetric care. The perceptions of the user may prevent her supplying an honest history. She may expect her attendants to be disapproving and critical. She may feel ashamed, or fear that disclosure will expose her to prosecution or possible removal of her baby after birth (in some jurisdictions, and circumstances, she may be right). Her recall of what she took and when she took it is likely to be incomplete, partly because of the very actions of the drugs themselves upon perception and memory.

### ANTENATAL CARE

In order to obtain the most accurate information, the history should be taken with a neutral attitude in a comfortable environment. Insisting upon a commitment to reduce or stop usage is regarded as counterproductive.[6]

Information about the partner's drug use should be sought. A sexual history should also be sensitively explored, including the potential history of prostitution. Further infectious disease testing may be indicated from the history.

The overall goal is to stop, or reduce, the use of the recreational substance. However, in some cases (*e.g.* heroin addiction), this may not be achievable, and the use of a substitute may be preferable. The English Department of Health recommends that: 'obstetric departments should develop good links with local drug specialists, GPs and the local social services'.[7]

As with other groups of antenatal patients with specialised health needs, substance abusers have been found to benefit from care by a liaison midwife, with specialised training in the management of substance abuse.[8]

These clinics would ideally comprise a consultant and trainee in obstetrics, a consultant and trainee in addiction medicine (generally from a psychiatry background, although general practitioners also specialise in this field), a psychologist, a health visitor (with particular training in the field), liaison midwives, social workers and a phlebotomist. The role of social workers is difficult: they can be of great help to patients with housing and other social benefits but their responsibility for the welfare of the child after birth (as well as any existing children) has the potential to conflict with the mother's actions and wishes. A consultation with an anaesthetist may be beneficial, as analgesia requirements in labour may differ from the non drug-using population.

Those undertaking ultrasound scans for fetal anomaly should be vigilant for structural anomalies. Further specialist ultrasound scanning for specific defects or syndromes (*e.g.* fetal alcohol syndrome) may be appropriate. Consideration should be given to serial growth scans and uterine artery Doppler ultrasonography.

## INTRAPARTUM CARE

These pregnancies require constant fetal monitoring during labour. Disturbances of fetal heart rhythm and rate have been observed with some drugs. Parenteral opioid use may be problematic in some drug abusers (especially heroin). Higher doses may be needed, which can fall outside usual maximum safe dosage regimens. For this reason, regional blockade may be preferable. A record should be kept of the umbilical cord vessel blood gas analyses.

## POSTNATAL CARE

Paediatricians should be notified about the history before delivery and careful neonatal assessment looking for evidence of birth defects or withdrawal effects should be performed soon after birth. Care on a transitional care unit is preferred. Occasionally, the mother's behaviour may have given concern about her fitness to care for the child. In these circumstances, early liaison with the social work team is vital. Symptoms of maternal withdrawal (restlessness, tremor, sweating) should be sought. Sedation or replacement therapy may then be indicated.

## SPECIFIC SUBSTANCES AND MANAGEMENT STRATEGIES

### ALCOHOL

Alcohol is one of the oldest of all recreational drugs, with evidence of production and inebriation in many of the world's ancient civilisations. Although long suspected, the excessive consumption of alcohol in pregnancy was finally accepted to be harmful by the scientific community during the early 1970s.[9] However, controversy remains over the effect of lower doses.

Heavy alcohol consumption is unmistakably connected with a specific disorder spectrum generally known as the fetal alcohol syndrome or fetal alcohol spectrum disorder. The characteristic features are:

1. Growth retardation (*in utero* and *ex utero*).

2. Neurodevelopmental problems, including behavioural problems.

3. Specific dysmorphic features – microcephaly, shortened flat philtrum, short palpebral fissures, elongated mid-face, small upturned nose and low-set asymmetrical ears.

4. Cardiac (ventriculoseptal and atrial septal defects) and joint anomalies.

The incidence of fetal alcohol syndrome is not clear. There is no simple diagnostic test and reported incidences vary enormously across geographic areas and racial subgroups.[10–13] Heavy consumption of alcohol does not invariably lead to fetal alcohol syndrome, raising the consideration of genetic susceptibility. Specific abnormalities have also been associated with heavy gestational alcohol consumption, namely brain abnormalities,[14] oral clefting[15] and childhood malignancies.[16]

Considerable controversy remains about 'safe' levels of alcohol consumption during pregnancy.[17] A recent systematic review compared low level use (up to 83 g/week) with abstinence and showed no consistent evidence of harmful effect. Though, as the authors pointed out, absence of evidence of harm does not equate to proof of safety.[18] The Royal College of Obstetricians and Gynaecologists acknowledges the difficulty for women trying to make an informed decision, but points out that 'the only way to be absolutely certain that your baby is not harmed by alcohol is not to drink at all during pregnancy or while you are trying for a baby'.[19] The English Department of Health appeared to be recommending abstinence in a press release of May 2007 by stating 'avoid alcohol if pregnant or trying to conceive', though tempered this line in the same statement later by advising 'women who do choose to drink, should have no more than one to two units per week'.

Epidemiological evidence[20] suggests that alcohol consumption in women of child-bearing age is increasing. In the UK, where alcohol misuse is high, at least 86% of women regularly consume alcohol (62% in the US). Of these, 42% had three or more 'standard' drinks per 'drinking' day (equivalent to 24 g of ethanol) and 9% had six or more drinks on one occasion at least twice weekly (48 g of ethanol). The proportion of British women aged 16–24 years drinking over 110 g of alcohol per week more than doubled from 1988/1989 to 2002/2003 (from 15% to 33%). The incidence of alcohol dependence (as defined by ICD10) in British women is estimated at 2.1%.

## Management of alcohol dependence

Fortunately, most women change their life-style when they become aware of their pregnancy, including cessation of, or serious reduction in, alcohol consumption. Motivation and the availability of support are important factors in this decision.

Alcohol-dependent women may benefit from co-ordinated care between maternity and psychiatric teams, perhaps at a combined antenatal clinic. Social circumstances, exposure to other recreational substances and domestic violence may all need to be addressed by the joint team. Attention to dietary deficiencies, especially the B vitamins, and to the possibility of hepatic compromise is important in heavy alcohol users. Acute withdrawal episodes appear to be safely managed by benzodiazepine use. Disulfiram is not recommended during pregnancy because of its teratogenic potential.[21]

## TOBACCO

Tobacco is perhaps the most commonly used recreational substance in pregnancy. Among all the recreational substances, tobacco smoke is the most complex because of its approximately 2000 individual constituents. The particulate phase (10%) contains nicotine and tar. Tar refers to the mixture of polycyclic aromatic hydrocarbons, such as phenols and benzenes, which are carcinogenic. The remaining 90% of gaseous compounds includes carbon dioxide, cyanides, aldehydes, organic acids and carbon monoxide. Nicotine is generally accepted as the compound responsible for the main pleasurable response, as well as the addictive action.[22]

The sight of antenatal patients smoking cigarettes at the entrances to maternity units is still all too familiar to obstetricians in the UK. An overall decrease in the smoking population, cessation classes and the novel use of tobacco substitutes, may be diminishing the incidence in the developed world. About a third of smokers reduce their smoking significantly, or cease, when they become aware of the pregnancy.[23]

A large observational study[24] examining over 87,000 pregnancies revealed a significant association between smoking and placental abruption (doubling of risk) as well as a smaller (36%), though significant, increase in risk of placenta praevia. Interestingly, the risks did not appear to be dose-dependent. There is also a link between smoking and the risk of still-birth, though it is unclear by what mechanism.[25]

Tobacco's association with intra-uterine growth restriction, first shown six decades ago,[26] is now widely accepted.[27] Unlike abruption and placenta praevia, the effect on birth weight and biometry does seem to be dose-dependent. Indeed, there is anecdotal evidence this action may be deliberately exploited by mothers wishing to have a small baby and 'easier' labour. Paradoxically, there are data to show that smoking in pregnancy decreases the incidence of hypertension/pre-eclampsia by about half.[28]

### Management of smoking in pregnancy

Unfortunately, public health campaigns illustrating the detrimental effects of smoking on the fetus do not appear to affect behaviour.[29] Most maternity units in the UK offer pregnant smokers referral to smoking cessation clinics. Women who attend these services often do well, mainly because they are well motivated to begin with. Unfortunately, only a minority of suitable women choose to attend these clinics, though their overall positive effect is significant.[30] The use of nicotine therapy remains controversial. However, many authors[31] advocate sparing use as preferable to tobacco, with its multiple constituents. The antidepressant bupropion has been employed with some encouraging results.[33]

## COCAINE

Cocaine inhibits the re-uptake of noradrenaline and dopamine (which gives its euphoric action) and so is a highly potent vasopressor and, therefore, especially fetotoxic. Its actions on maternal, placental and fetal vasculature can be profound. There is a strong association with placental abruption; in addition, subclinical retrochorial/retroplacental haemorrhage occurs with cocaine use, leading to impaired placental function and intra-uterine growth restriction, fetal hypoxic injury or fetal death. In a meta-analysis of 11 studies,[34] the pooled odds ratio for abruptio placentae and maternal cocaine use was 3.92 (95% confidence interval, 2.77–5.46).

Cocaine is used either as an intranasal inhalation of powder or as 'crack' cocaine. The latter involves mixing with an excipient such as bicarbonate of soda, before heating over a flame and smoking or intravenously injecting the resulting residue. Cocaine can result in personality changes, rendering the user more self-centred. The incidence of use is difficult to determine, and varies geographically.[35] Crack cocaine appears to be particularly hazardous to the fetus,[36] possibly because the heating process results in the formation of methylecgonidine (MEG) which has been shown to cause bronchoconstriction in guinea pigs[37] and cardiovascular changes in squirrel monkeys.[38] Adverse fetal and neonatal effects have been shown to be dose-dependent and remain even after other variables are controlled for.[39]

The vasopressive action of cocaine has also been held responsible for structural anomalies including renal, cardiac, gastrointestinal, ophthalmic, genitourinary, skeletal and respiratory defects.[40] By causing vasoconstriction, hypertension, and infarcts in any structure, cocaine exposure at specific times of development *in utero* has the potential to interrupt key moments of embryological development and thus cause a wide spectrum of disorders.[41]

Cocaine has also been associated with an increase in cerebral infarcts and hydrancephaly. A group of 74 infants exposed to cocaine *in utero* exhibited an incidence of major ultrasonic cerebral anomalies of 35.1%, significantly higher than the control incidence of 5.3%.[42] The term 'cocaine baby' became prevalent in the 1990s to describe an apparent pattern of neonatal behaviour in the offspring of cocaine-using mothers. However, this term has fallen out of favour, as it appeared to label many babies erroneously and did not encompass any specific syndrome – most fetuses are morphologically normal.

### Management of cocaine addicts

Although there is controversy as to whether cocaine or cigarette smoking is more addictive,[43] cocaine use is very habit-forming. Habitual users may benefit from care at a specialised multidisciplinary antenatal clinic.

## HEROIN/OPIATES

Heroin and other opiates have not been shown to be teratogenic. As with any drug, maternal massive overdosage, may lead to acute fetal demise. Their typical effects appear to be seen *ex utero*, and consist of two phases – an acute withdrawal phase and a longer term impairment of behaviour and mental function.[44]

However, these more subtle effects are notoriously difficult to distinguish from confounding factors such as poor parenting.

### Management of opiate addicts

Heroin is highly addictive and its euphoric effects diminish with repeated use, leading to tolerance and the use of increasing quantities. Women addicted to heroin benefit from care at multidisciplinary antenatal units where methadone substitution can be carefully managed. They will often seek help, especially to obtain further doses of methadone.[45]

Most UK centres seek to stabilise opiate levels in pregnancy, using methadone as a substitute. This provides greater stability of plasma concentrations and avoids other risks of heroin use, such as infection and reaction to impurities. The switch can be generally performed as an out-patient. Buprenorphine, a partial opiate agonist, is emerging as an alternative to methadone.

## AMPHETAMINES

These stimulants, like cocaine, are vasoconstrictive, although they stimulate the release of noradrenaline, rather than inhibit its re-uptake. They can be used intravenously, orally or smoked. They have an even greater potential than cocaine to alter the personality of the user. In addition to low birth-weight, microcephally, prematurity, still-birth, cerebral haemorrhage and hyperbilirubinaemia, amphetamine use has been reported in case series of various structural anomalies, including cleft lip, cardiac defects, biliary atresia and undescended testes. Animal models using rats, mice and rabbits show a clear teratogenic potential of amphetamines, with differing anomalies observed at specific gestational dosing times and dosages.[46] Interestingly, oral clefting was increased in pregnancies exposed in the first 56 days of amenorrhoea, which coincides with the period of embryonic development of the relevant structures.[47]

Amphetamines also have been associated with arrhythmias of fetal heart rhythm, namely bradycardia and tachycardia, although these effects appear to resolve.[48] Evidence from a Scandinavian cohort exposed during a period of drug legalisation suggested that amphetamine-exposed children suffered neurodevelopmental delay, and that boys became taller and heavier than controls; amphetamine-exposed girls were shorter and lighter.[49] This implies an effect upon the pituitary gland. However, in common with many observational reports, confounding factors such as the use of other substances during pregnancy and the upbringing of the children, prevents firm conclusions from these data.

### Management of pregnant amphetamine addicts

Amphetamine users appear to be less likely to present in the same way as heroin users. This poses a challenge for multidisciplinary pregnancy addiction units. The intravenous substitute, dexamphetamine, is rarely indicated.[6]

## OTHER RECREATIONAL SUBSTANCES

Data on many other drugs of abuse in pregnancy (animal and human) are scarce. These include:

- barbiturates
- benzodiazepines
- ketamine
- lysergic acid diethylamide (LSD)
- cannabis
- toluene
- glue or other inhaled chemicals.

Habitual users of these can also benefit from specialised care, led by a team with particular experience in this area.

---

## Key points for clinical practice

- Hard data and randomised controlled trials in this field are scarce and likely to remain so. The best available data are from human observational and animal studies. Conclusions from these must, therefore, be circumspect.

- There are wide ranges of recreational substances and their effective dosages. Multiple confounding factors and multiple substance usage are typical.

- The specific teratogenic effects appear to exhibit high temporal and dosage dependence.

- Harm to neurodevelopment is a particular problem with recreational substances because of their very neuro-activity and affinity.

- Drug users pose significant management challenges which can be better addressed in multidisciplinary antenatal units.

- Maternal disinhibition and personality alteration can further impair the welfare of the fetus.

- Vasoconstrictive agents, such as cocaine, have particular associations with vascular interference and placental abruption.

- Close liaison with neonatologists is useful in preparing for neonatal problems such as substance withdrawal.

- Long-term follow-up data on affected children are needed to appreciate more subtle neurological effects.

- Care of women abusing recreational substances can be exasperating, but is worthwhile. Although the mother's health needs must be met, the well-being and development of the fetus must not be neglected by her carers.

## References

1. Aristotle. *De Generatione Animalium*.
2. Morrison JJ, Chitty LS, Peebles D, Rodeck CH. Recreational drugs and fetal gastroschisis: maternal hair analysis in the peri-conceptional period and during pregnancy. *Br J Obstet Gynaecol* 2005; **112**: 1022–1025.
3. Hoyme HE, Higginbottom MC, Jones KL. The vascular pathogenesis of gastroschisis: intrauterine interruption of the omphalomesenteric artery. *J Pediatr* 1981; **98**: 228–231.
4. Fisher JE, Potturi RB, Collins M, Resnick E, Zimmerman EF. Cocaine-induced embryonic cardiovascular disruption in mice. *Teratology* 1994; **49**: 182–191.
5. Department of Health. *Annual Report of the Chief Medical Officer*. London: HMSO, 2004.
6. Wright A, Walker J. Drugs of abuse in pregnancy. *Best Pract Res Clin Obstet Gynaecol* 2001; **15**: 987–998.
7. Department of Health. *Guidelines on Clinical Management*, vol 79. London: HMSO, 1999.
8. Dawe S, Gerada C, Strang J. Establishment of a liaison service for pregnant opiate-dependent women. *Br J Addict* 1992; **87**: 867–871.
9. Jones KL, Smith DW. Recognition of the fetal alcohol syndrome in early infancy. *Lancet* 1973; **302**: 999–1001.
10. Sampson PD, Streissguth AP, Bookstein FL *et al*. Incidence of fetal alcohol syndrome and prevalence of alcohol-related neurodevelopmental disorder. *Teratology* 1997; **56**: 317–326.
11. Abel EL. An update on incidence of FAS: FAS is not an equal opportunity birth defect. *Neurotoxicol Teratol* 1995; **17**: 437–443.
12. May PA, Brooke L, Gossage JP *et al*. Epidemiology of fetal alcohol syndrome in a South African community in the Western Cape Province. *Am J Public Health* 2000; **90**: 1905–1912.
13. Bower C, Silva D, Henderson TR, Ryan A, Rudy E. Ascertainment of birth defects: the effect on completeness of adding a new source of data. *J Paediatr Child Health* 2000; **36**: 574–576.
14. Konovalov HV, Kovetsky NS, Bobryshev YV, Ashwell KWS. Disorders of brain development in the progeny of mothers who used alcohol during pregnancy. *Early Hum Dev* 1997; **48**: 153–166.
15. Lorente C, Cordier S, Goujard J *et al*. Tobacco and alcohol use during pregnancy and risk of oral clefts. Occupational Exposure and Congenital Malformation Working Group. *Am J Public Health* 2000; **90**: 415–419.
16. Menegaux F, Steffen C, Bellec S *et al*. Maternal coffee and alcohol consumption during pregnancy, parental smoking and risk of childhood acute leukaemia. *Cancer Detect Prev* 2005; **29**: 487–493.
17. O'Leary CM, Heuzenroeder L, Elliott EJ, Bower C. A review of policies on alcohol use during pregnancy in Australia and other English-speaking countries, 2006. *Med J Aust* 2007; **186**: 466–471.
18. Henderson J, Gray R, Brocklehurst P. Systematic review of effects of low–moderate prenatal alcohol exposure on pregnancy outcome. *Br J Obstet Gynaecol* 2007; **114**: 243–252.
19. The Royal College of Obstetricians and Gynaecologists. London: RCOG Press, 2006. http://www.rcog.org.uk/resources/public/pdf/alcohol_pregnancy_1206.pdf
20. Crome IB, Kumar MT. Epidemiology of drug and alcohol use in young women. *Semin Fetal Neonatal Med* 2007; **12**: 98–105.
21. Nora AH, Nora JI, Blue J. Limb reduction abnormalities in infants born to Disulfiram treated alcoholic mothers. *Lancet* 1977; **ii**: 644–646.
22. Grenhoff J, Svensson TH. Pharmacolog of nicotine. *Br J Addict* 1989; 84(5): 477–492
23. Adriaanse HP, Knottnerus JA, Delgado LR *et al*. Smoking in Dutch pregnant women and low birth weight. *Patient Educ Counsel* 1996; **28**: 25–30.
24. Ananth CV, Savitz DA, Luther ER. Maternal cigarette smoking as a risk factor for placental abruption, placenta previa, and uterine bleeding in pregnancy. *Am J Epidemiol* 1996; **144**: 881–889.
25. DiFranza JR, Lew RA. Effect of maternal cigarette smoking on pregnancy complications and sudden infant death syndrome. *J Fam Pract* 1995; **40**: 385–394.
26. Lowe CR. Effect of mothers' smoking habits on the birth weight of their children. *BMJ* 1959; **2**: 673–676.

27. Roquer JM, Figueras J, Botet F, Jimenez R. Influence on fetal growth of exposure to tobacco smoke during pregnancy. *Acta Paediatr* 1995; **84**: 118–124.

28. England L, Zhang J. Smoking and risk of preeclampsia: a systematic review. *Front Biosci* 2007; **12**: 2471–2483.

29. Campion P, Owen L, McNeil A, McGuire C. Evaluation of a mass media campaign on smoking and pregnancy. *Addiction* 1994; **89**: 1245–1254.

30. Lumley J, Oliver SS, Chamberlain C, Oakley L. Interventions for promoting smoking cessation during pregnancy. Cochrane Database System Rev 2004; (4): CD001055.

31. Dempsey DA, Benowitz NL. Risks and benefits of nicotine to aid smoking cessation in pregnancy. *Drug Safety* 2001; **24**: 277–322.

32. West R, McNeill A, Raw M. Smoking cessation guidelines for health professionals: an update. Health Education Authority. *Thorax* 2000; **55**: 987–999.

33. Chan B, Einarson A, Koren G. Effectiveness of bupropion for smoking cessation during pregnancy. *J Addict Dis* 2005; **24**: 19–23.

34. Hulse GK, Milne E, English DR, Holman CD. Assessing the relationship between maternal cocaine use and abruptio placentae. *Addiction* 1997; **92**: 1547–1551.

35. Shiono PH, Klebanoff MA, Nugent RP *et al.* The impact of cocaine and marijuana use on low birth weight and preterm birth: a multicenter study. *Am J Obstet Gynecol* 1995; **172**: 19–27.

36. Sprauve ME, Lindsay MK, Herbert S, Graves W. Adverse perinatal outcome in parturients who use crack cocaine. *Obstet Gynecol* 1997; **89**: 674–678.

37. Chen LC, Graefe JF, Shojaie J *et al.* Pulmonary effects of the cocaine pyloryisis product, methylecgonidine, in guinea pigs. *Life Sci* 1995; **56**: PL7–PL12.

38. Wood RW, Graefe JF, Fang CP *et al.* Generation of stable test atmospheres of cocaine base and its pyrolyzate, methylecgonidine, and demonstration of their biologic activity. *Pharmacol Biochem Behav* 1996; **55**: 237–248.

39. Chiriboga CA, Brust JC, Bateman D, Hauser WA. Dose-response effect of fetal cocaine exposure on newborn neurologic function. *Pediatrics* 1999; **103**: 79–85.

40. Hoyme HE, Jones KL, Dixon SD *et al.* Prenatal cocaine exposure and fetal vascular disruption. *Pediatrics* 1990; **85**: 743–747.

41. Plessinger MA, Woods Jr JR. Maternal, placental, and fetal pathophysiology of cocaine exposure during pregnancy. *Clin Obstet Gynecol* 1993; **36**: 267–278.

42. Dixon SD, Bejar R. Echoencephalographic findings in neonates associated with maternal cocaine and methamphetamine use: incidence and clinical correlates. *J Pediatr* 1989; **115**: 770–778.

43. Henningfield JE, Cohen C, Slade JD. Is nicotine more addictive than cocaine? *Br J Addict* 1991; **86**: 565–569.

44. Hutchings DE. Methadone and heroin during pregnancy: a review of behavioral effects in human and animal offspring. *Neurobehav Toxicol Teratol* 1982; **4**: 429–434.

45. Burns L, Mattick RP, Lim K, Wallace C. Methadone in pregnancy: treatment retention and neonatal outcomes. *Addiction* 2007; **102**: 264–270.

46. Plessinger MA. Prenatal exposure to amphetamines. Risks and adverse outcomes in pregnancy. *Obstet Gynecol Clin North Am* 1998; **25**: 119–138.

47. Milkovich L, van der Berg BJ. Effects of antenatal exposure to anorectic drugs. *Am J Obstet Gynecol* 1977; **129**: 637–642.

48. Oro AS, Dixon SD. Perinatal cocaine and methamphetamine exposure: maternal and neonatal correlates. *J Pediatr* 1987; **111**: 571–578.

49. Cernerud L, Eriksson M, Jonsson B, Steneroth G, Zetterstrom R. Amphetamine addiction during pregnancy: 14-year follow-up of growth and school performance. *Acta Paediatr* 1996; **85**: 204–208.

*James A. McIntyre*

**2**

# HIV and pregnancy – the African perspective

The prevention of mother-to-child transmission (MTCT) of HIV, as a result of the development and implementation of strategies for the care of HIV-positive pregnant women, has been one of the great successes in the response to the AIDS epidemic in well-resourced settings. In these programmes, the diagnosis or identification of HIV-infected pregnant women, the use of combination antiretroviral regimens and the avoidance of breast-feeding has reduced transmission rates to below 2%.[1,2] Despite this success in richer countries, an estimated 420,000 children (350,000–540,000) were estimated to be infected with HIV in 2007 world-wide, mostly through MTCT, and UNICEF estimates that a child dies every minute from HIV infection.[3,4]

In 2001, the United Nations General Assembly (UNGASS) set a goal of a 50% reduction in the number of infants infected with HIV by 2010.[5] This target now appears to be unachievable across Africa as a whole, and only likely to be achieved in a few settings globally: at the end of 2006, only eight out of 71 countries for which data were available appeared likely to meet the UNGASS target.[6] Although more than 100 countries across the world have implemented prevention of MTCT programmes, fewer than 10 provide antiretroviral prophylaxis to 40% or more of HIV-infected pregnant women, and only 11% of pregnant women in need of antiretroviral prophylaxis globally received it in 2005. In sub-Saharan Africa, this proportion ranged from 1% to 54% , while the coverage of HIV counselling and testing in pregnancy averaged 9.2%.[6] Africa bears the brunt of MTCT and paediatric AIDS. To put the transmission figures in context, of the average of around 1100 new infections globally in children each day, one occurs in the US or Europe, 100 in Asia and more than 1000 in Africa, and this occurs while almost 90% of women have no access to even the simplest prevention of MTCT intervention.

**James A. McIntyre** MBChB FRCOG
Executive Director, Perinatal HIV Research Unit, University of the Witwatersrand, PO Box 114, Diepkloof, Johannesburg 1864, South Africa
E-mail: mcintyre@pixie.co.za

## HIV IN PREGNANCY IN AFRICA

The AIDS epidemic is most marked in sub-Saharan Africa, where more than 22.5 million (20.9–24.3 million) people were living with HIV in 2007 and 60% of HIV-infected adults were women.[3] HIV prevalence rates in women of child-bearing age vary across African countries. HIV prevalence is considerably lower in North Africa, and the rates in women have remained stable in West Africa for several years. Infection rates are much higher in east and southern Africa, with the highest in the south. In southern Africa, adult HIV prevalence rates are higher than 15% in eight countries which collectively account for almost a third of the global epidemic. The highest prevalence rates in the world are in Swaziland, Botswana and Lesotho, whilst South Africa has the largest number of people living with HIV/AIDS.[1] There are some signs that prevalence rates in sub-Saharan Africa have begun to stabilize or decline, with reductions noted from 2006 in pregnant women in Kenya, Côte d'Ivoire, Zimbabwe and Malawi.[3]

## PREVENTION OF MTCT ADVANCES IN AFRICA

The World Health Organization (WHO) recommends a comprehensive approach to the prevention of MTCT of HIV, with four key areas: (i) primary prevention of HIV infection; (ii) the prevention of unintended pregnancies among women living with HIV; (iii) the prevention of HIV transmission from mothers living with HIV to their infants; and (iv) care, treatment and support for mothers living with HIV, their children and families.[7]

Research into strategies to reduce MTCT in low resource settings has demonstrated significant advances in the decade since 1994, when the PATCG 076 study was the first indication that antiretroviral prophylaxis could reduce the risk of MTCT.[8] At this time, the long and expensive zidovudine regimen appeared impossible to implement in poorer countries, and a series of studies in Africa and Asia investigated shorter and more feasible alternatives. Results from these studies, using short courses of zidovudine alone or zidovudine in combination with lamivudine or nevirapine, all showed a similar range of effectiveness in reducing transmission to around 10–15%.[9–14] The HIVNET 012 study, which used a single dose of nevirapine given to mothers at the onset of labour and a single dose to infants within 72 h of birth halved the risk of transmission, compared to a 1-week course of zidovudine in a Ugandan study.[15] This regimen (which was safe, feasible and affordable for women in high-prevalence, low-resource countries) provided the impetus to start prevention of MTCT programmes in many African countries.

The addition of the maternal and infant nevirapine doses to antepartum zidovudine, or zidovudine/lamivudine combination prophylaxis has been shown to reduce transmission further.[16] A study in Thailand, using a combination of zidovudine from 28 weeks of pregnancy, together with a single dose of nevirapine to mother and baby, demonstrated transmission rates of 2% or less in non-breast-feeding women,[17] equivalent to the rates seen with triple therapy prophylaxis. This has become the WHO's first-line recommendation for low-resourced settings, although expansion beyond single dose nevirapine has been slowly implemented.[18] Triple combination antiretroviral prophylaxis, similar to that used in high-resource countries, has also been shown to be effective and safe in some African research settings, with low rates of transmission reported in studies from Mozambique and Côte d'Ivoire.[19,20]

The effectiveness of prevention of MTCT programmes depends firstly on the identification of HIV-infected women during pregnancy. While the offer and uptake of HIV testing in antenatal care settings remains low, even the most effective interventions will be compromised. There are a number of factors which impact on the uptake of testing by pregnant women. These include fear of testing, stigma about HIV infection, inefficient service delivery and the judgmental attitudes of staff. A number of prevention of MTCT programmes have demonstrated that a routine offer of HIV testing to pregnant women (or 'provider initiated testing') can be very acceptable to women and can increase testing rates considerably. In Botswana, the proportion of HIV-infected pregnant women in public sector prevention of MTCT facilities who knew their status increased from 48% to 78% in the first 8 months following the introduction of routine testing in 2004, and has continued to rise since then to almost universal coverage.[21] Similar results are reported from Lilongwe, Malawi, where HIV testing uptake increased from 45% to 73% when rapid, same-day testing was instituted, and to 99% after opt-out testing was instituted.[22]

## PREVENTION OF TRANSMISSION THROUGH BREAST-FEEDING

Infection through breast-feeding remains one of the major challenges for prevention of MTCT in Africa. Avoidance of breast-feeding removes the further risk of transmission and has contributed to the reduction in infections in well-resourced settings. While replacement feeding has been successfully used in some African settings,[23,24] this is not feasible in many low-resourced settings, where the risks of replacement feeding may outweigh the risk of HIV transmission. Breast-feeding approximately doubles the risk of infection for an infant, continues to pose a risk throughout the period of breast-feeding and can add an additional 15–20% of risk if the mother breast-feeds for as long as 24 months, which has been common practice in many African settings. Transmission occurred after the first month of life in 42% of infected infants in the Breastfeeding and HIV International Transmission study (BHITS) meta-analysis,[27] while a study in Malawi showed that 85% of transmission to infants could have been avoided if women had weaned at 6 months.[28] The duration of breast-feeding is thus a major determinant of infection rates, but other factors such as advanced disease in mothers, high HIV viral load or low CD4 count, and the presence of mastitis also play a role.[25,29,30]

The risk of transmission through breast milk is also affected by the mode of feeding, with exclusive breast-feeding (without the addition of any other foods or liquids) carrying less risk than 'mixed' feeding in the first 6 months.[30,31] This forms the basis for the WHO's recommendations on infant feeding for HIV-positive mothers, which propose exclusive breast-feeding for the first 6 months of life unless replacement feeding is 'acceptable, feasible, affordable, sustainable and safe' – referred to as the 'AFASS' criteria.[32] This is not easy to implement in practice, as 'mixed' feeding is most common in most settings, and achieving exclusive breast-feeding requires additional education and support services. Increasing evidence has also demonstrated the risks of weaning at or before 6 months, regardless of feeding modality prior to this, with severe morbidity or mortality from the use of replacement feeding in unsafe circumstances, which may exceed the HIV risk.[30,33–35] In these settings, continued breast-feeding, with additional complementary feeds, may be safer for overall HIV-free survival.

The application of the 'AFASS' principles has proved difficult for prevention of MTCT programmes, as the requirements for safe use of replacement feeding depend predominantly on the socio-economic status of mothers and their communities.[36] Health workers also find it difficult to provide non-judgmental guidance for HIV-positive women on feeding choices, and clearer decision-making tools are needed. A South African study demonstrated that three factors were associated with successful replacement feeding, even in very poor environments, and these could be used to guide infant feeding decisions. They were: (i) the availability of electricity or gas as fuel; (ii) the availability of piped water; and (iii) disclosure of maternal HIV status.[37] Using criteria such as these can help to avoid inappropriate feeding choices, either for or against replacement feeding, and reduce transmission and improve survival.

Since transmission through breast milk continues to be a major source of infection, even despite exclusive breast-feeding interventions,[38] other alternative approaches to preserve the benefits of breast-feeding with a reduced risk of transmission are needed and are being investigated. A promising approach is to provide antiretroviral prophylaxis – either given directly to breast-fed infants or by providing antiretroviral therapy to breast-feeding mothers.[25,39] Where mothers have not received antiretroviral prophylaxis, post-exposure prophylaxis given to the infants has been shown to reduce transmission.[40,41] Extending nevirapine dosing to infants for a longer period of 6–14 weeks has also been shown to reduce transmission risk and improve survival. In the PEPi-Malawi study, giving breast-fed infants nevirapine (extNVP)or a combination of nevirapine and zidovudine (extNVP/AZT) for 14 weeks resulted in transmission rates at 14 weeks of 5.2% and 6.4%, respectively, in infants uninfected at birth compared to 10.6% in those who only received single dose nevirapine. Combined infections and mortality rates at 9 months were 11% (extNVP) and 12% (extNVP/AZT), compared to 17% for infants in the single-dose nevirapine control group.[42] The Six Week Extended Nevirapine (SWEN) study combined data from three similarly designed trials in Ethiopia, Uganda and India, and showed that infants who received the additional 6 weeks of nevirapine had a 50% lower risk of infection at 6 weeks of age than those receiving single-dose nevirapine (2.5% versus 5.27%). By 6 months, this difference was less marked, with around 20% less transmission (7% versus 9%), and no longer statistically significant, but the combined risk of infection or death at 6 months remained significantly lower at 8% compared to 11.6%.[43] These results suggest that extended nevirapine to infants may be a useful additional intervention in breast-fed infants.

Several observational trials of maternal antiretroviral treatment have shown success in reducing transmission during breast-feeding.[44,45] In a study in Kisumu, Kenya, the provision of triple antiretroviral therapy to breast-feeding mothers for the first 6 months postpartum resulted in 3.5% transmission attributable to breast-feeding at 12 months.[46] If randomized trials currently in progress confirm the success of this approach in reducing transmission, and the safety of interrupted treatment in this manner for mothers, this could be a powerful option to reduce MTCT where access to antiretrovirals is available. However, in high prevalence African settings, the feasibility may be limited by the affordability and infrastructure demands required to deliver antiretroviral treatment to large numbers of women, and the social implications of providing this treatment.

## MATERNAL MORTALITY AND HIV

A narrow focus on preventing MTCT can sometimes mask the medical needs of HIV-infected pregnant women for their own health. Maternal mortality also has a major additional impact on child survival, with children more likely to die if their mothers die,[47–49] which may reverse any gains in survival of children achieved by prevention of MTCT interventions.

While AIDS is now a rare cause of maternal death in well-resourced countries, it remains a significant contributing cause of maternal mortality in high-prevalence African settings.[50–53] Although follow-up cohort data on the effect of pregnancy and progression of disease are limited in Africa, there is some evidence of a higher HIV-related mortality risk linked to pregnancy and in the first year postpartum. In the 1990s, prior to the availability of antiretroviral treatment, the maternal mortality rates in HIV-infected women in Zaire were 10 times those of HIV-negative women[54] with 22% of HIV-infected mothers dying during a 3-year follow-up period. In a prospective study in Malawi, the maternal mortality rate was 370 per 100,000 women and the mortality rate between 6 weeks and 1 year postpartum was 341 per 100,000 live births, with AIDS and anaemia the major causes of post-pregnancy mortality.[55]

The Report on the Confidential Enquiry into Maternal Deaths (CEMD) in South Africa – 2002–2004 considered 3406 maternal deaths in the 3 years covered by the study. HIV status was unknown in 53.7% of women, 10.3% were HIV negative and 36.7% were known to be HIV positive, suggesting an under-reporting of HIV-related causes of death. Despite this, the impact of HIV is reflected in the statistics: non-pregnancy related infections were the most common cause of death, responsible for 37.8% of deaths. AIDS was the single biggest cause of death at 20.1% of all deaths, higher than any direct obstetric cause.[56]

A number of factors may influence HIV progression during and after pregnancy, including nutritional and maternal genetic factors, and other infections such as tuberculosis. Progression post-pregnancy has been described as more rapid in women who have anaemia during pregnancy,[57] while multivitamin supplements delayed progression in a Tanzanian study.[58] Where HIV is prevalent, increased AIDS-related mortality in young women may have the opposite effect on maternal mortality rates, if more women die before becoming pregnant. A study in the Congo showed a 32-times higher mortality rate in HIV-infected women than uninfected, but a higher relative increase in non-pregnant than pregnant women.[59] As antiretroviral treatment becomes more accessible in Africa, and expanded, more comprehensive prevention of MTCT programmes are strengthened, reductions should be achieved in AIDS-related maternal mortality.

## MANAGEMENT IN PREGNANCY

The approach to management of HIV-positive pregnant women is not determined by geography, but by the available resources and services. Where resources permit, the management of a pregnant HIV-positive woman should follow guidelines and practices which are recommended in high-resource countries such as the US and UK.[60,61] These include preconception counselling for known HIV-positive women, identification of previously undiagnosed women as early as possible in pregnancy, the provision of triple combination antiretroviral therapy for prophylaxis of MTCT, elective caesarean section and the avoidance of breast-feeding. In some settings in Africa, women may have access to this standard of care, through privately funded health care, or in well-equipped facilities in major urban areas. Some country-wide prevention of MTCT programmes, including those in Botswana and Rwanda, have indicated that they intend to move towards the use of triple antiretroviral therapy for all pregnant women in the state-funded programmes. Where resources do not permit this, the WHO has recommended the provision of a 'public health approach' to treatment and care of HIV-infected women. This aims to provide access to high-quality services within public health facilities, balancing the best proven standard of care with what is feasible on a large scale where resources are scarce. These recommendations form the core of an approach to the care of HIV-infected pregnant women and the prevention of MTCT which can be rolled out in many African settings.

Once a pregnant woman is found to be HIV-infected, her clinical stage should be assessed, and a $CD4^+$ cell count obtained to enable decisions on future treatment. Where CD4 counts are not available, clinical staging alone can be used to guide treatment, but this will be less accurate in determining prognosis. Clinical staging may be complicated in pregnancy, where the key condition of weight loss may be masked by pregnancy-related weight gain. Other laboratory investigations will be determined by what is available in the service or facility, but should include haemoglobin estimation and syphilis testing as a minimum. Screening for symptoms of tuberculosis, with follow-up investigations where necessary is an important addition in African settings.[62]

### WOMEN WHO REQUIRE ANTIRETROVIRAL TREATMENT FOR THEIR OWN HEALTH

All maternity services should strive to identify HIV-infected women who require antiretroviral therapy for their own health, and to ensure that they receive this. Pregnancy is not an obstacle to the use of effective antiretroviral treatment regimens, but the regimen used may need to be adapted because of potential teratogenic or side effects of the drugs on the fetus or infant, the physiological changes of pregnancy or the possible side effects of the drugs in the mother, which may be worse in pregnancy.[60,63] The benefits of antiretroviral therapy during pregnancy outweigh the potential side effects or risks to mother or baby, on the available evidence.[64,65] The major concern with regard to drug choice is about the use of efavirenz in pregnancy, due to an association with neural tube defects in animal studies and a small number of reports of neural tube defects and the Dandy–Walker malformation in human infants.[66] Although the causal relationship is not completely established, efavirenz is now classified as US Food and Drug Administration (FDA) Pregnancy Category D on the basis of potential fetal harm, and it should not be used in the first trimester of pregnancy or in women of child-bearing potential without ensuring the provision of adequate contraception. The antiretroviral pregnancy register has accumulated a large quantity of data on the use of antiretrovirals in pregnancy, providing sufficient re-assuring data that zidovudine, lamivudine, nevirapine, abacavir and nelfinavir are not teratogenic.[60] Stavudine and didanosine should not be used together in pregnant women, unless the potential benefits outweigh the risks, due to an increased risk of lactic acidosis. A further concern is around nevirapine-containing antiretroviral regimens in women with higher CD4 counts (more than 250 cells/mm$^3$), following a US FDA advisory and a change to the manufacturer's product package insert in early 2005. This reported on an increased risk of hepatic adverse events, which may be fatal and are often associated with rash, in women with pre-treatment CD4$^+$ cell counts greater than 250 cells/mm$^3$.[67] Although there has not been additional evidence for an increased risk in pregnancy, pregnant women are more likely to receive antiretrovirals at these higher CD4$^+$ counts, in line with the recommendations above.

Pregnant women who need antiretroviral treatment should start this as soon as possible in pregnancy, and those women already on antiretroviral treatment when they become pregnant should continue with a triple antiretroviral regimen, although the drugs used may need to be adjusted.[18,60,61] Antiretroviral treatment is primarily aimed at benefiting the mother but will also significantly reduce the risk of MTCT of HIV, and benefit the longer term survival of the mother and child. Women who are immunocompromised with low CD4 cell counts are more likely to transmit HIV to their babies,[68] more likely to have detectable NNRTI-resistant virus following the use of nevirapine monotherapy,[69] and their infants are more likely to die,[48,49] all of which can be improved by access to ARV treatment.

While the CD4$^+$ cell count level for initiating therapy in most well-resourced settings is 350 cells/mm$^3$, treatment is not generally available above a CD4 count of 200 cells/mm$^3$ in most African settings. In general, the criteria for initiating antiretroviral therapy in pregnant women are similar to those for all adults. However, the WHO 2006 guidelines for the management of HIV-infected pregnant women recommend starting antiretroviral therapy in pregnancy at CD4 cell counts of 350 cells/mm$^3$ for women with clinical stage 3 disease, for all women with stage 4 disease irrespective of CD4$^+$ cell count, and for women in clinical stage 1 and 2 with CD4$^+$ cell counts less than 200/mm$^3$.[18] This is on the basis that starting antiretroviral treatment at this higher CD4$^+$ cell count will benefit maternal health and will avoid the potential adverse effect of the selection of nevirapine resistance following simpler nevirapine containing regimens.

As CD4$^+$ cell counts drop during pregnancy, and increase again postpartum, it has been suggested, from work in Abidjan, that the use of a CD4 percentage could be a more accurate indication of when to start treatment. In this study, when a combination of the CD4+ cell count and WHO clinical stage was used, the proportion of women who met the WHO 2006 criteria for initiating antiretroviral therapy was 28.3% at baseline but dropped to 17.2% at 4 weeks after delivery.[70] The CD4+ cell count experienced increased significantly post delivery but the CD4 percentage remained unchanged. While this should be borne in mind, most treatment guidelines have continued to use CD4+ cell counts rather than percentage measures.

A number of reports have now demonstrated the safety and success of using antiretroviral treatment regimens in African settings, where antiretroviral treatment access has expanded dramatically in the past few years. While the use of antiretroviral therapy in pregnant women in Africa has predominantly been for treatment of the mother rather than as MTCT prophylaxis, this is likely to change in the future as access improves. A report from Abidjan showed a low rate of toxicity and no transmissions in women receiving antiretroviral therapy.[71] In Mozambique, the DREAM project has demonstrated successful use of antiretroviral therapy with a transmission rate of 4% in infants reported at 4 weeks of age,[72] while a study in Kisumu has demonstrated low rates of side effects and reduced transmission rates with antiretroviral treatment in pregnancy and during breast-feeding.[46]

## WOMEN WHO DO NOT YET REQUIRE ANTIRETROVIRAL TREATMENT FOR THEIR OWN HEALTH

For women with higher CD4+ cell counts and at earlier stages of HIV disease, the best available antiretroviral prophylactic regimen should be provided. In some settings this would be a triple antiretroviral regimen, similar to that used in well-resourced centres, but this may be more complicated in African treatment programmes where nevirapine is a key component of first-line combination regimens, but would not be recommended for women with higher CD4+ cell counts. The use of a protease inhibitor, most commonly lopinavir/ritoinavir, is the most wide-spread alternative.

In most African settings this level of care is not yet attainable, and a shorter, more feasible regimen is recommended. The first choice in the WHO 2006 guidelines is provision of zidovudine (ZDV, AZT) 300 mg twice daily, from 28 weeks' gestation or as soon after as possible, to the mother, a single 200 mg dose of nevirapine to the mother at the onset of labour, a single 2 mg/kg dose of nevirapine to the baby after birth and zidovudine 4 mg/kg twice a day for 7 days to the baby. These guidelines also recommend the use of 7 days of zidovudine (300 mg twice daily) and lamivudine (150 mg twice daily) to mothers to reduce the risk of nevirapine resistance, starting in labour.[18] Where mothers have received less than 4 weeks of antenatal zidovudine, an extended regimen of 4 weeks of zidovudine can be given to the infant. Where even this simpler regimen is not available, or mothers have not accessed it, the single dose of nevirapine to mother and baby regimen remains an option.

Nevirapine is a highly potent antiretroviral, with a long half-life, which remains in detectable concentrations for up to 21 days after a single maternal dose. Unfortunately, only a single point mutation in the viral genome is needed to confer resistance to the non-nucleoside reverse transcriptase family of drugs. The long half-life of the drug, leading to effective prolonged nevirapine monotherapy, and the low genetic barrier for viral resistance, contribute to the high rates of selection of resistant viral variant, reported to range from 15% to 75% using standard population sequencing techniques following a single-dose nevirapine alone.[69,73–77] This selection of resistant virus has also been described with the addition of intrapartum nevirapine to zidovudine, in around 30% of mothers.[78,79] The major concern about this selection of resistance has been the possible adverse effect on response to nevirapine-containing antiretroviral therapy regimens after pregnancy, with some evidence that mothers are more likely to fail a first-line regimen if started within 6 months of prevention of MTCT dosing, and that this is even more likely in exposed infants.[80]

The use of a 'tail-cover' regimen to counteract the long half-life of the single dose of nevirapine is recommended. This was first shown to be effective using a 4-day or 7-day regimen of zidovudine and lamivudine (AZT/3TC) to mothers[81] and, more recently, the addition of a single dose of tenofovir and emtricitabine to the labour dose of nevirapine has been shown to reduce selection of resistance effectively, in women who had also received antenatal zidovudine.[82]

With all of the possible antiretroviral regimens, infant feeding options and choices should be discussed with the mother antenatally, and she should be supported in her choice of feeding regimen. New information on the effectiveness of extended nevirapine to infants and of antiretroviral therapy for breast-feeding mothers may result in a change in these guidelines to include one or other of these strategies in the future.

---

## Key points for clinical practice

- All mothers should have a routine offer of an HIV test in pregnancy.

- HIV-infected pregnant women should be assessed for clinical stage and CD4+ cell count.

- Women who need antiretroviral therapy for their own health should initiate this as soon as possible in their pregnancy.

- Where antiretroviral treatment is not yet required, HIV-infected pregnant women should receive the best available prophylactic antiretroviral regimen to reduce the risk of transmission to the infant.

- Where circumstances permit, this should be a triple combination antiretroviral regimen during pregnancy.

- Where this is not available, a combination of zidovudine from 28 weeks and single dose intrapartum nevirapine to mothers, and single-dose nevirapine and 1 week of zidovudine to infants is the recommended prevention of a mother-to-child treatment (MTCT) regimen.

**Key points for clinical practice** *(continued)*

- Where even this cannot be provided, single-dose nevirapine provides some protection against transmission.

- Selection of nevirapine resistant virus is common following nevirapine use in non-virologically suppressive prevention of MTCT regimens, and can be reduced by the use of 'tail-cover' with either 1 week of zidovudine and lamivudine to mothers or a single dose of tenofovir and emtricitabine.

- Breast-feeding contributes to almost half of infant infections. Where replacement feeding is safe and feasible, this should be an option. Where not, exclusive breast-feeding for the first 6 months reduced the risk of transmission compared to 'mixed' feeding. Women should be counselled on the risks and benefits of infant feeding options and supported in their choice.

- Care of HIV-infected women during pregnancy should focus both on maternal health and on reducing the risk of transmission to the infant.

## References

1. UNAIDS. *2006 Report on the Global AIDS Epidemic*. Geneva: UNAIDS, 2006.
2. Townsend C, Cortina-Borja M, Peckham C, de Ruiter A, Lyall H, Tookey P. Very low risk of mother-to-child transmission in women on HAART who achieve viral suppression. The UK and Ireland, 2000 to 2006 15th Conference on Retroviruses and Opportunistic Infections, February 2008. Boston, MA: Abstract 653.
3. UNAIDS. *AIDS epidemic update: December 2007*. Joint United Nations Programme on HIV/AIDS (UNAIDS) and World Health Organization (WHO). Geneva: 2007.
4. The United Nations Children's Fund (UNICEF). *A Call To Action: Children, the missing face to AIDS*. The Global Campaign on Children and AIDS: Unite for Children. Unite against. New York: UNICEF, 2005.
5. United Nations General Assembly. *Final declaration of commitment on HIV/AIDS* (A/s-26/L.2). New York: 2001.
6. Global Partners Forum. *Achieving Universal Access To Comprehensive prevention of MTCT Services*. 2007.
7. World Health Organization. *Strategic approaches to the prevention of HIV infection in infants*. Report of a WHO meeting, Morges, Switzerland, 20–22 March 2002. Geneva: WHO, 2002.
8. Connor EM, Sperling RS, Gelber R *et al*. Reduction of maternal–infant transmission of human immunodeficiency virus type 1 with zidovudine treatment. Pediatric AIDS Clinical Trials Group Protocol 076 Study Group. *N Engl J Med* 1994; **331**: 1173–1180.
9. Shaffer N, Chuachoowong R, Mock PA *et al*. Short-course zidovudine for perinatal HIV-1 transmission in Bangkok, Thailand: a randomised controlled trial. Bangkok Collaborative Perinatal HIV Transmission Study Group. *Lancet* 1999; **353**: 773–780.
10. Wiktor SZ, Ekpini E, Karon JM *et al*. Short-course oral zidovudine for prevention of mother-to-child transmission of HIV-1 in Abidjan, Côte d'Ivoire: a randomised trial. *Lancet* 1999; **353**: 781–785.
11. The Petra Study Team. Efficacy of three short-course regimens of zidovudine and lamivudine in preventing early and late transmission of HIV-1 from mother to child in Tanzania, South Africa, and Uganda (Petra study): a randomised, double- blind, placebo-controlled trial. *Lancet* 2002; **359**: 1178–1186.

12. Guay LA, Musoke P, Fleming T *et al*. Intrapartum and neonatal single-dose nevirapine compared with zidovudine for prevention of mother-to-child transmission of HIV-1 in Kampala, Uganda: HIVNET 012 randomised trial. *Lancet* 1999; **354**: 795–802.

13. Moodley D, Moodley J, Coovadia H *et al*. A multicenter randomized controlled trial of nevirapine versus a combination of zidovudine and lamivudine to reduce intrapartum and early postpartum mother-to-child transmission of human immunodeficiency virus type 1. *J Infect Dis* 2003; **187**: 725–735.

14. Leroy V, Sakarovitch C, Cortina-Borja M *et al*. Is there a difference in the efficacy of peripartum antiretroviral regimens in reducing mother-to-child transmission of HIV in Africa? *AIDS* 2005; **19**: 1865–1875.

15. Guay L, Musoke P, Fleming T *et al*. Intrapartum and neonatal single-dose nevirapine compared with zidovudine for prevention of mother-to-child transmission of HIV-1 in Kampala, Uganda: HIVNET 012 randomised trial. *Lancet* 1999; **354**: 795–802.

16. Dabis F, Bequet L, Ekouevi DK *et al*. Field efficacy of zidovudine, lamivudine and single-dose nevirapine to prevent peripartum HIV transmission. *AIDS* 2005; **19**: 309–318.

17. Lallemant M, Jourdain G, Le Coeur S *et al*. Single-dose perinatal nevirapine plus standard zidovudine to prevent mother-to-child transmission of HIV-1 in Thailand. *N Engl J Med* 2004; **351**: 217–228.

18. World Health Organization. *Antiretroviral drugs for treating pregnant women and preventing HIV infection in infants in resource-limited settings: towards universal access. Recommendations for a public health approach.* Geneva: WHO, 2006.

19. Marazzi CM, Germano P, Liotta G *et al*. Implementing anti-retroviral triple therapy to prevent HIV mother-to-child transmission: a public health approach in resource-limited settings. *Eur J Pediatr* 2007; **166**: 1305–1307.

20. Tonwe-Gold B, Ekouevi DK, Viho I *et al*. Antiretroviral treatment and prevention of peripartum and postnatal HIV transmission in West Africa: evaluation of a two-tiered approach. *PLoS Med* 2007; **4**: e257.

21. Creek TL, Ntumy R, Seipone K *et al*. Successful introduction of routine opt-out HIV testing in antenatal care in Botswana. *J Acquir Immune Defic Syndr* 2007; **45**: 102–107.

22. Moses A, Zimba C, Kamanga E *et al*. Prevention of mother-to-child transmission: program changes and the effect on uptake of the HIVNET 012 regimen in Malawi. *AIDS* 2008; **22**: 83–87.

23. Leroy V, Sakarovitch C, Viho I *et al*. Acceptability of formula-feeding to prevent HIV postnatal transmission, Abidjan, Côte d'Ivoire: ANRS 1201/1202 Ditrame Plus Study. *J Acquir Immune Defic Syndr* 2007; **44**: 77–86.

24. Coetzee D, Hilderbrand K, Boulle A, Draper B, Abdullah F, Goemaere E. Effectiveness of the first district-wide programme for the prevention of mother-to-child transmission of HIV in South Africa. *Bull World Health Organ* 2005; **83**: 489–494.

25. Kourtis AP, Jamieson DJ, de Vincenzi I *et al*. Prevention of human immunodeficiency virus-1 transmission to the infant through breastfeeding: new developments. *Am J Obstet Gynecol* 2007; **197**: S113–S122.

26. Newell ML. Current issues in the prevention of mother-to-child transmission of HIV-1 infection. *Trans R Soc Trop Med Hyg* 2006; **100**: 1–5.

27. Breastfeeding and HIV International Transmission Study Group. Late postnatal transmission of HIV-1 in breast-fed children: an individual patient data meta-analysis. *J Infect Dis* 2004; **189**: 2154–2166.

28. Taha TE, Hoover DR, Kumwenda NI *et al*. Late postnatal transmission of HIV-1 and associated factors. *J Infect Dis* 2007; **196**: 10–14.

29. John-Stewart GC. Breast-feeding and HIV-1 transmission: how risky for how long? *J Infect Dis* 2007; **196**: 1–3.

30. Coovadia HM, Rollins NC, Bland RM *et al*. Mother-to-child transmission of HIV-1 infection during exclusive breastfeeding in the first 6 months of life: an intervention cohort study. *Lancet* 2007; **369**: 1107–1116.

31. Coutsoudis A, Pillay K, Spooner E, Kuhn L, Coovadia HM. Influence of infant-feeding patterns on early mother-to-child transmission of HIV-1 in Durban, South Africa: a prospective cohort study. South African Vitamin A Study Group. *Lancet* 1999; **354**: 471–476.

32. World Health Organization. *New data on the prevention of mother-to-child transmission of*

*HIV and their policy implications: conclusions and recommendations*. WHO Technical Consultation on behalf of the UNFPA/UNICEF/WHO/UNAIDS inter-Agency Task Team on Mother-to-Child Transmission of HIV. October 11–13, 2000. WHO/RHR/01.28ed. Geneva: WHO, 2001

33. Creek T, Arvelo W, Kim A *et al*. Role of infant feeding and HIV in a severe outbreak of diarrhea and malnutrition among young children, Botswana, 2006. 14th Conference on Retroviruses and Opportunistic Infections, Los Angeles, 25–28 February 2007. Abstract 770.

34. Thior I, Lockman S, Smeaton L *et al*. Breast-feeding with 6 months of infant zidovudine prophylaxis vs formula-feeding for reducing postnatal HIV transmission and infant mortality: a randomised trial in Southern Africa. 12th Conference on Retroviruses and Opportunistic Infections, Boston, 22–25 February 2005. Abstract 75LB.

35. Sinkala M, Kuhn L, Kankasa C *et al*. No benefit of early cessation of breastfeeding at 4 months on HIV-free survival of infants born to HIV-infected mothers in Zambia: The Zambia Exclusive Breastfeeding Study. 14th Conference on Retroviruses and Opportunistic Infections, Los Angeles, 25–28 February 2007. Abstract 74.

36. Chopra M, Rollins N. Infant feeding in the time of HIV: Assessment of infant feeding policy and programmes in four African countries scaling up prevention of mother to child transmission programmes. *Arch Dis Child* 2007; Epub.

37. Doherty T, Chopra M, Jackson D, Goga A, Colvin M, Persson LA. Effectiveness of the WHO/UNICEF guidelines on infant feeding for HIV-positive women: results from a prospective cohort study in South Africa. *AIDS* 2007; **21**: 1791–1797.

38. Becquet R, Bland R, Leroy V *et al*. Duration and pattern of breastfeeding and postnatal transmission of HIV: pooled analysis of individual data from a West and South African cohort study. 15th Conference on Retroviruses and Opportunistic Infections, 3–6 February 2008. Boston, MA: Abstract 46.

39. Gaillard P, Fowler MG, Dabis F *et al*. Use of antiretroviral drugs to prevent HIV-1 transmission through breast-feeding: from animal studies to randomized clinical trials. *J Acquir Immune Defic Syndr* 2004; **35**: 178–187.

40. Gray GE, Urban M, Chersich MF *et al*. A randomized trial of two postexposure prophylaxis regimens to reduce mother-to-child HIV-1 transmission in infants of untreated mothers. *AIDS* 2005; **19**: 1289–1297.

41. Taha TE, Kumwenda NI, Hoover DR *et al*. Nevirapine and zidovudine at birth to reduce perinatal transmission of HIV in an African setting: a randomized controlled trial. *JAMA* 2004; **292**: 202–209.

42. Taha T, Thigpen M, Kumwenda N *et al*. Extended infant post-exposure prophylaxis with antiretroviral drugs significantly reduces postnatal HIV transmission: the PEPI-Malawi Study, 15th Conference on Retroviruses and Opportunistic Infections, 3–6 February 2008. Boston, MA: Abstract 42LB.

43. Sastry J, The Six Week Extended Dose Nevirapine (SWEN) Study Team. Extended-dose nevirapine to 6 weeks of age for infants in Ethiopia, India, and Uganda: a randomized trial for prevention of HIV transmission through breastfeeding. 15th Conference on Retroviruses and Opportunistic Infections, 3–6 February 2008. Boston, MA: Abstract 43.

44. Arendt V, Ndimubanzi P, Vyankandondera J *et al*. AMATA study: effectiveness of antiretroviral therapy in breastfeeding mothers to prevent post-natal vertical transmission in Rwanda. Cross-track Session: 4th IAS Conference on HIV Pathogenesis, Treatment and Prevention, Sydney, 22–25 July 2007. Abstract TUAX102.

45. Kilewo C, Karlsson K, Ngarina M *et al*. Prevention of mother-to-child transmission of HIV-1 through breastfeeding by treating mothers prophylactically with triple antiretroviral therapy in Dar es Salaam, Tanzania – the MITRA PLUS study. 4th IAS Conference on HIV Pathogenesis, Treatment and Prevention. Sydney, 22–25 July 2007. Abstract TUAX101.

46. Thomas T, Masaba R, Ndivo R *et al*. Prevention of mother-to-child transmission of HIV-1 among breastfeeding mothers using HAART: The Kisumu Breastfeeding Study, Kisumu, Kenya, 2003–2007. 15th Conference on Retroviruses and Opportunistic Infections, 3–6 February 2008. Boston, MA: Abstract 45aLB.

47. Zaba B, Whitworth J, Marston M *et al*. HIV and mortality of mothers and children: evidence from cohort studies in Uganda, Tanzania, and Malawi. *Epidemiology* 2005; **16**: 275–280.

48. Newell ML, Coovadia H, Cortina-Borja M, Rollins N, Gaillard P, Dabis F. Mortality of infected and uninfected infants born to HIV-infected mothers in Africa: a pooled analysis. *Lancet* 2004; **364**: 1236–1243.

49. Taha TE, Miotti P, Liomba G, Dallabetta G, Chiphangwi J. HIV, maternal death and child survival in Africa. *AIDS* 1996; **10**: 111–112.

50. Lema VM, Changole J, Kanyighe C, Malunga EV. Maternal mortality at the Queen Elizabeth Central Teaching Hospital, Blantyre, Malawi. *East Afr Med J* 2005; **82**: 3–9.

51. Majoko F, Chipato T, Iliff V. Trends in maternal mortality for the Greater Harare Maternity Unit: 1976 to 1997. *Cent Afr J Med* 2001; **47**: 199–203.

52. Oyieke JB, Obore S, Kigondu CS. Millennium development goal 5: a review of maternal mortality at the Kenyatta National Hospital, Nairobi. *East Afr Med J* 2006; **83**: 4–9.

53. Fawcus SR, van Coeverden de Groot HA, Isaacs S. A 50-year audit of maternal mortality in the Peninsula Maternal and Neonatal Service, Cape Town (1953–2002). *Br J Obstet Gynaecol* 2005; **112**: 1257–1263.

54. Ryder RW, Nsuami M, Nsa W *et al.* Mortality in HIV-1-seropositive women, their spouses and their newly born children during 36 months of follow-up in Kinshasa, Zaire. *AIDS* 1994; **8**: 667–672.

55. McDermott JM, Slutsker L, Steketee RW, Wirima JJ, Breman JG, Heymann DL. Prospective assessment of mortality among a cohort of pregnant women in rural Malawi. *Am J Trop Med Hyg* 1996; **55**: 66–70.

56. Department of Health, South Africa. *Saving Mothers – Report on Confidential Enquiries into Maternal Deaths in South Africa 2002–2004*. Pretoria: Department of Health, 2006.

57. O'Brien ME, Kupka R, Msamanga GI, Saathoff E, Hunter DJ, Fawzi WW. Anemia is an independent predictor of mortality and immunologic progression of disease among women with HIV in Tanzania. *J Acquir Immune Defic Syndr* 2005; **40**: 219–225.

58. Fawzi W, Msamanga G, Spiegelman D, Hunter DJ. Studies of vitamins and minerals and HIV transmission and disease progression. *J Nutr* 2005; **135**: 938–944.

59. Le Coeur S, Khlat M, Halembokaka G *et al.* HIV and the magnitude of pregnancy-related mortality in Pointe Noire, Congo. *AIDS* 2005; **19**: 69–75.

60. Perinatal HIV Guidelines Working Group. Public Health Service Task Force Recommendations for Use of Antiretroviral Drugs in Pregnant HIV-Infected Women for Maternal Health and Interventions to Reduce Perinatal HIV Transmission in the United States. November 2, 2007.

61. British HIV Association and Children's HIV Association. *BHIVA and CHIVA guidelines for the management of HIV infection in pregnant women 2008*: Consultation draft. 2007.

62. Kali PB, Gray GE, Violari A, Chaisson RE, McIntyre JA, Martinson NA. Combining prevention of MTCT with active case finding for tuberculosis. *J Acquir Immune Defic Syndr* 2006; **42**: 379–381.

63. Newell ML. Routine provision of nevirapine to women of unknown serostatus: at best a temporary solution to prevent MTCT. *Bull World Health Organ* 2005; **83**: 228–229.

64. Thorne C, Newell ML. The safety of antiretroviral drugs in pregnancy. *Expert Opin Drug Saf* 2005; **4**: 323–335.

65. Tuomala RE, Watts DH, Li D *et al.* Improved obstetric outcomes and few maternal toxicities are associated with antiretroviral therapy, including highly active antiretroviral therapy during pregnancy. *J Acquir Immune Defic Syndr* 2005; **38**: 449–473.

66. De Santis M, Carducci B, De Santis L, Cavaliere AF, Straface G. Periconceptional exposure to efavirenz and neural tube defects. *Arch Intern Med* 2002; **162**: 355.

67. US Food and Drug Administration. FDA Public Health Advisory for Nevirapine (Viramune) 2005.

68. Thorne C, Newell ML. Prevention of mother-to-child transmission of HIV infection. *Curr Opin Infect Dis* 2004; **17**: 247–252.

69. Martinson N, Morris L, Gray G *et al.* HIV resistance and transmission following single-dose nevirapine in a prevention of MTCT cohort. 11th Conference on Retroviruses and Opportunistic Infections, San Francisco, 8–11 February 2004. Abstract 38.

70. Ekouevi DK, Inwoley A, Tonwe-Gold B *et al.* Variation of CD4 count and percentage during pregnancy and after delivery: implications for HAART initiation in resource-limited settings. *AIDS Res Hum Retroviruses* 2007; **23**: 1469–1474.

71. Tonwe-Gold B, Ekouevi D, Rouet F et al. Highly active antiretroviral therapy for the

prevention of perinatal HIV transmission in Africa.: mother-to-child HIV transmission plus, Abidjan, Côte d'Ivoire, 2003–2004. 12th Conference on Retroviruses and Opportunistic Infections, Boston, 22–25 February 2005. Abstract 785.

72. Palombi L, Germano P, Liotta G *et al.* HAART in pregnancy: safety, effectiveness, and protection from viral resistance: results from the DREAM cohort. 12th Conference on Retroviruses and Opportunistic Infections, Boston, 22–25 February 2005. Abstract 67.

73. Eshleman SH, Jones D, Guay L, Musoke P, Mmiro F, Jackson JB. HIV-1 variants with diverse nevirapine resistance mutations emerge rapidly after single dose nevirapine: HIVNET 012. XII International HIV Drug Resistance Workshop: Basic principles and clinical implications. July 2003, Cabo San Lucas, Mexico. 2003; Abstract.

74. Eshleman SH, Guay LA, Mwatha A *et al.* Characterization of nevirapine resistance mutations in women with subtype A vs. D HIV-1 6-8 weeks after single-dose nevirapine (HIVNET 012). *J Acquir Immune Defic Syndr* 2004; **35**: 126–130.

75. Eshleman SH, Guay LA, Mwatha A *et al.* Comparison of nevirapine (NVP) resistance in Ugandan women 7 days vs. 6-8 weeks after single-dose NVP prophylaxis: HIVNET 012. *AIDS Res Hum Retroviruses* 2004; **20**: 595–599.

76. Eshleman SH, Hoover DR, Chen S *et al.* Resistance after single-dose nevirapine prophylaxis emerges in a high proportion of Malawian newborns. *AIDS* 2005; **19**: 2167–2169.

77. Chaix ML, Ekouevi DK, Peytavin G *et al.* Impact of nevirapine (NVP) plasma concentration on selection of resistant virus in mothers who received single-dose NVP to prevent perinatal human immunodeficiency virus type 1 transmission and persistence of resistant virus in their infected children. *Antimicrob Agents Chemother* 2007; **51**: 896–901.

78. Chaix ML, Dabis F, Ekouevi D *et al.* Addition of 3 days of ZDV+3TC postpartum to a short course of ZDV+3TC and single-dose NVP provides low rate of NVP resistance mutations and high efficacy in preventing peri-partum HIV-1 transmission: ANRS DITRAME Plus, Abidjan, Côte d'Ivoire. 12th Conference on Retroviruses and Opportunistic Infections, Boston, 22–25 February 2005, Abstract 72LB.

79. Jourdain G, Ngo-Giang-Huong N, Le Coeur S, Bowonwatanuwong C, Kantipong P, Leechanachai P, et al. Intrapartum exposure to nevirapine and subsequent maternal responses to nevirapine-based antiretroviral therapy. *N Engl J Med* 2004; **351**: 229–240.

80. Lockman S, Shapiro RL, Smeaton LM *et al.* Response to antiretroviral therapy after a single, peripartum dose of nevirapine. *N Engl J Med* 2007; **356**: 135–147.

81. McIntyre JA, Martinson N, Gray GE *et al.* Addition of short course Combivir to single dose Viramune for the prevention of mother to child transmission of HIV-1 can significantly decrease the subsequent development of maternal and paediatric NNRTI-resistant virus. 3rd IAS Conference on HIV Pathogenesis and Treatment, Rio de Janeiro, 24–27 July 2005. Abstract TuFoO2O4.

82. Chi BH, Sinkala M, Mbewe F *et al.* Single-dose tenofovir and emtricitabine for reduction of viral resistance to non-nucleoside reverse transcriptase inhibitor drugs in women given intrapartum nevirapine for perinatal HIV prevention: an open-label randomised trial. *Lancet* 2007; **370**: 1698–1705.

*Robert Fraser*

**3**

# Management of gestational diabetes

As recently as 2003 in a Cochrane systematic review,[1] it was stated that: 'it is uncertain whether intensive treatment of gestational diabetes can influence birth-weight and reduce perinatal morbidity, *i.e.* is there any benefit to treating women with GDM [gestational diabetes mellitus] in pregnancy?' Obviously, in the absence of evidence of therapeutic benefit, the principal justification for screening would be absent; indeed, later that same year in the Antenatal Care Guidelines produced by the National Institute for Health and Clinical Excellence,[2] the following was included: 'there is an absence of evidence to support routine screening for gestational diabetes mellitus and, therefore, it is not recommended'.

This review principally concentrates on evidence published since the end of 2003 and addresses the question: is gestational diabetes mellitus (GDM) a disease capable of causing adverse perinatal outcomes and, if so, is there effective treatment available and are there effective screening protocols?

## IS GESTATIONAL DIABETES A DISEASE?

At the time of writing, publication of the Hyperglycaemia and Pregnancy Outcome (HAPO) study is awaited. This is an international study in which more than 23,000 women had a 75-g glucose tolerance test performed between 24–32 weeks' gestation.[3] Those with frank diabetes were unblinded but the remaining results were kept confidential pending the outcomes of the pregnancy. Preliminary results of the HAPO study suggest that, in the four principal outcomes – caesarean delivery, fetal macrosomia, neonatal hypoglycaemia, and fetal hyperinsulinism (measured by cord C-peptide levels) – there was a continuum producing an increase in each of these

**Robert Fraser** MD FRCOG
Reader, Reproductive & Developmental Medicine, University of Sheffield, Level 4, The Jessop Wing, Tree Root Walk, Sheffield S10 2SF, UK
E-mail: r.b.fraser@sheffield.ac.uk

complications with both increasing levels of fasting, and 1-h, and 2-h glucose levels. It seems likely that the HAPO study will result in a lowering of the glycaemic levels either on fasting or post load which are currently required to make the diagnosis of GDM. Certainly, earlier suppositions that there was limited adverse pregnancy outcome associated with impaired glucose tolerance (*i.e.* a 2-h value between 7.8–11 mmol/l) have not been confirmed by the preliminary results of this study.

The 2005 publication of the ACHOIS trial (*Effective Treatment of Gestational Diabetes on Pregnancy Outcomes*) was a landmark in relation to both confirming the fact that gestational diabetes has an adverse effect on perinatal outcomes and that treatment is effective in reducing those outcomes.[4] The study was a double-blind, randomised study of treatment versus no treatment in women with GDM (or impaired glucose tolerance 2-h level on oral glucose-tolerance test of 7.8–11.1 mmol/l of glucose) and addressed the question 'does treatment of women with screened detected impaired glucose tolerance in pregnancy reduce perinatal morbidity without increasing maternal physical and psychological morbidity?' The study was double-blind in that those in the routine care group were not aware that they had an abnormal glucose tolerance test nor were the obstetricians responsible for their care. In the intervention group, the results were revealed and those women were referred to routine diabetes/antenatal joint care for the remainder of their pregnancies. In this intervention group, the rate of serious perinatal complications by a composite measure was 1% whereas it was 4% in the routine care group, a relative risk of 0.33 (95% confidence interval, 0.14–0.70). Labour induction was more common in the intervention group and the rate of large-for-gestational-age (macrosomic) infants was 13% in the intervention group but 22% in the routine care group, a result which was also significant. There was no excess of caesarean deliveries in the intervention group although earlier, non-randomised, cohort studies had suggested that caesarean delivery might be more common in women who had been labelled as GDM. Measures of physical and mental well-being performed in a subgroup of the women following delivery showed a reduction in all adverse outcomes in the intervention group including a halving of diagnosed cases of postnatal depression from 17% down to 8%.

The authors concluded that treatment of gestational diabetes reduces serious perinatal morbidity and may also improve the women's health-related quality of life. On this basis, and accepting the results of this trial, it can be concluded that treatment is beneficial and, therefore, screening for GDM is justified.

## HOW SHOULD SCREENING BE PERFORMED?

The traditional use of risk factors for screening for gestational diabetes may still be appropriate for populations with a low prevalence (< 2%). The traditional risk factors – obesity (body mass index > 30 kg/m$^2$) family history of diabetes, previous pregnancy failure and previous macrosomia– will identify about 40% of the antenatal population in most clinics. If women with risk factors go on to diagnostic testing, the overall sensitivity is 69%, the specificity 68% and the positive predictive value is 5%.[5] For populations with intermediate or higher prevalence rates (above 2%), two-stage screening using the 50-g glucose challenge test is probably a pragmatic approach. In this test, originally described by O'Sullivan and co-workers in 1973,[6] the unprepared subject at 24–28 weeks' gestation is administered a 50-g glucose load in 150 ml of water. A spot plasma glucose test 1 h later above 7.8 mmol/l is an indication for a formal oral glucose-tolerance test. This approach has a sensitivity of 79%, a specificity of 87%, and a positive predictive value of 15%. The disadvantage, however, is in relation to the logistics of performing two provocative tests and the fact that patient acceptability may fall dramatically with such a demanding schedule.

In a population known to have a relatively high prevalence of gestational diabetes (4% or above), diagnostic screening by a modified 75-g oral glucose-tolerance test after an overnight fast may be appropriate.[7] In this study, women were visited, usually at home, by midwives and were given a 75-g glucose load first thing in the morning and had a 2-h blood glucose value measured on a portable glucose meter which was interpreted according to World Health Organization criteria.[8]

The number of women subjected to any of the above screening protocols might be reduced by identifying women at low risk of gestational diabetes as recommended by the American Diabetes Association.[9] That group consists of those women who are aged less than 25 years, of normal body weight, and from a low prevalence ethnic group.

## DOES GDM CAUSE AN INCREASE IN CONGENITAL MALFORMATIONS?

The relationship between pre-existing (Types 1 or 2) diabetes and major congenital malformations is well understood; in our own audit in Sheffield, major malformations were detected in 7.6% of such women but in only 2.0% of women with GDM. The latter figure is not significantly different from the non-diabetic population. Despite this, it is widely held that an increase in congenital malformations can be expected with GDM. The Californian group of Schaefer-Graf[10] showed that the likelihood of major malformations was related to the initial fasting level of glucose on diagnostic testing. Amongst the group who had no malformations (numbering more than 3800 women), the initial fasting plasma glucose was $6.4 \pm 2.0$ mmol/l; in those with major malformations (numbering 143), the initial fasting plasma glucose was $8.0 \pm 3.1$ mmol/l. In a small group of infants with aneuploidies, an abnormality not thought to be related to periconceptional hyperglycaemia, the fasting plasma glucose level was not significantly different from the group with no malformations. In a New Zealand study by Farrell and colleagues,[11] major congenital malformations were reported in 5.9% of women with Type 1 diabetes, 4.4% of women with Type 2 diabetes but only 1.4% of women with GDM, again not significantly different from the non-diabetic hospital population. In this study, however, 13% of the 1822 women with gestational diabetes had a diagnosis of new Type 2 diabetes on follow-up oral glucose-tolerance test. A retrospective analysis of this group showed a congenital malformation rate of 4.6%. The conclusion from these two studies is that periconceptional hyperglycaemia is the pathological mechanism in structural congenital malformation. Whilst this is not a feature of reversible GDM, it certainly does appear to be a feature of previously unrecognised Type 2 diabetes.

There is a clinical point here which emphasises the importance of both short- and long-term follow-up of women with GDM who may be planning a pregnancy in the future, as they should be advised to attend for preconceptional counselling and assessment of glycaemic control where possible.

## CAN GDM MANAGEMENT BE MORE EFFECTIVE?

Whilst the finding of newborn macrosomia is numerically more likely in women with diabetes, many studies have revealed the absence of a direct correlation between levels of glycaemia experienced in pregnancy and absolute birth-weight. Data from our own unit for women with pre-existing diabetes showed no relationship between the birth-weight ratio and the mean $HbA_{1C}$ averaged over three trimesters of pregnancy. The points of interest are that, in the offspring of women with diabetes: (i) the mean birth-weight is about 20% higher than that seen in the non-diabetic population; (ii) some of the bigger babies are born to some of the best controlled women; and (iii) some of the smaller babies are born to those women who have the highest levels of mean $HbA_{1C}$ during the pregnancy. We, therefore, suggest that birth-weight as a surrogate measure of quality of diabetes control is of interest but should not be judged to be the gold standard. We would recommend instead the use of a laboratory-based measurement of fetal insulinisation either based on amniotic fluid insulin or cord blood insulin measured at or around the time of delivery (Fig. 1).[12] The two measurements are highly correlated but the amniotic fluid insulin is less subject to hour-to-hour variability and is a more robust reflection of the metabolic perturbation to which the fetus has been exposed during the second half of pregnancy. In Figure 1, the amniotic fluid insulin levels are

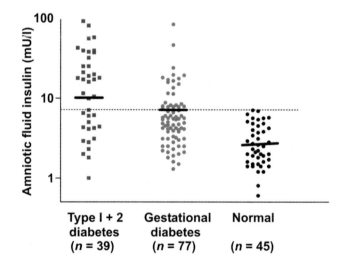

**Fig. 1** Amniotic fluid insulin levels (mU/l) at delivery in women with Types 1 or 2 diabetes and women with GDM, compared to a non-diabetic group. Bars represent geometrical means of each distribution; the dotted line is the upper limit of amniotic fluid insulin levels measured in non-diabetic women.

reported from women who had all been treated in a joint antenatal/diabetes clinic where attempts were made to control their glycaemia with diet and insulin. It can be seen that about a third of women with gestational diabetes at the end of pregnancy continue to have relatively hyperinsulinaemic fetuses; this illustrates the reason why perinatal complications are still seen in this group, and perhaps present a target for improvement of maternal glycaemic control.

There is evidence from the work of Weiss and colleagues[13] in Austria that, having diagnosed fetal hyperinsulinaemia by amniocentesis from 28 weeks' gestation onwards, targeted insulin therapy can correct fetal hyper-insulinaemia in cases of gestational diabetes and prevent expected levels of fetopathy. This technique, however, has not found general favour and, in our experience, there is considerable resistance from pregnant women to late amniocentesis although it is a safe procedure.

In offering any therapeutic regimen to women with GDM, the importance of diet should not be forgotten. The recommendations of organisations such as the American Diabetes Association and Diabetes UK[14] are a good starting point with particular emphasis on increasing carbohydrate sources from foods with low glycaemic indices. In an important publication from the DIAGEST group in Lille,[15] there was an inverse relationship between the proportion of large-for-gestational-age infants in diet-treated women with gestational diabetes and the percentage of calories from carbohydrate sources. There were no large-for-gestational-age babies in the two highest quintiles of carbohydrate intake but, in the lowest three quintiles, the rates were between 12–37%. The benefit, in terms of reducing the number of large-for-gestational-age infants, did not result in any detectable increase in small-for-gestational-age infants.

When considering hypoglycaemic therapy (which is usually insulin), guidance from the classic, randomised, controlled trial of Persson et al.[16] is still relevant. In this study, two groups of 97 and 105 women were randomised to diet and routine use of insulin for gestational diabetes or diet with insulin only if there was hyperglycaemia despite dietary adherence. In the diet alone group, 14% required additional insulin usually for a post-prandial plasma glucose level above 6.5 mmol/l. In this study, there were no significant differences in mean birth-weight rates, or small-for-gestational-age or large-for-gestational-age babies or in triceps skinfold thicknesses. Common neonatal morbidities such as respiratory distress syndrome, hypoglycaemia, hyperbilirubinaemia and polycythaemia were all similar in the group who had universal prescription of insulin compared to the group who had selective prescription of insulin. This study, therefore, justifies the selective use of insulin and suggests that the number of women and their offspring who would benefit from insulin is about 1 in 6.

This approach was refined by Kjos and colleagues[17] who used ultrasound parameters of abdominal circumference growth as a trigger for insulin, as well as maternal plasma glucose measurements in 98 women with GDM who had a fasting plasma glucose between 5.8–6.7 mmol/l. The experimental group were only given insulin if the abdominal circumference was above the 70th centile or plasma glucose exceeded 6.7 mmol/l post-prandially. The control group all received insulin with glycaemic targets of a pre-prandial level below 5 mmol/l of glucose and a 2-h post-prandial level below 6.7 mmol/l. The outcomes were that insulin was only prescribed in 62% of the experimental group, birth-weights were: controls, 3.27 ± 0.5 kg; experimental group, 3.37 ± 0.5 kg. Birth-weights above the 90th centile were 6.3% versus 8.3%, and neonatal morbidity present in 25% versus 25%. On the basis of this study, it was felt that ultrasound parameters of fetal growth were a useful addition to glycaemic parameters for judging those women who would benefit most from an insulin regimen.

The most useful study, however, addressed to this question is that of de Veciana and colleagues.[18] They performed a randomised, controlled trial of women with GDM diagnosed before 30 weeks' gestation who were judged to require an insulin prescription because of relative hyperglycaemia despite diet. They were split into a preprandial group in whom insulin was adjusted to keep the fasting glucose between 3.3–5.0 mmol/l and the preprandial glucose between 3.3–5.9 mmol/l, and a post-prandial group who had insulin adjusted to keep the fasting glucose between 3.3–5.0 mmol/l and the 1-h post prandial glucose < 7.8 mmol/l. The target levels were met by > 85% of both groups of women but the insulin dose at an average of 100 units/day was 25% higher in the post-prandial group. This was accompanied by a significant reduction of third trimester $HbA_{1C}$ measurement which was 6.5 ± 1.4% in the post-prandial group but 8.1 ± 2.2% in the preprandial group. In relation to maternal outcomes, there were no significant differences in rates of pre-eclampsia or gestational age at delivery. There was a non-significant trend towards a higher rate of caesarean section and a higher rate of third-degree tears in the preprandial group. In neonatal outcomes, mean birth-weights were 3.47 kg in the post-prandial group and 3.85 kg in the preprandial group, which was a highly significant difference as was the proportion of large-for-gestational age babies (12% versus 42%). Shoulder dystocia occurred in 1% of the post-prandial group and 6% of the preprandial group and neonatal hypoglycaemia (glucose < 1.6 mmol/l) in 3% of the post-prandial and 21% of the preprandial group. However, perhaps because of the small number of subjects in the study, these latter two trends were not statistically significant.

Although the use of oral hypoglycaemics has not found general favour in the management of GDM, principally because of concerns about possible teratogenesis and increased risks of neonatal hypoglycaemia, recent randomised studies do not support these concerns. A large scale study of Glyburide (Glibenclamide) compared to insulin in women with gestational diabetes has been performed in the US by Langer and colleagues.[19] A total of 404 women were randomised either to Glyburide 2.5 mg daily rising to 20 mg daily, or insulin. In the Glyburide group, insulin was prescribed if Glyburide did not maintain subjects within the set glycaemic parameters and 4% of women in this group required additional insulin. The percentage $HbA_{1C}$ in the two groups at 5.5% and 5.4% were not significantly different and the proportion of large-for-gestational-age babies at 12% in the Glyburide group and 13% in the insulin group were again not statistically significant. Cord serum insulin measurements at 15 µU/l in both groups of babies were identical. In relation to neonatal outcomes (respiratory distress syndrome/ transient tachypnoea of the newborn rates, hypoglycaemia requiring intravenous dextrose, the proportion of babies admitted to special care, and the proportion with congenital anomalies), no significant differences emerged between infants of the Glyburide-treated and insulin-treated women.

Sulphonylureas, therefore, represent an alternative to insulin in the majority of women with GDM who required hypoglycaemic therapy; it may soon become clear that this is an alternative which is cheaper and more acceptable to women than self-injection with insulin.

Also keenly awaited are the imminent results from the Metformin in Gestational Diabetes (MiG) study. In this study, randomisation to insulin or metformin to achieve glycaemic control in a group of 750 women with gestational diabetes has been performed. If the results support the use of metformin, then it probably has some theoretical advantages over the sulphonylureas for this group of women many of whom are obese and insulin resistant.

## TIMING OF DELIVERY

Timing of delivery in gestational diabetes remains somewhat controversial; some have suggested that the earlier delivery secured in the ACHOIS trial rather than the day-to-day management of maternal glycaemia was a more important factor in the observed reduction in adverse perinatal outcomes. Only one randomised, controlled trial of expectant versus elective delivery in gestational diabetes has been published.[20] In this study, 200 women (187 of whom had insulin-treated GDM) were randomised to an active group who had induction of labour within 5 days of reaching 38 completed weeks of gestation and an expectant group who were managed with twice weekly CTGs and weekly ultrasound estimates of amniotic fluid volume until spontaneous labour. There was a highly significant difference in birth-weights above the 90th centile (active group 10%, expectant group 23%) and, counter intuitively, the caesarean section rate was lower in the actively managed group although the difference was not significant (25% versus 31%). There were no cases of shoulder dystocia in the actively managed group but 3% were reported in the expectant group. There was a doubling of the spontaneous labour rate to 44% in the expectant group but this without any detectable benefit and some suggestion of harm.

This study seems to be sufficiently robust to be a basis for management recommendations and further studies addressed to this question may not be ethical. Since approximately 25% of still-births occurring in pregnancy and associated with maternal diabetes occur after 37 weeks of completed gestation, this would be another reason to follow the active management regimen, although, of course, the study reported did not have sufficient power to detect this.

## FOLLOW-UP

Because at least 12%, and in some populations up to 20%, of women diagnosed with gestational diabetes have, in fact, a new diagnosis of Type 2 diabetes or impaired glucose tolerance, a follow-up diagnostic glucose tolerance test is of considerable value. Even women who fail to attend for this test should be registered for appropriate follow-up through primary care. Initially, life-style and dietary interventions should be suggested which might reduce their risk of Type 2 diabetes later in life. An annual fasting plasma glucose should be performed to identify that group of women who have developed Type 2 diabetes since their pregnancy. This type of follow-up would also enable the identification of those women who would benefit from prepregnancy glycaemic control, to reduce the risk of congenital malformation in subsequent pregnancies. It also seems likely that, in addition to life-style and dietary changes, pharmacological approaches to prevention of Type 2 diabetes may be on the near horizon; if so, the diagnosis of gestational diabetes may identify a group of women who would benefit in terms of their long-term health from avoiding diabetes by suitable and timely pharmacological intervention.

## CONCLUSIONS

From a position of uncertainty about the significance of gestational diabetes and the value of systematic screening for this condition as recently as 2003, recent publications have confirmed that gestational diabetes is a disease with adverse perinatal outcomes and is susceptible to effective management. Screening is justified and should be based on expected prevalence of GDM in the unit which the woman attends. Both gestational diabetes and new-onset Type 2 diabetes are increasing dramatically on a world-wide basis and will come to have an increasingly important contribution to the workload of obstetricians in the years to come.

---

### Key points for clinical practice

- Gestational diabetes should be identified by screening and treated.
- Screening methods will very in their practical effectiveness and acceptability depending on local population prevalence of GDM.
- Treatment should be initially by high carbohydrate low glycaemic index diet.
- Insulin or oral hypoglycaemic therapy should be considered in women with incipient fetal macrosomia – despite apparently adequate glycaemic control.
- Elective delivery should be offered after 38 completed weeks of gestation.
- Women with GDM should have an annual fasting glucose performed for life and referred for pre-pregnancy counselling if contemplating a further pregnancy.

---

### References

1. Tuffnell DJ, West J, Walkinshaw SA. Treatments for gestational diabetes and impaired glucose tolerance in pregnancy. The Cochrane Database of Systematic Reviews 2003: Issue 3, CD003395.
2. National Institute for Health and Clinical Excellence. *NICE Clinical Guideline 6: Antenatal Care. Routine care for the healthy pregnant woman*. London: NICE, 2003; 96–99.
3. HAPO Study Cooperative Research Group. The Hyperglycaemia and Adverse

Pregnancy Outcome (HAPO) study. *Int J Gynaecol Obstet* 2002; **78**: 69–77.

4. Crowther CA, Hiller JE, Moss JR, McPhee AJ, Jeffries WS, Robinson JS. Effect of treatment of gestational diabetes mellitus on pregnancy outcomes. *N Engl J Med* 2005; **352**: 2477–2486.

5. Helton MR, Arndt J, Kebede M, King M. Do low risk prenatal patients really need a screening glucose challenge test? *J Fam Pract* 1997; **44**: 556–561.

6. O'Sullivan JB, Mahan CM, Charles D, Dandrow RV. Screening criteria for high-risk gestational diabetic patients. *Am J Obstet Gynecol* 1973; **116**: 895–900.

7. Åberg A, Rydhstroem H, Frid A. Impaired glucose tolerance associated with adverse pregnancy outcome. A population-based study in Southern Sweden. *Am J Obstet Gynecol* 2001; **184**: 77–83.

8. Alberti KG, Zimmett PZ. Definition, diagnosis and classification of diabetes mellitus and its complications. Part 1: diagnosis and classification of diabetes mellitus: provisional report of a WHO consultation. *Diabet Med* 1998; **15**: 539–553.

9. American Diabetes Association. Gestational Diabetes Mellitus. *Diabetes Care* 2004; **27 (Suppl 1)**: 588–590.

10. Schaefer-Graf UM, Buchanan TA, Xiang A *et al*. Patterns of congenital anomalies and relationship to initial maternal fasting glucose levels in pregnancies complicated by Type 2 and gestational diabetes. *Am J Obstet Gynecol* 2000; **182**: 313–320.

11. Farrell T, Neale L, Cundy T. Congenital anomalies in the offspring of women with Type 1, Type 2 and gestational diabetes. *Diabet Med* 2002; **19**: 322–326.

12. Fraser RB, Bruce C. Amniotic fluid insulin levels identify the fetus at risk of neonatal hypoglycaemia. *Diabet Med* 1999; **16**: 568–572.

13. Weiss PAM, Hofman H. Intensified conventional insulin therapy for the pregnant diabetic patient. *Obstet Gynecol* 1984; **64**: 629–637.

14. Nutrition Subcommittee of the Diabetes Care Advisory Committee of Diabetes UK. The implementation of nutritional advice for people with diabetes. *Diabet Med* 2003; **20**: 786–807.

15. Romon M, Nuttens MC, Vambergue A *et al*. Higher carbohydrate intake is associated with decreased incidence of newborn macrosomia in women with gestational diabetes. *J Am Dietet Assoc* 2001; **101**: 897–902.

16. Persson B, Stangenberg M, Hansson U, Norlander E. Gestational diabetes mellitus (GDM). Comparative evaluation of two treatment regimens, diet versus insulin and diet. *Diabetes* 1985; **34 (Suppl 1)**: 101–105.

17. Kjos SL, Schaeffer-Graf U, Sardesi S *et al*. A randomised controlled trial using glycaemic plus fetal ultrasound parameters versus glycaemic parameters to determine insulin therapy in gestational diabetes with fasting hyperglycaemia. *Diabetes Care* 2001; **24**: 1904–1910.

18. De Viciana M, Major CA, Morgan MA *et al*. Postprandial versus preprandial blood glucose monitoring in women with gestational diabetes mellitus requiring insulin therapy. *N Engl J Med* 1995; **333**: 1237–1241.

19. Langer O, Conway DL, Berkus MD, Xenakis EM, Gonzales O. A comparison of Glyburide and insulin in women with gestational diabetes mellitus. *N Engl J Med* 2000; **343**: 1134–1138.

20. Kjos SL, Henry OA, Montoro M, Buchanan TA, Mestman JH. Insulin-requiring diabetes in pregnancy: a randomised trial of active induction of labor and expectant management. *Am J Obstet Gynecol* 1993; **169**: 611–615.

*Susana Aguilera  Peter Soothill*

# 4

# Abnormalities of the fetal urinary tract

Anomalies of the urinary tract are the largest group of fetal abnormalities diagnosed by ultrasound in pregnancy, corresponding to 20–25% of all antenatally diagnosed anomalies using ultrasonography,[1,2] and with a reported prevalence ranging from 1 in 250 to 1 in 1000 deliveries.[3] At about 90%, the detection sensitivity is high even in low-risk populations when compared to postnatal examination and scans.[4,5] However, most genito-urinary abnormalities are asymptomatic and so are not detected at birth unless the kidneys and bladder have been carefully visualised during obstetrical ultrasound screening.

With modern high-resolution scanning, it is possible to evaluate the fetal kidneys in detail at 12 weeks of pregnancy,[6] when they appear as homogeneous structures on each side of the spine. The fetal urinary bladder can usually be identified at 13 weeks and is often seen earlier. The kidneys and bladder can almost always be identified by 16 weeks with a transabdominal approach. In longitudinal section, the kidneys are seen as bilateral elliptical structures; in transverse section, they have a circular appearance adjacent to the lumbar spine. Between 18–24 weeks, the medulla becomes hypo-echogenic and is distinguishable from the echogenic renal cortex. Normally, the ureters are not visible on scanning. After the 16th week of gestation, almost all of the amniotic fluid arises from fetal urine as evidenced by profound oligo- or anhydramnios by 18 weeks in cases of bilateral renal agenesis. A normal amount of amniotic fluid implies the presence of at least one functioning kidney and a patent urinary conduit to the amniotic cavity. The fetal kidney

**Susana Aguilera** MBBS
Clinical Research Fellow, Centro de Referencia Perinatal Oriente (CEPO), Hospital Luis Tisné Brousse, Av Las Torres 5150, Peñalolén, Santiago, Chile
E-mail: susag29i@gmail.com

**Peter Soothill** MBBS BSc MD FRCOG (for correspondence)
Emeritus Professor of Maternal and Fetal Medicine, University of Bristol, Bristol, UK
Consultant in Fetal Medicine, St Michael's Hospital, Southwell Street, Bristol BS2 8EG, UK
E-mail: peter.soothill@bristol.ac.uk

produces hypotonic urine from the fifth to ninth weeks and the volume increases throughout gestation up to a rate of about 50 ml/h. The fetal kidneys grow throughout pregnancy but the ratio of kidney circumference to abdominal circumference remains relatively constant at 0.27–0.30.

The severity of fetal renal tract disorders ranges between lethal disorders (with genetic syndromes or chromosomal defects) to transient, mild, renal, pelvic dilatation in an otherwise normal fetus and an excellent prognosis. Overall, abnormalities of the fetal urinary tract have been associated with chromosomal abnormalities in about 12% of cases[7] but the rate will be much lower in cases where the urinary tract defect is isolated or when a decision is made not to undertake an invasive procedure. A complete absence of amniotic fluid during the critical time of lung development (16–24 weeks) usually leads to pulmonary hypoplasia not compatible with extra-uterine life. Oligohydramnios also results in a characteristic group of clinical findings known as Potter sequence including low-set and flattened ears, short and snubbed nose, deep eye creases, micrognathia and deformity of extremities such as club foot.

In this chapter, we consider the range of diagnoses and effects in anatomical order from the renal tissue to the genitalia.

## RENAL TISSUE ABNORMALITIES

### ABNORMALITIES OF NUMBER

#### Renal agenesis

Renal agenesis may affect one or both kidneys and bilateral cases are fatal. The use of high-resolution sonography and colour Doppler of the renal artery help with the diagnosis. However, the adrenal gland can appear similar to a kidney especially when scanning is difficult in the absence of amniotic fluid. When severe oligohydramnios is associated with no visible renal tissue or bladder, bilateral agenesis is likely. It is our practice to use the term 'no functioning renal tissue' to avoid causing distress to the parents should a small amount of renal tissue be subsequently found at post-mortem. The prognosis of unilateral disease is good (usually normal) but other associated anomalies may be found subsequently, for example genital malformations in Mayer–Rokintansky–Küstner–Hauser syndrome.

#### Duplex kidney

A duplex kidney has a single renal parenchyma drained by two pyelocaliceal systems that are associated with bifid or duplicated ureters. The upper ureter enters the bladder in a more caudal and medial position and ectopically outside of the trigone. The upper part of the kidney often has some degree of outflow obstruction and parenchymal dysplasia. On scanning, the parts of the kidney are seen to have their own renal pelvises and sometimes a ureterocele will be seen in the bladder which should be carefully examined (see below).

### ABNORMALITIES OF POSITION

#### Ectopic kidneys

When kidneys are abnormally positioned, they are usually displaced caudally.

One or both kidneys may be involved and this is usually an asymptomatic condition, although postnatally renal tract infection may be more common.

Sometimes, the two kidneys may join, usually at their lower poles. This is conventionally called a 'horseshoe' kidney. On scan, the lower poles of the kidneys may not be delineated clearly or the kidneys may look abnormally small. Usually, these children are asymptomatic, but the condition can be associated with other renal problems, such as pelvi-ureteric junction obstruction (present in 35% of cases). Rarely, horseshoe kidneys can be associated with chromosomal abnormalities such as Turner syndrome and trisomy 18.

## ABNORMALITIES OF THE SIZE AND STRUCTURE

### Multicystic dysplasia of the kidney (MCDK, Potter II)
Multicystic dysplasia is the most common cause of an abdominal mass in the newborn period and the most common cystic malformation of the kidney in infancy. MCDK can be uni- or bilateral and is a form of renal dysplasia characterised by the presence of multiple cysts of varying size in the kidney. The condition is associated with ureteric or ureteropelvic atresia and the affected kidney is non-functional.[8,9] Unilateral incidence is reported as 1 in 4300 live births, being slightly more common in males (ratio 1.48:1) and on the left side (55%). Two theories have been proposed to explain the aetiology of this disease:

1. *Primary abnormality of kidney development.* The metanephric blastema differentiates into the renal parenchyma under the influence of the ampulla of the ureteric bud. An abnormal induction of the metanephric blastema by the migrating ureteric bud may result in a MCDK.

2. *Early obstruction of the urinary tract.* Obstruction can damage fetal kidneys and the earlier and more complete the obstruction, the more profound the effect. When obstruction occurs early, the result can be a cystic, non-functioning kidney including MCDK. Later obstructive events such as at the pelvi-ureteric junction or ureterovesical obstruction can also produce cysts and renal dysplasia but may allow preservation of some degree of renal function.

Both of the above probably occur but the difference in aetiology cannot be distinguished at present. MCDK usually is a sporadic problem but associations have been reported with mendelian and chromosomal conditions and exposure to teratogens like cocaine.[10] Moreover, the condition has been associated with several genetic syndromes including Beckwith Wiedemann, Joubert, Branchio-oto-renal, Williams's syndrome, VACTERL association and also with trisomy 18.

### Diagnosis
The ultrasound appearances included enlarged, echogenic renal tissue with multiple cysts of varying sizes (Potter 2a; Fig. 1). The outline of the kidney and the parenchyma between the cysts tends to be lost and in some cases involution results in a small or undetectable 'absent' kidney (Potter 2b). The appearances of MCKD can be hard to distinguish from a large hydronephrotic

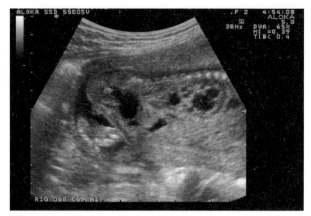

**Fig. 1** Multicystic dysplasia of the kidney.

kidney. However, the latter is usually still reniform in contour, while the parenchyma is present around the cysts (which are dilated calices). The size of the cysts is more uniform.

The contralateral kidney needs to be assessed, bilateral disease occurs in about 20% of cases. Many MCDK cases have other urological problems,[11,12] such as contralateral vesico-ureteral reflux, hydronephrosis secondary to pelvi-ureteric junction obstruction or a duplicated collecting system, agenesis of the contralateral kidney, ectopic pelvic kidney and ureterocele. Doppler assessment of blood flows in the renal artery of the affected kidney may demonstrate a lower blood velocity than normal.[13] Associated non-renal anomalies include gastrointestinal, neurological, cardiovascular, spinal and cranial abnormalities.[14] Fetal karyotyping should be considered when other anomalies are found.

### Management

Treatment of the fetus is not possible and the affected kidney will not function. Termination of pregnancy should be discussed in bilateral disease and a post-mortem examination should be recommended in order to confirm the diagnosis, determine additional features and thus assess the risk of recurrence. For unilateral disease, observation of the contralateral kidney during pregnancy should be followed by postnatal investigation. Follow-up is important in order to reduce the risks of injury to the normal kidney by events such as urinary tract infection.

In the absence of other abnormalities, unilateral MCDK disease has an excellent prognosis. MCDK may remain static without any change, may increase in size or may undergo spontaneous involution: the last is most common. Symptoms after birth are uncommon but can include abdominal or flank pain, urinary tract infections, hypertension and, very rarely, malignant degeneration. The role of nephrectomy in MCDK is controversial but, at present, these kidneys are not being removed in most centres.

### POLYCYSTIC KIDNEY DISEASE

Polycystic disease includes two different forms of inherited bilateral renal disease – autosomal recessive polycystic kidney disease (ARPKD; previously known as infantile polycystic kidney disease) and autosomal dominant polycystic kidney disease (ADPKD; previously known as adult polycystic kidney disease). However, both conditions can involve the presence of renal cysts at any time during an affected person's life, from the prenatal period to adolescence or adulthood.

## AUTOSOMAL RECESSIVE DISEASE (POTTER I)

Autosomal recessive disease is characterised by bilateral cystic dilatation of the renal collecting ducts associated with hepatic abnormalities of varying severity including biliary dysgenesis combined with periportal hepatic fibrosis. The incidence is 1 in 20,000 live births.[15] Males and females are affected equally. The frequency of heterozygous gene carriers is estimated to be 1 in 70. Mutations in the same gene (PKDHD1) are responsible for all typical forms of the disease. This gene is localised in the short arm of chromosome 6 and encodes for a ciliary protein called fibrocystin which is expressed on the cilia of renal and bile duct epithelial cells. Because of the recessive pattern of inheritance, both parents are unaffected and the recurrence risk in subsequent pregnancies is 25%.

### Diagnosis

On ultrasound, recessive polycystic kidneys appear as bilaterally enlarged echogenic kidneys with a reniform shape (Fig. 2). Cysts are not usually seen prenatally because the abnormality is in the collecting ducts and the cysts usually measure less than 3 mm. The degree of renal enlargement is directly proportional to the number of dilated ducts. There is loss of corticomedullary differentiation, although there may be a thin rim of hypo-echoic parenchyma at the periphery that is presumed to be compressed cortex. Macrocysts may become evident over time as they tend to become larger and more numerous.[16] Usually, the bladder is small or not visible. The disease is not commonly associated with other anomalies but MRI has been used in cases of maternal obesity and severe oligohydramnios.[17]

The differential diagnosis of the kidney's appearance includes autosomal dominant polycystic kidney disease, but in that condition the corticomedullary

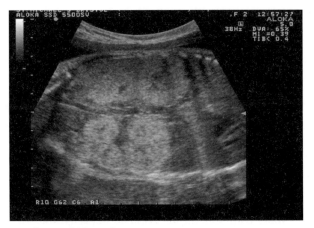

**Fig. 2** Recessive polycystic kidney disease.

differentiation tends to be preserved and usually the amniotic fluid is normal. Furthermore, one of the parents will be affected in 90% of cases. Meckel Gruber syndrome can also give the appearances of polycystic kidney disease but, in addition, one would usually see the other features of that condition such as encephalocele or post axial polydactyly in addition to enlarged echogenic kidneys. In asphyxiating thoracic dysplasia, a narrow thorax and rhizomelic limb shortening would also be seen. In trisomy 13 holoprosencephaly, cardiac or facial defects and postaxial hexadactyly are also found.

A haplotype-based diagnostic test has been developed for at-risk pregnancies.[18] At least one mutation is identified in 92–98% of cases when a prenatal diagnostic genetic test is performed. Haplotype-based molecular analysis needs at least one index case in the patient's family. Linkage analysis can be used when no mutation has been identified.[18,19]

### Prognosis

The severity of the disease varies depending of the number of collecting ducts affected (10–90%), resulting in varying degrees of renal function impairment and in amniotic fluid related pulmonary hypoplasia. Frequently, these infants die from pulmonary complications after birth. It is estimated that 20–30% of patients die, primarily from respiratory insufficiency due to pulmonary hypoplasia, however, longer term hepatic interstitial fibrosis is also important. In an American follow-up multicentre study,[20] 74.7% of the patients were alive after a median age of 5.4 years, 40.5% of patients required ventilation, 11.6% developed chronic lung disease and chronic renal insufficiency was reported in 40% of patients.

## AUTOSOMAL DOMINANT DISEASE (POTTER III)

This is the most common inherited kidney disease in humans with an estimated prevalence of about 1 in 1000 people. There is a wide clinical spectrum ranging from severe fetal renal impairment with similar presentation to ARPKD to asymptomatic cysts found incidentally at autopsy after death of an adult. The majority of fetuses show normal renal function at birth. The condition is characterised by progressive bilateral cystic dilatation developing anywhere along the nephron with variable extrarenal manifestations. In adults with this condition, cysts can occur in liver, pancreas, spleen, lungs, and ovaries as well as cerebral aneurysms but these are not seen in fetuses. This condition is not commonly associated with other abnormalities. Three genes are responsible for ADPKD (PKD1, PKD2 and PKD3) and, in 90% of patients, the affected gene is localised on the short arm of chromosome 16. In the remaining 10%, the disease arises from a spontaneous mutation.[21] The PKD genes encode for polycystyn proteins which are expressed in the developing kidney.

Because of the dominant inheritance of the disease, one of the parents is usually affected and the risk of recurrence is, therefore, 50%. The clinical manifestations vary from completely asymptomatic to severe neonatal disease. However, the most common presentation is hypertension and progressive renal failure occurring during the third or fourth decades of life.

## Diagnosis

On fetal ultrasound, enlarged echogenic kidneys with conserved cortico-medullary differentiation may be observed but cysts tend not to be seen at all until late pregnancy. In adults, the classical appearance is multiple bilateral macrocysts of different sizes usually smaller than 2 cm. Amniotic fluid volume is usually normal but the findings may be indistinguishable from ARPKD cases. The diagnosis is easy when renal cysts are found in one of the parents and parental renal ultrasound examinations may, therefore, be helpful. While a prenatal diagnostic test is available in 85% of cases following gene sequence analysis,[22] this presents an ethical dilemma in relation to a disease which is usually of late onset. For example, the child could be treated differently and medical insurance availability may be limited. It is also important to explain to the parents that normal fetal kidney ultrasound appearances do not exclude the chance of a later presentation.

The differential diagnosis is recessive polycystic renal disease (see above).

# RENAL PELVIS

## RENAL PELVIS DILATATION

About half of the urinary tract abnormalities detected prenatally are dilated renal pelvises or hydronephrosis which occurs in 1–2% of pregnancies.[23,31] If the problem were not detected prenatally, some of these children would present later in life with pyelonephritis, flank or abdominal pain, renal calculi, hypertension, or even renal failure. Renal pelvis dilatation (RPD) can be the result of non-obstructive processes: 79–84% of isolated hydronephrosis is caused by physiological dilatation of the developing ureter. However vesico-ureteral reflux, pathological mega-ureter without reflux or obstruction, and prune belly syndrome are also possible causes. On the other hand, the problem may be the result of obstructive processes: (i) pelvi-ureteric junction obstruction; (ii) ureterovesical obstruction; or (iii) lower urinary tract obstruction.

A hypothesis as to how obstruction induces dysplasia is that increased renin–angiotensin–aldosterone may produce vasoconstriction, interstitial fibrosis, ischaemic atrophy and induction of apoptosis in the obstructed kidney, resulting in cysts and renal dysplasia.[24] Early relief of the obstructive process has been reported to be followed by significant haemodynamic recovery.[25] However, others have reported that only a small percentage of the damage is relieved by early intervention.[26] Candidates for antenatal treatment are, therefore, those fetuses who have an obstructive uropathy giving rise to a significant threat of neonatal death (oligohydramnios and subsequent pulmonary hypoplasia). Even so, there is controversy about the efficacy of therapeutic intervention.[27,28]

## Diagnosis

The maximum anterior–posterior diameter of the renal pelvis is the measurement used to assess RPD but different cut-off values have been applied.[29] We use 5 mm to define RPD until 32 weeks of pregnancy.

The term pyelectasis is used for a mild degree of renal pelvis dilatation not including the renal calices and the term hydronephrosis is for more severe

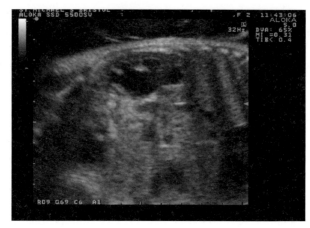

**Fig. 3** Fetal hydronephrosis.

dilatation with caliceal dilatation (Fig. 3). Renal parenchyma is considered thinned when it is less than 3 mm thick.

The Society for Fetal Urology has developed a grading system:

Grade 0      No dilatation (*i.e.* normal).

Grade I      Slight renal pelvis dilatation without calices visible.

Grade II     Renal pelvis dilatation with a few calices visible.

Grade III    Renal pelvis and calices dilated.

Grade IV     Features of grade III with parenchymal thinning.

There is a correlation between the degree of renal pelvic dilatation and the risk of obstruction. Coplen *et al.*[30] reported that renal pelvic dilatation greater than 15 mm will identify obstruction in about 80% of fetuses (sensitivity, 73%; specificity, 82%). In a retrospective study, Wollenberg *et al.*[31] reported that none of 20 children with a prenatal diagnosis of mild renal pelvis dilatation (7–9.9 mm) during the third trimester experienced a urinary tract infection or underwent surgery. In contrast, 5 out of 22 (23%) children with moderate hydronephrosis (10-14.9 mm) and 23 out of 36 (64%) children with severe hydronephrosis (≥ 15 mm) had either a UTI or required surgery (*P* < 0.001).

## Management

The risk of associated abnormalities (such as Down's syndrome) has been controversial. According to a meta-analysis published in 2001,[32] the presence of isolated renal pelvis dilatation has a sensitivity of 0.02 (95% CI, 0.01–0.06) for the diagnosis of fetuses with Down's syndrome at the time of second trimester ultrasound; it would, therefore, be necessary to screen 30,404 women in order to diagnose one case. The UK national screening committee recommends that the risk of Down's syndrome should not be recalculated up or down due to the presence or absence of a single ultrasound marker of less predictive power than that of an increased nuchal fold. In the absence of other findings, isolated pyelectasis is not a justification for the performance of amniocentesis.

Isolated bilateral RPD should be monitored and the baby referred for postnatal assessment. Very rarely and in the severest cases associated with obstruction, the kidney can rupture into the retroperitoneal space and urine can be seen around the kidney, confined within Gerota's facia, forming a urinoma.

## PELVI-URETERIC JUNCTION OBSTRUCTION

Pelvi-ureteric junction (PUJ) obstruction is the commonest cause of hydronephrosis in paediatric practice. The reported incidence is 1 in 1000–2000 newborns. At birth, this pathology is most common in males (2:1) and on the left side (67%) but it is bilateral in 10% of cases. It is thought to be caused by inadequate recanalisation of the ureteric bud in this area. Several growth factors and transcriptional factors like Pax 2, NO and neuropeptide Y have been suggested as causes of abnormal ureteric innervation.[33] The condition may also result from external compression or in association with ureteric duplication.

### Management
Bilateral lesions with oligohydramnios but adequate renal function have occasionally been treated by ultrasound-guided pelvi-ureteric amniotic shunting. The aim is to avoid the development of pulmonary hypoplasia from the oligohydramnios as well as to preserve renal function.

## URETER

Dilatation of the ureter can result from four different causes:
1. Ureterocele (discussed in bladder section).
2. Congenital megalo-ureter/ureterovesical junction stenosis.
3. Prune belly syndrome.
4. Lower urinary tract obstruction (discussed in bladder section).

## CONGENITAL MEGALO-URETER/URETEROVESICAL JUNCTION STENOSIS

Congenital megalo-ureter means a dilated ureter without reflux and with a normal bladder. It can be the result of a dysfunction at the ureterovesical junction. This is more common in males and on the left side and may regress spontaneously. The only way for the condition to be distinguished from reflux is by performing a voiding cysto-urethrogram in the newborn period and so is not a diagnosis that can be made prenatally. Ureterovesical junction stenosis is extremely rare.

## PRUNE BELLY SYNDROME

Prune belly syndrome is the term used to describe a newborn's abnormally lax and severely wrinkled abdominal wall resulting from a severe and early dilatation of the fetal urinary bladder. Characteristically, there would be dilatation of the bladder and ureters with bilateral hydronephrosis and oligohydramnios but this term may be used in the absence of a postnatally identifiable obstructive lesion. In such cases, it seems likely that there had been an early obstruction which had resolved spontaneously but had left the after effects.[34] The condition is strongly associated with pulmonary hypoplasia and a high perinatal mortality.

## BLADDER

The most important pathologies of the bladder are:

1. Ureterocele.
2. Bladder extrophy/cloacal malformations.
3. Lower urinary tract obstruction: posterior urethral valves, urethral atresia.
4. Megacystis microcolon syndrome.

### URETEROCELE

Ureterocele is a cystic dilatation of the portion of the ureter inside the bladder. The Urologic Section of the American Academy of Pediatrics classifies the condition as: (i) intravesical (the ureterocele is completely contained inside the bladder); or (ii) extravesical or ectopic (part of the cyst extends to the urethra or bladder neck).

Of cases, 80% are associated with the upper pole of a complete duplication and 60–80% are ectopic or extravesical. The incidence of ureterocele has been reported to lie between 1 in 5000 and 1 in 12,000 general paediatric admissions.[35] The malformation is observed almost exclusively in Caucasians and females are affected 4 times more frequently than males. Left and right side are equally affected and 10% are bilateral. In females 95% and in males 44% are associated with a duplex system. There can be dysplasia or obstructive nephropathy affecting the upper pole or the kidney drained by the ureterocele, suggesting that this is due to obstruction. The contralateral urinary tract is duplex in 30–40% of cases without a contralateral ureterocele.

The aetiology is unknown but possible causes include obstruction of the ureteric orifice, incomplete muscularisation of the intramural ureter and excessive dilation of the intramural ureter during the development. The most commonly accepted factor is a delayed and incomplete re-absorption of the membrane that separates the ureteric bud from the mesonephric duct in the embryo resulting in prolapse of the ureteric epithelium into the bladder.

On prenatal ultrasound examination, ureteroceles appear as thin-walled cyst-like structures within the bladder (Fig. 4). The detection of a ureterocele has been associated with postnatal confirmation of a duplex kidney in 78% of cases.[36] This finding becomes urgent prenatally when the prolapse is sufficient to block the urethra and cause a lower urinary tract obstruction. After birth, the most common clinical presentation is urinary tract infection.

### Management

There is no need for the management of pregnancy to be changed unless there is evidence of lower urinary tract obstruction. Although uncommon, a large prolapsing ureterocele may cause bladder outlet obstruction and a risk of bilateral renal damage. Options for treatment include the placement of a

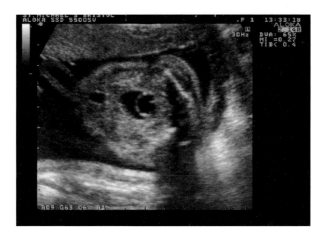

**Fig. 4** Ureterocele.

vesico-amniotic shunt and cystoscopically or ultrasound-guided laser incision to perforate the ureterocele[37] allowing collapse and relief of obstruction

## BLADDER EXTROPHY

Bladder extrophy is a lower abdominal wall defect that leads to malformation of the bladder and urethra, in which the bladder is turned 'inside out'. The bladder does not form into its normal round shape but instead is flattened and exposed on to the lower abdominal wall. As an isolated abnormality, it has a prevalence of 1 in 30,000 births and it is more common in males than females (ratio 2:1). The diagnosis is suspected when the fluid-filled intrapelvic bladder is not seen during a prolonged scanning period, the amniotic fluid volume is normal and a soft tissue mass is seen within the lower abdominal wall. Bladder extrophy is associated with urogenital anomalies (epispadias) and diastasis of pelvic bone as well as being part of a cloacal malformation including omphalocele, extrophy, imperforate anus, and spina bifida called OEIS syndrome. The cause is unknown and the condition most commonly occurs as an isolated sporadic birth defect with a low recurrence risk. However, familial clusters have been reported.[38] An isolated defect is surgically correctable at birth using a three-stage reconstruction procedure; in the UK, the care of these children is centralised to two services.

Cloacal malformation is described when the genital, urinary and gastrointestinal tracts are fused into a single common channel. It occurs in about 1 in 20,000 live births and is almost exclusively described in females. The cloaca is usually a transient structure, occurring during embryonic development until 5 weeks' gestation and a persistent cloaca results from failure of development of the urorectal septum. It can be associated with bladder extrophy, which involves an anterior abdominal wall defect (1 in 100,000 live births) and spinal defects. The commonest signs detected by ultrasound are a pelvic cystic structure (corresponding to a dilated vagina), inability to visualise the bladder, bilateral hydronephrosis, normal or reduced amniotic fluid and, in some cases, ambiguous genitalia and growth retardation.[39] Repairing this defect represents a serious technical challenge.

Procedures should be performed in specialised centres by paediatric surgeons dedicated to the care of these patients. Success rates vary, depending upon the complexity of the abnormality.

## LOWER URINARY TRACT OBSTRUCTION (LUTO)

The majority of affected individuals are males. However, females may demonstrate bladder outlet obstruction from a cloacal malformation, ureterocele (see above) or urethral atresia. In males, the most common cause is posterior urethral valves (PUVs).

## POSTERIOR URETHRAL VALVES

Posterior urethral valves are the commonest cause of bladder outlet obstruction in males. The prevalence reported is 1 in 5000–8000 live births and it accounts for 10% of all urological anomalies detected prenatally. It results from a thin membrane of tissue that obstructs normal bladder emptying. The aetiology is not known but the condition is thought to arise due to an abnormally anterior insertion of the Wolffian duct into the cloaca prior to its division into the urogenital sinus and the anorectal canal. Obstruction then increases the voiding pressure and may alter normal development of the fetal bladder and kidney; for example, vesico-ureteral reflux is present in one-half of patients. The perinatal mortality is around 30–50%.

### Diagnosis

PUVs are suspected when there is persistent urinary bladder dilatation often with a thickened (> 3 mm) over-trabeculated bladder wall. The dilated bladder can become very large  filling the abdomen; the dilated proximal urethra often resembles a keyhole extending from the bladder toward the fetal perineum (Fig. 5). Oligohydramnios is usually found. If the amniotic fluid volume is normal, there may be a partial obstruction but other diagnoses should be considered. The upper renal tract often becomes dilated as well due to vesico-ureteral reflux induced by the high intravesical pressure. In severe obstruction, the bladder may spontaneously decompress following rupture, resulting in fetal urinary ascites.

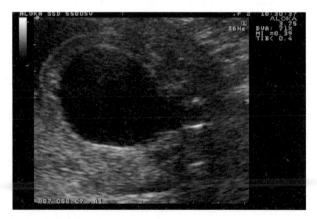

**Fig. 5** Keyhole sign in fetal LUTO.

## Management

There is controversy about whether early fetal therapy improves the prognosis. Serial vesicocentesis has been performed as early as the first trimester, but its efficacy remains unclear.[40] Vesico-amniotic shunting bypassing the congenital urethral obstruction could potentially improve the fetal outcome as a result of either reducing renal tissue damage or improving fetal lung development. A double pigtail catheter[41] can be inserted through a cannula with the distal end placed into the dilated bladder and the proximal end in the amniotic cavity. This reduces the pressure in the urinary tract to amniotic fluid pressure, and allows fetal urine to form amniotic fluid.

The appropriate selection of fetuses that could benefit from this procedure is probably the most important issue. The aim should be to identify fetuses without already established irreversible renal impairment or pulmonary hypoplasia, when shunting will not help. It is also important to exclude cases that will have good outcome in any event, to avoid a greater risk from the procedure than from the disease itself. At present, there are no large prospective randomised studies assessing the risks and benefits of this intervention. For this reason, a multicentre randomised controlled trial is under way (PLUTO).[42] The intention is to recruit 200 singleton pregnancies with ultrasound evidence of LUTO in order to evaluate the safety and effectiveness of *in utero* shunting compared to conservative management. Potential complications include preterm labour or spontaneous abortion, shunt blockage or displacement, fetal trauma, hydrops fetalis and urinary ascites. Fetal cystoscopy with endoscopic destruction of posterior urethral valves has also been described as a possible approach to management in some centres,[43] but the results have not demonstrated a clear benefit.

Until the results of such studies are available, clinicians will need to continue to make the best possible clinical judgements in relation to these complex issues. Parents must be informed of the uncertainty surrounding the efficacy of the available procedures and must be permitted a considerable degree of choice.[44]

## URETHRAL ATRESIA

The appearances obtained in cases of urethral atresia are similar to those of PUVs. However, with atresia, the features develop very early in pregnancy and are very severe, perhaps because the obstruction in PUVs may be partial. Atresia is seen in both sexes, but is more frequent in males and is usually associated with profound oligohydramnios after 16 weeks. Survival is very unlikely; if there is a patent urachus, vesicocutaneous fistula or if a vesico-amniotic shunt has been placed, long-term survival has been reported.[45]

## ASSESSMENT OF FETUSES WITH OBSTRUCTIVE UROPATHY

Therapy *in utero* is restricted to fetuses with bladder outlet obstruction, some with bilateral PUJ obstruction, and a few with a large prolapsing ureterocele causing bladder outlet obstruction. Moreover, the ultrasound appearances of the renal cortex are important (presence of cysts and parenchymal echogenicity); in cases of severe oligohydramnios, the ratio of the cardiac/thoracic circumference can be used as a guide to possible lung hypoplasia. The presence of associated anomalies is also important: they may be found in about 17–30% of cases. Knowledge of the fetal gender may contribute to the diagnosis as different conditions affect males, females and both sexes. However, the genitalia may be abnormal and maternal blood free fetal DNA sexing may be useful (see below). For chromosomal analysis when oligohydramnios and megacystis are present, it is usually easier to obtain fetal urine than amniotic fluid, with a success rate of 96% with the combination of the traditional cytogenetic analysis and FISH (95% success for traditional and 65% for FISH).[46] This can easily be combined with urine aspiration for biochemistry.

Fetal renal function may be assessed by biochemical analysis of the fetal urine. A healthy fetus produces hypotonic urine which becomes isotonic in the presence of progressive renal damage that impairs proximal tubular function. Muller et al.[47] established reference ranges for different biochemical markers according to gestational age (Fig. 6). A good outcome can be anticipated if urinary sodium and $\beta_2$-microglobulin are below the 95th percentile. It is possible that urine within the fetal bladder could have been produced some time previously and so may reflect conditions before kidney damage progressed. Therefore, results from the first sample of urine may be less reliable than those obtained when the procedure is repeated and newly produced urine is collected. One management option is that, if the initial sample indicates good renal function, decisions are made without further vesicocentesis; if values are abnormal, a second sample may be taken within 48 h.[48] Another option is to perform a fetal blood sample to assess values of $\beta_2$-microglobulin.[49] This has the advantages of requiring a single invasive procedure and obtaining faster karyotype results.

Some have used the placement of a vesico-amniotic shunt as a diagnostic test, reasoning that, if the shunt is correctly sited and the amniotic fluid does not return to normal, renal failure can be assumed and termination of pregnancy offered. However, this is a major procedure and such an approach needs detailed explanation of the options to parents in order to obtain informed consent.

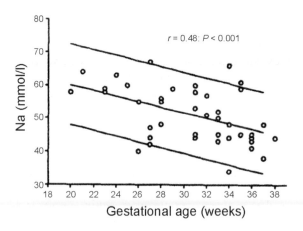

Fig. 6 Reference ranges for fetal urinary sodium according to gestational age.[47]

## MEGACYSTIS MICROCOLON INTESTINAL HYPOPERISTALSIS SYNDROME (MMIHS)

MMIHS is a rare condition resulting in decreased muscle tone in the urinary tract and intestine without obstruction. The intestinal hypoperistalsis causes a pseudo-obstruction, which antenatally leads to a shortened and malrotated microcolon. It is suspected when there is a large dilated bladder but no keyhole sign (see above), with variable degrees of upper urinary tract dilatation and bowel dilatation. It has an autosomal recessive inheritance but no genetic locus has yet been identified. Females are more affected than males (ratio, 4:1). Prenatal diagnosis is complicated because the bowel usually appears normal at 20 weeks and becomes dilated late in second or third trimesters. Differential diagnoses in females are hydrocolpos and ovarian cyst; however, the presence of an enlarged bladder, hydronephrosis and normal or increased liquor volume in a female fetus makes MMIHS a diagnosis that should be considered.[50] This condition is usually lethal in the first year of life.

## GENITALIA

### HYPOSPADIAS

Hypospadias is a condition in which the urethral meatus opens on the ventral aspect of the penis. Prenatal diagnosis is not possible unless it is associated with a condition called chordee, which results in angulation of the corpora cavernosa. On scanning, these cases are seen to have a short or bent penis. Surgical repair in an otherwise healthy child is usually performed at 6–12 months of age.

### VIRILISATION OF FEMALE FETUSES

This occurs in congenital adrenal hyperplasia including 21-hydroxylase deficiency. They are autosomal recessive conditions in which a defect in hydrocortisone biosynthesis is present with consequent over-production of ACTH and secondary adrenal hyperplasia. Rather than hydrocortisone, the adrenals produce excess sex hormone precursors that do not require 21-hydroxylation for their synthesis. Once secreted, these hormones are further metabolised to the active androgens (testosterone and dihydrotestosterone) and, to a lesser extent, oestrogens (oestrone and oestradiol). The effect of androgen production may be prenatal virilisation of female fetuses but is without effects in male fetuses before birth. The most important aspects of virilisation are urogenital closure and a phallic urethra, malformations which occur at 8–12 weeks' gestation. It is possible to prevent the virilisation by administering glucocorticoids to the mother during the pregnancy but it is preferable to avoid potentially hazardous medication during pregnancy when there is no possible gain. Therefore, knowledge of the fetal sex early in pregnancy is useful in order to prevent unnecessary therapy in pregnancies with male fetuses. The fetal sex can be determined by CVS at 11 weeks with a risk of miscarriage of 1% related to this procedure. However, this would be too late to avoid the risks of medication inducing malformation in pregnancy. A new option is to use a blood sample from the mother as early as 6 weeks' gestation to detect Y chromosome genes such as SRY or DYS 14 by PCR. A positive signal for male fetuses would allow steroid treatment to be stopped.[51]

## TESTICULAR FEMINISATION

Testicular feminisation is an X-linked recessive condition, in which the fetus lacks the receptor for dihydrotestosterone. Although cytogenetically male, the fetus develops female external genitalia, but has testes instead of ovaries and the vagina or uterus do not develop normally. The diagnosis should be suspected when a 46 XY karyotype is obtained in a fetus with apparently normal female external genitalia.

*References*

## Key points for clinical practice

- The family history is important including postnatal follow-up information about previously affected children in order to assess the risk of inherited disease.

- A check list of structures to be examined in an obstetric scan should be used in order to screen systematically. When a urinary tract abnormality is found, a specialised fetal medicine scan should be performed to look for other abnormalities including detailed assessment of the contralateral kidney.

- Consider fetal karyotyping, especially when additional problems are found in association with urinary tract abnormalities.

- Enlarged echogenic kidneys are likely to indicate polycystic kidney disease, whereas cysts of different sizes are usually due to multicystic dysplastic kidney.

- Unilateral defects, especially with normal amniotic fluid volume, are usually associated with good renal function and good prognosis.

- Renal pelvis dilatation > 15 mm is most likely due to an obstructive process and is associated with high probability of postnatal infections or need for surgery.

- Prenatal therapeutic interventions are restricted to Lower urinary tract obstruction, bilateral pelvi-ureteric junction obstruction, some ureteroceles and their efficacy remains uncertain.

- Termination of pregnancy should be considered in severe cases and post-mortem examination recommended.

- The organisation of perinatal management and follow-up should be planned with nephrologists/urologists and paediatricians.

1. Valentin L, Marshal K. Does the prenatal diagnosis of fetal urinary tract anomalies affect perinatal outcome? *Ann NY Acad Sci* 1998; **847**: 59–73.
2. Levi S, Grandjean H, Lebrun T. *Eurofetus Study report. Cost-effectiveness of antenatal screening for fetal malformation by ultrasound*, Vol 1. Brussels: European Union, Direction Generale XII, 1995.
3. Dommergues M. Fetal genitourinary abnormalities. In: James DL, Steer PJ, Weiner CP, Gonik B. (eds) *High risk pregnancy. Management options*. Philadelphia, PA: Pergamon, 2006; 399–421.
4. Levi S. Mass screening for fetal malformation: the Eurofetus study. *Ultrasound Obstet Gynecol* 2003; **22**: 555–558.
5. Carrera JM, Torrents M, Mortera C *et al* .Routine prenatal ultrasound screening for fetal abnormalities: 22 year's experience. *Ultrasound Obstet Gynecol* 1995; **5**: 174–179.
6. Rosati P, Guariglia L. Endovaginal sonographic diagnosis of the fetal urinary tract anomalies in early pregnancy. *Arch Gynecol Obstet* 2001; **265**: 1–6.
7. Nicolaides KH, Cheng HH, Abbas A, Snijders RJ, Gosden C. Fetal renal defects: associated malformations and chromosomal defects. *Fetal Diagn Ther* 1992; **7**: 1–11.
8. Robson WL, Thomason MA, Minette LJ. Cystic dysplasia of the testis associated with multicystic dysplasia of the kidney. *Urology* 1998; **51**: 477–479.
9. Robson WL, Rogers RC, Leung AK. Renal agenesis, multicystic dysplasia, and ureteropelvic junction obstruction – a common pathogenesis? *Am J Med Genet* 1994; **53**: 302.
10. Greenfield SP, Rutigliano E, Steinhardt G, Elder JS. Genitourinary tract malformations and maternal cocaine abuse. *Urology* 1991; **37**: 455–459.
11. Atiyeh B, Husmann D, Baum M. Contralateral renal abnormalities in multicystic dysplastic kidney disease. *J Pediatr* 1992; **121**: 65–67.
12. Damen-Elias HA, Stoutenbeek PH, Visser GH, Nikkels PG, de Jong TP. Concomitant anomalies in 100 children with unilateral multicystic kidney. *Ultrasound Obstet Gynecol* 2005; **25**: 384–388.
13. Iura T, Makinoda S, Miyazaki S *et al*. Prenatal diagnosis of the hemodynamics of fetal renal disease by color Doppler ultrasound. *Fetal Diagn Ther* 2003; **18**: 148–153.
14. Dungan JS, Fernandez MT, Abbitt PL *et al*. Multicystic dysplastic kidney: natural history of prenatally detected cases. *Prenat Diagn* 1990; **10**: 175–182.
15. Zerres K, Muecher G, Becker J *et al*. Prenatal diagnosis of autosomal recessive polycystic kidney disease (ARPKD): molecular genetics, clinical experience, and fetal morphology. *Am J Med Genet* 1998; **76**: 137–144.
16. Lonergan GJ, Rice RR, Suarez ES. Autosomal recessive polycystic kidney disease: radiologic-pathologic correlation. *Radiographics* 2000; **20**: 837–855.
17. Liu Y-P, Cheng S-J, Shih S-L, Huang J-H. Autosomal recessive polycystic kidney disease: appearance on fetal MRI. *Pediatr Radiol* 2006; **36**: 169.
18. Bergmann C, Senderek J, Schneider F *et al*. PKHD1 mutations in families requesting prenatal diagnosis for autosomal recessive polycystic kidney disease (ARPKD). *Hum Mutat* 2004; **23**: 487–495.
19. Bergmann C, Senderek J, Windelen E *et al*. Clinical consequences of PKHD1 mutations in 164 patients with autosomal-recessive polycystic kidney disease (ARPKD). *Kidney Int* 2005; **67**: 829–848.
20. Guay-Woodford LM, Desmond RA. Autosomal recessive polycystic kidney disease: the clinical experience in North America. *Pediatrics* 2003; **111**: 1072–1080.
21. Deltas CC. Mutations of the human polycystic kidney disease 2 (PKD2) gene. *Hum Mutat* 2001; **18**: 13–24.
22. Rossetti S, Chauveau D, Walker D *et al*. A complete mutation screen of the ADPKD genes by DHPLC. *Kidney Int* 2002; **61**: 1588–1599.
23. Sairam S, Al-Habib A, Sasson S, Thilaganathan B. Natural history of fetal hydronephrosis diagnosed on mid-trimester ultrasound. *Ultrasound Obstet Gynecol* 2001; **17**: 191–196.
24. Chevalier RL. Growth factors and apoptosis in neonatal ureteral obstruction. *J Am Soc Nephrol* 1996; **7**: 1098–1105.
25. Chevalier RL, Chung KH, Smith CD *et al*. Renal apoptosis and clustering following ureteral obstruction: the role of maturation. *J Urol* 1996; **156**: 1474–1479.
26. Josephson S. Suspected pyelo-ureteral junction obstruction in the fetus: when to do

what? II. Experimental viewpoints. *Eur Urol* 1991; **19**: 132–138.

27. Freedman AL, Johnson MP, Gonzalez R. Fetal therapy for obstructive uropathy: past, present and future? *Pediatr Nephrol* 2000; **14**: 167–176.

28. Makino Y, Kobayashi H, Kyono K, Oshima K, Kawarabayashi T. Clinical results of fetal obstructive uropathy treated by vesicoamniotic shunting. *Urology* 2000; **55**: 118–122.

29. John U, Kähler C, Schulz S *et al.* The impact of fetal renal pelvic diameter on postnatal outcome. *Prenat Diagn* 2004; **24**: 591–595.

30. Coplen D, Austin P, Yan Y, Blanco V, Dicke J. The magnitude of fetal renal pelvic dilatation can identify obstructive postnatal hydronephrosis, and direct postnatal evaluation and management. *J Urol* 2006; **176**: 724–727.

31. Wollenberg A, Neuhaus TJ, Willi UV, Wisser J. Outcome of fetal renal pelvic dilatation diagnosed during the third trimester. *Ultrasound Obstet Gynecol* 2005; **25**: 483–488.

32. Smith-Bindman R, Hosner W, Feldstein V, Deeks J, Goldberg J. Second trimester ultrasound to detect fetuses with Down syndrome: a meta-analysis. *JAMA* 2001; **285**: 1044–1055.

33. Dressler GR, Wilkinson JE, Rothenpieler UW *et al.* Desregulation of Pax-2 expression in transgenic mice generates severe kidney abnormalities. *Nature* 1993; **362**: 65–67.

34. Carroll SG, Soothill PW, Tizard J, Kyle PM. Vesicocentesis at 10–14 weeks of gestation for treatment of fetal megacystis. *Ultrasound Obstet Gynecol* 2001; **18**: 366–370.

35. Merlini E, Chiesa PL. Obstructive ureterocele – an ongoing challenge. *World J Urol* 2004; **22**: 107–114.

36. Whitten SM, McHoney M, Wilcox DT, New S, Chitty LS. Accuracy of antenatal fetal ultrasound in the diagnosis of duplex kidneys. *Ultrasound Obstet Gynecol* 2003; **21**: 342–346.

37. Soothill PW, Bartha JL, Tizard J. Ultrasound-guided laser treatment for fetal bladder outlet obstruction resulting from ureterocele. *Am J Obstet Gynecol* 2003; **188**: 1107–1108.

38. Boyadjiev SA, Dodson JL, Radford CL *et al.* Clinical and molecular characterization of the bladder extrophy–epispadias complex: analysis of 232 families. *BJU Int* 2004; **94**: 1337–1343.

39. Warne S, Chitty LS, Wilcox DT. Prenatal diagnosis of cloacal anomalies. *BJU Int* 2002; **89**: 78–81.

40. Liao AW, Sebire NJ, Geers L *et al.* Megacystis at 10–14 weeks of gestation: chromosomal defects and outcome according to bladder length. *Ultrasound Obstet Gynecol* 2003; **21**: 338–341.

41. Rodeck CH, Fisk NM, Fraser DI, Nicolini U. Long term *in utero* drainage of fetal hydrothorax. *N Engl J Med* 1988; **319**: 1135–1138.

42. PLUTO Collaborative Study Group. PLUTO: the percutaneous shunting for lower urinary tract obstruction trial. *Br J Obstet Gynaecol* 2007; **114**: 904–905.

43. Quintero RA, Hume R, Smith C *et al.* Percutaneous fetal cystoscopy and endoscopic fulguration of posterior urethral valves. *Am J Obstet Gynecol* 1995; **172**: 206–209

44. National Institute for Health and Clinical Excellence. London N1173,2006. <www.nice.org.uk/IPG202distributionlist>.

45. Gonzalez R, De Filippo R, Jednak R, Barthold JS. Urethral atresia: long-term outcome in 6 children who survived the neonatal period. *J Urol* 2001; **165**: 2241–2244.

46. Donnefeld AE, Lockwood D, Custer T, Lamb AN. Prenatal diagnosis from fetal urine in bladder outlet obstruction: success rates for traditional cytogenetic evaluation and interphase fluorescence *in situ* hybridization. *Genet Med* 2002; **4**: 444–447.

47. Muller F, Dommergues M, Bussieres L *et al.* Development of human renal function: reference intervals for 10 biochemical markers in fetal urine. *Clin Chem* 1996; **42**: 1855–1860.

48. Johnson MP, Corsi P, Bradfield W *et al.* Sequential urinalysis improves evaluation of fetal renal function in obstructive uropathy. *Am J Obstet Gynecol* 1995; **173**: 59–65.

49. White SM, Chamberlain P, Hitchcock R, Sullivan PB, Boyd PA. Megacystis-microcolon-intestinal hypoperistalsis syndrome: the difficulties with antenatal diagnosis. Case report and review of the literature. *Prenat Diagn* 2000; **20**: 697–700.

50. Dommergues M, Muller F, Ngo S *et al.* Fetal serum $\beta_2$-microglobulin predicts postnatal renal function in bilateral uropathies. *Kidney Int* 2000; **58**: 312–316.

51. Bartha JL, Finning K, Soothill PW. Fetal sex determination from maternal blood at 6 weeks of gestation when at risk for 21-hydroxylase deficiency. *Obstet Gynecol* 2003; **101**: 1135–1136.

*Alaa El-Ghobashy  WanLye Haw*
*Chris Brewer  Derek Tuffnell*

**5**

# Causes and management of suspected fetal macrosomia

Fetal macrosomia is variously defined as a birth-weight of either more than 4 kg or 4.5 kg and complicates more than 10% of all pregnancies. It is associated with increased risks of caesarean section and trauma to the birth canal and the fetus. Fetal macrosomia is difficult to predict, and clinical and ultrasonographic estimates of fetal weight are prone to error. Elective caesarean section for suspected macrosomia results in a high number of unnecessary procedures, and early induction of labour to limit fetal growth may result in a substantial increase in the caesarean section rate because of failed inductions.

In this review, the causes of macrosomia and the accuracy of various methods of prediction of macrosomia will be assessed. The efficacy of different interventions to manage the macrosomic baby will be appraised on the light of currently available evidence.

## DEFINITION AND INCIDENCE

The way in which a large infant or a large fetus is classified has been variously described. Several definitions of fetal macrosomia exist, the most common

**Alaa El-Ghobashy** MD MRCOG (for correspondence)
Specialist Registrar in Obstetrics and Gynaecology, Department of Obstetrics and Gynaecology, St James's University Hospital, Leeds, UK
E-mail: ghobashy@doctors.org.uk

**WanLye Haw** BMedSci MRCOG
Specialist Registrar in Obstetrics and Gynaecology, Department of Obstetrics and Gynaecology, St James's University Hospital, Leeds, UK

**Chris Brewer** MBBCh
Specialist Registrar in Obstetrics and Gynaecology, Department of Obstetrics and Gynaecology, St James's University Hospital, Leeds, UK

**Derek Tuffnell** FRCOG (for correspondence)
Honorary Visiting Professor in Obstetrics, Bradford University and Consultant Obstetrician and Gynaecologist, Department of Obstetrics and Gynaecology, Bradford Royal Infirmary, Duckworth Road, Bradford BD9 6RJ, UK.  E-mail: Derek.Tuffnell@bradfordhospitals.nhs.uk

include:

- an absolute birth-weight of greater than 4000 g

- an absolute birth-weight of greater than 4500 g

- a birth-weight greater than the 90th centile for gestational age.

These definitions are based on measurements of the infant after delivery – a retrospective diagnosis. The American College of Obstetricians and Gynecologists (ACOG) defines macrosomia as an infant with an absolute birth-weight greater than 4500 g irrespective of gestational age or other demographic variables. The different definitions are useful when used in different contexts. Definitions based on absolute birth-weight are most useful when determining the effects on parturition. Conversely, using birth-weight in comparison to a centile chart for gestational age is more appropriate when determining fetal growth or neonatal outcomes. In such cases, gestational age has a significant confounding effect. The diagnosis or suspicion of fetal macrosomia or 'large for dates' in an antenatal setting is based on anthropomorphic measurements and estimates of fetal weight. Clearly, the definitions that use birth-weight as a determinant of macrosomia are more robust. This form of retrospective diagnosis is less useful when planning antenatal care.

A grading system of macrosomia has been described. This grading system has been used in the research setting to determine maternal and neonatal outcomes associated with fetal macrosomia. First described by Boulet et al.,[1] macrosomic infants are sub-classified into three groups:

| | |
|---|---|
| Grade 1 | 4000–4499 g |
| Grade 2 | 4500–4999 g |
| Grade 3 | ≥ 5000 g |

It has been shown that maternal and neonatal outcome becomes progressively worse from grade 1 to grade 3.[1,2] It could be envisaged that a grading system similar to the one outlined by Boulet et al.[1] could be used for risk stratification in cases of fetal macrosomia.

The incidence of fetal macrosomia has increased over the course of the last few decades in both Europe and the US. Mean birth-weight has increased and proportionally more infants are being born with birth-weights of more than 4000 g.[3–5]

Fetal macrosomia occurs with an incidence of approximately 8–10% in developed countries.[6] This may be a conservative estimate as higher incidence rates have been described in some Scandinavian reports. In Sweden in the mid-1970s, approximately 17% of infants had a birth-weight greater than 4000 g but, by the beginning of the 1990s, the incidence of fetal macrosomia in Sweden had increased to 20%.[7] Similarly, in a Danish study, rates of fetal macrosomia (defined as birth weight greater than 4000 g) increased from 16.7% to 20.0% during the 1990s.[5]

## CAUSES

Birth-weight is influenced by a variety of maternal, fetal, metabolic and genetic factors. A fetus may be constitutionally programmed to become macrosomic or may develop macrosomia secondary to a growth-promoting environment *in utero*. Risk factors for fetal macrosomia are well-documented in the literature. There is, however, substantial variation in the relative importance of individual risk factors and the strength of influence on the development of fetal macrosomia.

Factors that have been shown to increase the probability of developing fetal macrosomia include gestational age, maternal diabetes mellitus, maternal obesity, multiparity, previous macrosomic infant, maternal birth-weight, maternal age, maternal height and ethnicity or race.[1,8]

Many of the risk factors for developing fetal macrosomia overlap with those for the development of gestational diabetes. Much research has been devoted to determining the relative contribution of these individual factors in the development of fetal macrosomia. Strong associations have been demonstrated between maternal obesity, gestational weight gain, increasing maternal age or parity and the development of fetal macrosomia independent of gestational diabetes.[8] Indeed, maternal constitutional factors, such as obesity, have been strongly associated with fetal macrosomia and it has been suggested that such factors have a stronger predictive value for the development of macrosomia when compared to gestational diabetes.[9–11]

## GESTATIONAL AGE

Intuitively, gestational age has a significant impact on absolute birth-weight. Pre-term infants will tend to weigh less and so-called 'post-mature' infants will tend to weigh more.

A Danish study of 24,093 non-diabetic women with singleton pregnancies demonstrated that a gestational age of more than 42 weeks was associated with more than twice the risk of delivering an infant weighing more than 4000 g, when compared to those delivered at 40 weeks (OR, 2.36; 95% CI, 2.17–2.56).[11]

Similarly, Stotland *et al.*[2] studied 146,526 'mother–infant pairs' and found that one-third of infants with a gestational age greater than 41 weeks had an absolute birth-weight of greater than 4000 g. Births at a gestational age over 41 weeks had a 3-fold increased risk of macrosomia (birth-weight > 4000 g), adjusted OR 3.39 (95% CI, 3.14–3.66). In addition to this, the risk of delivering a more severely macrosomic infant is increased. The risk of delivering a Grade 2 macrosomic infant (4500–4999 g) is increased 4-fold.[2]

Clearly, gestational age has a significant impact on absolute birth-weight. However, when analysed against gestational age percentile charts, the proportion of 'macrosomic' infants is decreased. The relevance of this depends on outcomes measured. However, absolute birth-weight is highly relevant when considering the effects upon parturition.

## MATERNAL AGE

Advanced maternal age has been associated with adverse pregnancy outcomes such as increased perinatal mortality, pre-term delivery and low birth-weight.[12] Advanced maternal age has been shown to be associated with an increased incidence of fetal macrosomia.

A study of risk factors for fetal macrosomia in California demonstrated that women aged 30–39 years had elevated rates of fetal macrosomia.[2] A small study of women with very advanced maternal age, defined as greater than 45 years, showed markedly increased rates of macrosomia. This study demonstrated increased rates of macrosomia in this subgroup of women when compared to US national birth-weight statistics. Using the grading scale of macrosomia described by Boulet et al.,[1] advanced maternal age was associated with an increased incidence of macrosomia in all three groups (Table 1).

Table 1 Maternal age as a risk factor for fetal macrosomia

| Macrosomia grade | Age greater than 45 years | US national birth-weight statistics |
| --- | --- | --- |
| Grade 1 (4000–4499 g) | 19.8% | 10.7% |
| Grade 2 (4500–4999 g) | 4.9% | 1.7% |
| Grade 3 (> 5000 g) | 3.7% | 0.2% |

Other studies have shown that advanced maternal age is more strongly associated with a low birth-weight.[13] Therefore, the value of age as a predictor of fetal macrosomia is unclear. However, it would be prudent to recall the findings of the above studies when caring for pregnant women greater than 35 years of age.

## PARITY

It has been suggested that multiparity is associated with an increased probability of fetal macrosomia. A large UK study of 350,311 completed singleton pregnancies investigating macrosomia demonstrated that a parity of greater than four was associated with a 2-fold increased risk of delivering a macrosomic infant (> 4000 g or a birth-weight greater than the 90th percentile for gestational age).[10]

Similarly, a study of 874,163 births in Sweden between 1992–2001 showed that parity influenced the probability of delivering a macrosomic infant. The odds of delivering a macrosomic infant increased with parity. A parity of two was associated with a 2-fold increased risk (OR, 2.19), whereas a parity of greater than five was associated with a 3-fold increased risk (OR, 3.23).[7]

## SMOKING

Smoking is negatively associated with macrosomia. Demographic studies have found that, whilst rates of macrosomia have increased over a 20-year period, the rates of obesity and of smoking have declined over the same time. The reduction in prevalence of daily smoking in the obstetric population has been tentatively linked to the increasing trend towards macrosomia.[7]

A Canadian case-control study investigating the relative importance of given risk factors in the development of fetal macrosomia demonstrated a negative correlation between smoking and the probability of delivering a macrosomic infant.[8]

## PREVIOUS MACROSOMIC INFANT

A factor strongly associated with developing fetal macrosomia is the birth-weight of infants in previous pregnancies. A Canadian case-control study found a history of previous macrosomia to be a powerful predictor of macrosomia in subsequent pregnancies. The risk of fetal macrosomia is increased 9-fold (OR, 9 95%; 95% CI, 5.8–14.2).[8]

Similarly, a Dutch study of sibling birth-weight in type 1 diabetes mellitus found that the birth-weight of the second-born infant was significantly related to the birth-weight of the first-born (R = 0.737; $R^2$ = 0.544; $P < 0.001$).[14]

The same findings have been demonstrated in the non-diabetic population.[15,16] One study suggested that women with a previous delivery of a macrosomic infant are 10 times more likely to develop fetal macrosomia in subsequent pregnancies.[15]

## FETAL GENDER

Fetal macrosomia has been reported to occur more frequently in the male fetus, occurring in a 2:1 male to female ratio.[17]

## RACE AND ETHNICITY

The incidence of fetal macrosomia has been shown to vary in different ethnic populations or races. There exists considerable disagreement in the literature regarding which sub-population of women are at most risk of delivering a macrosomic infant. An interesting outcome of the research into race and macrosomia is the interplay of race/ethnicity and other concomitant risk factors.

Despite disagreement in the literature, the majority of studies place white and Hispanic women at increased risk of fetal macrosomia.[2,10,18,19] In the non-diabetic population, there appears to be increased rates of macrosomia among white women. In studies including diabetic women, both white women and Hispanic women appear to be at greater risk of developing fetal macrosomia.

An American study of 146,526 births found that the rate of fetal macrosomia (> 4000 g) in white women was 16% compared to 11% in the non-white population ($P < 0.001$). Likewise, for a birth-weight greater than 4500 g, the rate among white women was 2.9% compared to 2% in non-whites ($P < 0.001$). It should be noted, however, that 'non-white' was defined as black or Asian. Hispanics did not show statistically significant different rates from white women.[2]

It has been shown elsewhere that Hispanic ethnicity is independently associated with fetal macrosomia.[20] It should be noted that Hispanic women are at increased risk of developing gestational diabetes.[18,19,21] Several studies have found that, in the presence of other risk factors, certain ethnic groups have an elevated risk of fetal macrosomia. In a study of 22,658 women, obesity was found to increase the incidence of macrosomia significantly in white, Hispanic and Asian women by 3-fold, but not in African-Americans.[10] Other studies demonstrated that obesity exerts a profound effect on Hispanic women in particular. In that, Hispanic women are at markedly increased risk of delivering a macrosomic infant.[19,21]

## WEIGHT

A universal finding among all studies of fetal macrosomia is the profound effect that maternal weight imparts upon the birth-weight of the infant.[2,7,9–11,19] A UK-based study of 350,311 women demonstrated that maternal body mass index (BMI) was a strong risk factor for developing fetal macrosomia. It was found that if the maternal BMI was greater than 30 kg/m² then there was a 2-fold increased risk of fetal macrosomia (> 4000 g or greater than 90th percentile for gestational age). Conversely, the study demonstrated that a BMI < 20 kg/m² was significantly associated with a reduced risk of fetal macrosomia by either definition.[10]

A Swedish population based study investigating the trend for increasing birth-weight demonstrated that increasing BMI was associated with an increasing risk of fetal macrosomia in a 'dose-dependent' type relationship. Using women with a normal BMI (20.0–24.9 kg/m²) as a reference, they found that overweight women (BMI 25–29.9 kg/m²) had a 2-fold increased risk of delivering a macrosomic infant; furthermore, obese women (BMI > 30 kg/m²) had a 3-fold increased risk of macrosomia.[7] A strong predictor of fetal macrosomia is pre-gravid weight. In a Danish study of macrosomia, a pre-gravid weight greater than 80 kg was associated with a 2-fold increased risk of fetal macrosomia.[11] Similar to BMI, the risk of macrosomia increases with an increase in pre-gravid weight. Spellacy et al.[17] demonstrated that a pre-gravid weight of greater than 90 kg was associated with a 3.7-fold increased risk of delivering a macrosomic infant; women with a pre-gravid weight of greater than 112.5 kg were shown to have a 5.8-fold increased risk of macrosomia.

An 'excessive' gestational weight gain has been associated with a significantly increased risk of fetal macrosomia.[7–9] It has been shown that overweight and obese women tend to gain more weight in pregnancy.[22] Therefore, pre-gravid BMI and gestational weight gain could well be compound risk factors for the development of fetal macrosomia. Brown et al.[23] demonstrated that birth-weight was most directly influenced by first trimester weight gain.

It has also been demonstrated that maternal birth-weight is a predictor of the birth-weights of their progeny. Thus, women who were born macrosomic are at an elevated risk of developing fetal macrosomia.[24]

## DIABETES MELLITUS

Maternal diabetes, pre-pregnancy or gestational, has long been associated with fetal macrosomia. It has been suggested that fetal macrosomia is produced by fetal hyperinsulinaemia in response to maternal hyperglycaemia. Diabetic mothers with poor glycaemic control are at an elevated risk of delivering a macrosomic infant. It has been shown that tight glycaemic control in type 1 diabetic mothers decreases the rates of macrosomia.[25] Similarly, intensive management of gestational diabetes was found to reduce the rates of macrosomia significantly when compared to conventionally managed gestational diabetics.[26]

In a UK-based study of 350,311 pregnancies, it was found that pre-existing diabetes was associated with an increased risk of delivering a macrosomic infant, almost 2-fold (OR 1.81) increased risk of an infant greater than 4000 g and almost 7-fold (OR 6.97) increased risk of delivering an infant with birth-weight greater than the 90th centile for gestational age. Likewise, gestational diabetes was associated with an increased risk of macrosomia: a 1.5-fold (OR 1.51) increased risk of delivering an infant greater than 4000 g and an almost 3-fold (OR 2.77) increased risk of delivering an infant greater than the 90th percentile for gestational age.[10] Other studies have demonstrated a similar effect, gestational diabetes being associated with a 3-fold increase in risk of delivering a macrosomic infant.[7,17]

Interestingly, the perinatal mortality rate in gestational diabetes has decreased but there has been little change in the rates of macrosomia in these patients.[25] Macrosomia remains prevalent in diabetic mothers despite good glycaemic control. The rates of fetal macrosomia have been shown to be high even in a population of diabetic mothers with near normal $HbA_{1C}$ levels. This would imply that $HbA_{1C}$ levels are very poor predictors for the development of macrosomia in diabetics.[14,27]

As in the non-diabetic population, obesity increases the risk of fetal macrosomia. Obese diabetics are at a significantly higher risk of developing fetal macrosomia.[9,25] A study of risk factors for macrosomia in gestational diabetics found that for each increase of 10 BMI units the chance of fetal macrosomia increased 2-fold (OR 2.46).[25]

## PATHOPHYSIOLOGY

The normal growth of a fetus is a delicate balance of several factors. The genetic drive for growth, environmental factors *in utero* and the supply of growth substrates to the fetus. Perturbations to this balance may result in growth restriction or accelerated growth. Two growth pathways have been described – fetal hormone dependent growth and substrate-limited growth. It should be noted that the supply of substrate to the fetus is regulated by maternoplacental factors. Insulin and insulin-like growth factors are important regulators of fetal growth. Insulin has been shown to be present in the fetus from 8–10 weeks of pregnancy but remains inactive until 20 weeks, when a response to glucose levels becomes evident. Glucose in the fetal circulation is transferred from the maternal compartment via the placenta. The fetal glucose concentration is approximately 80% of the maternal level. Clearly, as maternal blood glucose increases, so will fetal blood glucose.[28] Such changes in glucose concentration are monitored by the fetal β-cells.

Normal pregnant women have reduced insulin sensitivity, tending towards a state of hyperglycaemia to provide substrates for the fetus.[29,30] It is well documented that obesity reduces insulin sensitivity and increases insulin resistance.[7,10] Likewise, increasing age is associated with an increasing insulin resistance. The factors may compound the already suppressed insulin sensitivity of pregnancy leading to a state of increased carbohydrate intolerance, increasing the amount of glucose available for maternofetal transport, thus driving fetal hyperinsulinaemia and accelerated intra-uterine growth.

Additionally, insulin resistance perturbs metabolism and increases the substrate availability to the fetus. Increased flux of nutrients across the placenta causes fetal hyperinsulinaemia and accelerated fetal growth. Insulin resistance is associated with higher fasting triglyceride concentrations.

Triglycerides are energy-rich and placental lipases can cleave them and transfer free fatty acids into the fetal circulation. This increases energy and substrate delivery to the fetus and may further increase insulin levels.[10]

Fetal hyperinsulinaemia may also be driven by insulin secretogogues present in the maternal circulation, which may be transferred to the fetus via the placenta. Certain amino acids, such as leucine, stimulate the secretion of insulin. Insulin resistance is associated with a greater leucine turnover. It can be envisaged that this may help to promote fetal growth by increasing fetal insulin levels.

The above factors may well combine in obese, older and diabetic women to promote the development of macrosomia by increasing hormone-dependent growth and the availability of substrates for growth. The exact mechanisms by which fetal macrosomia develops have yet to be elucidated fully. However, the above factors may account for the phenomenon in certain at-risk groups.

## MATERNAL AND FETAL COMPLICATIONS

There is little doubt that fetal macrosomia is associated with an increased risk of maternal and neonatal morbidity and mortality. Certain obstetric complications such as prolonged labour, labour augmentation with oxytocin, caesarean delivery, postpartum haemorrhage and infection occur with greater frequency during the births of macrosomic infants compared to infants of normal birth-weight. However, the extent to which prophylactic caesarean delivery reduces the likelihood of poor outcomes in high birth-weight infants had not been fully explored. In the *6th Annual Report of the Confidential Enquiry into Stillbirths and Deaths in Infancy* (CESDI) in 1997, a detailed investigation of the mortality of high birth-weight infants demonstrated that, when compared to infants weighing 2500–3999 g, infants with birth-weights $\geq$ 4000 g were less likely to die during the first year of life but were more likely to die from intrapartum-related factors. A recent study by Boulet *et al.*[31] using national data indicated that an increased risk of death among large infants was not evident until fetal birth-weights exceeded 5000 g. However, infants in the highest birth-weight category (> 5000 g) are 3 times as likely as normosomic infants to die during the neonatal period.[1] These findings lend support for a growing consensus that, although macrosomic infants experience an increased risk of birth complications, a trial of labour is not contra-indicated for women without diabetes in whom the estimated fetal weight is < 5000 g. However, as recognised in the most recent practice guidelines prepared by ACOG, these recommendations are based primarily on limited, and often inconsistent, scientific evidence.

ACOG emphasises that an increase risk of caesarean delivery is the primary maternal risk factor associated with macrosomia. Results from cohort studies demonstrate that the risk of caesarean section in women attempting a vaginal delivery at least doubles when the fetal weight is estimated to be more than 4500 g. Conversely, when this group of women achieve vaginal delivery, the risk of severe perineal trauma increases. Baskett and Allen[32] reported an increase of third or fourth degree laceration by 5-fold in this high-risk group.

The major fetal complication associated with delivery of a macrosomic fetus is birth trauma such as clavicle fracture and subsequent brachial plexus injury from a difficult vaginal delivery. Irrespective of aetiology or body composition, an increased risk of shoulder dystocia and of hypoxia in macrosomic fetus continues to be a reality, as demonstrated by the 1990 data from Scandinavia. Operative vaginal delivery by itself or in combination with an abnormal course of labour may predispose to shoulder dystocia in the case of fetal macrosomia.[33] Thus, it is necessary to be very cautious when selecting an operative vaginal delivery to correct the disorders of descent or cervical dilatation in the presence of fetal macrosomia, even though the sensitivity of these clinical parameters in the predicting shoulder dystocia is low. Besides shoulder dystocia, other adverse outcomes include meconium aspiration, perinatal asphyxia, hypoglycaemia and fetal death.[34] The risk of shoulder dystocia rises sharply from 3% for birth-weights < 4000g to 10.3% and 23.9% for the ranges of birth-weights between 4000–4500 g and > 4500 g, respectively.[35] In diabetic women, when birth-weights are > 3500 g, the incidence of shoulder dystocia generally doubles compared to non-diabetic patients for similar birth-weights. Thus, the combination of macrosomia and diabetes places the patient at a high risk for shoulder dystocia.[36] Gross et al.[37] reported that asphyxia and brachial palsy occurred in up to 42% of infants with true shoulder dystocia. Gherman et al.[38] indicated that 25% of infants with shoulder dystocia experience brachial plexus or facial injury or fractures of humerus or clavicle. The increased risk of clavicle fracture and brachial plexus injury is approximately 10-fold and 20-fold, respectively, although neonatal fractures almost invariably heal with simple supportive therapy.[39] However, brachial plexus injuries are of much greater consequence, with possibilities of surgery and permanent disability, even after rehabilitation.[40] Because fetal macrosomia greatly increases the risk of shoulder dystocia, it has been recommended that ultrasonography should be used to predict macrosomia and to indicate elective caesarean section to prevent shoulder dystocia if macrosomia is diagnosed.[41] Reports stratifying risk by birth-weight have consistently demonstrated that macrosomic infants born after shoulder dystocia are at higher risk of brachial plexus injury relative to non-macrosomic infants, although the relative risk (1.2–2.6%) and absolute risk (6–35%) varied across studies.[42,43] Rouse et al.[44] estimated the probability that shoulder dystocia would result in, or be associated with, a brachial plexus injury to be 9%, 18%, and 26% for infants with birth-weights of less than 4000 g, 4000–4499 g, and ≥ 4500 g, respectively. Although this complication is rare, severe shoulder dystocia may also result in a hypoxic baby.[45] Shoulder dystocia usually occurs unexpectedly. It would be ideal if shoulder dystocia could be anticipated and thus could be avoided in pregnancies at risk for this condition; however, in general, fetal weight estimation and pelvimetry are poor predictors of cephalopelvic disproportion or birth trauma.

## ESTIMATING FETAL SIZE AND GROWTH

The next step in the management of patients at risk for fetal macrosomia at term is estimating fetal weight. This can be done by clinical assessment and/or ultrasound examination. Making and understanding the distinction between fetal size and growth is fundamental to the interpretation of different methods of quantification. Estimation of fetal weight by clinical examination of symphysiofundal height is usually inaccurate, especially at the extremes of fetal sizes. The volume of amniotic fluid, the size and the configuration of the uterus and maternal body habitus complicate estimation of the size of the fetus by palpation through the abdominal wall. Several studies have documented mean errors of about 300 g.[46,47] The correlation between correctly determined symphysiofundal height (SFH) measurements and fetal weight means that customised fetal weight standards can be applied to entire antenatal populations resulting in more appropriate use of antenatal monitoring resources.[48] These observational studies are interesting and represent an important advance in our understanding of the importance of birth-weight development but there are, as yet, no published randomised trials upon which to recommend or discourage the introduction of these methods into clinical practice.

Ultrasonography provides a more accurate means of obtaining an estimated fetal weight (EFW). Measurements of several fetal parameters have been described for the estimation of fetal weight. Formulae incorporating measures of the fetal head and abdominal circumference (AC) are the most predictive.[49] There will inevitably be an inherent error of ± 15% in ultrasonographic estimation of fetal weight, which will vary according to the size of the fetus, gestational age and quality of measurements. Delpapa and Muller-Heubach[50] found that 48% of ultrasonographically estimated fetal weights among a cohort of macrosomic fetuses were within 500 g of the actual birth-weight. Of the women allowed a trial of labour, 72% were able to deliver vaginally and five cases of shoulder dystocia were identified. No birth trauma occurred, and the authors suggested that caesarean delivery based on an ultrasonographic diagnosis of macrosomia would not reduce infant morbidity significantly. These limitations need not deter the clinicians from employing estimated fetal weight in clinical practice but it is essential that decision-making takes account of the range of error that is inherent in the practice.

Altman and Chitty[51] recommended key criteria for designing a study aiming to establish size standards constructed from cross-sectional data. Few published references range for ultrasound fetal biometry fulfil these criteria and, together with the poor performance of fetal size estimation in the prediction of important measures of perinatal outcomes, this limits the clinical value of estimating fetal size in the third trimester. It appears that Hadlock's formula utilising the abdominal circumference (AC) and femur length (FL) provides the best estimation of birth-weight of macrosomic fetuses.[51] The formula is:

$$Log_{10} (weight) = 1.304 + 0.05281\ AC + 0.1938\ FL - 0.004\ AC \times FL$$

where weight is measured in grams, AC (abdominal circumference) in centimetres, and FL (femur length) in centimetres.

Review of the literature concerning sensitivity and specificity revealed that there were many differences in the study methods, including study populations, formulae for fetal weight estimation, and definitions of macrosomia.[53,54] These differences precluded direct comparisons and simple data extrapolation. However, the data suggest that the sensitivity is around 60%, with a higher specificity of about 90%.[44] Results reviewed by Reece et al.[55] reporting on a variety of fetal measurements suggested sensitivities varying from 24–88% and specificities from 60–98%. In diabetic pregnancies, abdominal circumference, especially measured serially during the third trimester of pregnancy, is the best single sonographic measurement for the detection of the macrosomic fetus.[56] The main problems with using ultrasonography for assessing fetal macrosomia are that fetal body composition and fetal shoulder width cannot be reliably assessed. In pregnancies at risk of fetal macrosomia, serial ultrasound examinations (every 3–4 weeks) for EFW and AC starting at 32 weeks of gestation may be helpful in detecting the condition.[53] There have been reports in the literature of the use of MRI to estimate fetal weight as well as shoulder width. The mean shoulder circumference was significantly greater when shoulder dystocia subsequently complicated delivery. The fetal bisacromial diameter was well correlated with the ultrasonographically measured circumferences of the fetal chest and arm. Thus, the relationship between fetal chest circumference and other fetal parameters (such as head circumference or abdominal circumference) may be potentially useful in predicting shoulder dystocia in pregnancies at risk for this condition. However, current data are inadequate to provide an accurate estimate of the usefulness of fetal ultrasonography or MRI for shoulder width and EFW. Further studies in this area should refine the ability to diagnose macrosomia incorporating all the required parameters.

## PREVENTION OF MACROSOMIA

The major obstacle in reducing the perinatal morbidity and mortality associated with fetal macrosomia has been the inability to predict with certainty which fetuses will sustain birth injury prior to delivery. To minimise the adverse perinatal and maternal outcomes associated with this problem, it is important to have a well-planned management scheme for patients with fetal macrosomia, recognising that there is currently no perfect solution. With the exception of optimal blood glucose management in pregnancies complicated by diabetes, little is known about the prevention of macrosomia. Obesity and pregestational diabetes are independently associated with an increased risk of macrosomia. Results from large cohort studies have confirmed that excessive weight gain during pregnancy is also associated with fetal macrosomia. The association between maternal weight, weight gain during pregnancy and macrosomia has led to a proposal that the optimisation of maternal weight before pregnancy and limitation of weight gain during pregnancy would be useful strategies.[24]

## MANAGEMENT OF SUSPECTED MACROSOMIA

In attempting to establish a coherent plan of management for large infants, it must be acknowledged that the professional preferences of individual doctors may directly influence the method of delivery. However, few studies have examined the impact of non-medical factors on the mode of delivery of this population. Sandmire and DeMott[57] identified individual and group caesarean rates and found that groups with higher rates of caesarean section were not associated with better neonatal outcomes. In a prospective cohort study, Naylor et al.[58] compared the rates of caesarean delivery and macrosomia among women with untreated borderline gestational diabetes, women with treated overt gestational diabetes and women who remained normoglycaemic. Treated patients demonstrated a significantly increased rate of caesarean delivery compared to normoglycaemic women after controlling for a number of risk factors. The authors suggested that the doctor's awareness of gestational diabetes might have contributed to a lower threshold for surgical delivery.

Blackwell et al.[59] conducted a retrospective study to assess factors that might be predictive of the mode of delivery among diabetic women. The investigators concluded that non-medical factors might have influenced the risk of caesarean delivery within the study population. Accurate monitoring of fetal growth is one of the most critically important components of antenatal care. The ramifications of abnormal fetal growth have short-term and long-term sequelae for early neonatal life and beyond. Although not perfectly accurate, ultrasound and other monitoring technologies have markedly improved the ability to follow abnormalities of fetal growth and to decide if early intervention or early delivery is necessary. It is clear that perinatal morbidity and mortality can be reduced when such at risk fetuses are closely monitored.

## EXPECTANT MANAGEMENT

The management of patients with fetal macrosomia is controversial. Although expectant management has been suggested as a valid option in the management of macrosomic fetuses, elective caesarean delivery and early labour induction have also been proposed as interventions to prevent maternal and perinatal complications.[60] Despite the current controversy concerning the optimal mode of delivery for macrosomic infants, relatively few authors appear to have assessed birth outcomes related to the method of delivery. Nasser et al.[61] reported a statistically non-significant increase in the incidence of fetal injuries among infants weighing > 4500 g who were delivered vaginally as compared to infants of the same weight who were delivered by caesarean section (7.7% versus 1.6%, respectively). Diani et al.[62] examined outcomes associated with the delivery of fetuses weighing ≥ 4000 g and reported that normal vaginal delivery occurred in 79% of the cases. The most frequent neonatal complication was clavicle disruption. No perinatal deaths were reported. The investigators concluded that expectant management of low-risk macrosomic infants was a viable option. In a study published in 1995, Lipscomb et al.[45] reported no increase in birth asphyxia, perinatal mortality or permanent injury associated with the vaginal delivery of infants weighing > 4500 g. Kolderup et al.[63] found that forceps delivery was associated with a 4-fold risk of persistent injury compared to spontaneous vaginal or caesarean delivery. On the other hand, it has been estimated that more than 3600 caesarean deliveries need to be performed in non-diabetic patients with suspected macrosomia (≥ 4500 g) to prevent a single permanent neonatal injury.[44] Thus, the authors suggested that elective caesarean section for the sole indication of suspected macrosomia could not be justified.

One randomised clinical trial comparing elective induction of labour with expectant management in women with suspected fetal macrosomia has been reported.[64] The trial showed that induction of labour did not decrease the rate of caesarean section or reduce neonatal morbidity. Although several observational studies[53,65,66] have also been published, none was of sufficient size to evaluate properly such an infrequently occurring event.

A systematic review carried out by Sanchez-Ramos et al.[67] included 2700 women with fetal macrosomia who were managed expectantly. The results suggested that, for suspected fetal macrosomia at term, expectant management led to a reduced proportion of caesarean deliveries without compromising perinatal outcomes.

More recently, a Yorkshire medical staff survey on the management of suspected macrosomia revealed that the majority of consultants (15 of 21; 71.4%) and middle-grade doctors (45 of 61; 73.7%) would not offer induction of labour or lower segment caesarean section when the predicted fetal weight was over 4 kg. When asked about the management options when the estimated fetal weight was over 4.5 kg, only 10 out of 21 consultants (47.6%) and 25 of 61 middle-grade doctors (40.9%) did not recommend elective intervention. A similar trend of conservative management (60.3% versus 30.4%) was found in responses from more junior doctors (SHOs) when questioned similarly about the management of suspected fetal macrosomia.[68]

## ELECTIVE CAESAREAN SECTION

The role of caesarean delivery in suspected fetal macrosomia remains controversial. It has been shown that the rate of caesarean delivery increases directly with increasing birth-weight.[1,69] While the risk of birth trauma with vaginal delivery is higher with increased birth-weight, caesarean delivery reduces, but does not eliminate, this risk. However, the favourable outcome for most women who undergo a trial of labour implies that a large number of unnecessary caesarean sections would have to be performed to prevent a single bad outcome in the pregnancy complicated by suspected fetal macrosomia.[44,45] Further analysis by Rouse et al.[44] suggests that. for the 97% of pregnant women at term who are not diabetic, a policy of using ultrasound to predict macrosomia and then performing elective caesarean section would be medically and economically unsound. In practice, macrosomic infants are more likely to be delivered by emergency caesarean section and less likely to be delivered by elective caesarean section than normosomic infants.[6,10,70] However, the incidences of hypoglycaemia, transient tachypnoea of the newborn and longer stay in the nursery have been shown to be significantly higher among macrosomic infants delivered by caesarean section.[61]

A study by Lim et al.[71] showed that 57% of macrosomic infants delivered by caesarean section were admitted to special care baby unit. Gregory et al.[72] compared the rates of maternal and neonatal complications among infants weighing > 4000 g delivered by caesarean section with and without a trial of labour with those among infants weighing > 4000 g delivered vaginally. Asphyxia occurred with greater frequency among macrosomic infants delivered vaginally and by caesarean section after trial of labour compared to normosomic infants. Long-bone injuries were more frequent in infants of high birth-weight delivered vaginally and by caesarean section without a trial of labour than in infants of normal birth-weight. The rates of postpartum haemorrhage and shoulder dystocia were higher among women who delivered infants weighing at least 4000 g by caesarean section after trial of labour compared to women delivering normosomic infants. In contrast, no significant differences were noted in the rates of maternal complications in women delivering macrosomic infants by caesarean section without labour compared to normal birth-weight infants.[73] Blickstein et al.[74] found that a policy of caesarean delivery for all infants with birth-weights > 4200 g would result in a 5–6-fold increase in the caesarean section rate.

In addition, Gonen et al.[75] investigated the effects of a policy of routine caesarean delivery for suspected macrosomia among non-diabetic mothers and found that fetal macrosomia was correctly predicted in only 18% of the cases despite the use of both clinical and ultrasonographic estimates. Using the observed 3% risk for brachial plexus injury, the authors estimated that 74 caesarean deliveries would be necessary in order to avert one case of brachial plexus injury. Rouse et al.[44] investigated the outcomes and cost-effectiveness of a policy of elective caesarean delivery following the ultrasonographic diagnosis of macrosomia. They concluded that, for non-diabetic women, a minimum of 2345 caesarean deliveries at a cost of at least $4 million would be required to avert one permanent brachial plexus injury. Furthermore, the investigators concluded that risk associated with caesarean deliveries would increase maternal morbidity and mortality with one maternal death occurring for every 3.2 permanent brachial plexus injuries. Thus, they concluded that for 97% of non-diabetic women, caesarean delivery for suspected macrosomia diagnosed by ultrasound was medically and economically unsound. In 1999, Rouse et al.[44] applied more recent data to their decision analytical framework, re-affirmed the findings of the earlier study and proposed that the management of shoulder dystocia be optimised in order to reduce birth injury effectively.

Conversely, in pregnancies complicated by diabetes, elective caesarean section for ultrasonographically diagnosed fetal macrosomia, appears to be a more medically and economically tenable policy. Conway and Langer[76] found that, after instituting a protocol supporting elective caesarean delivery among diabetic mothers with ultrasonographically diagnosed fetal weights of > 4250 g, the rate of shoulder dystocia was significantly decreased without a clinically meaningful increase in the caesarean section rate. In 2002, Conway[73] further commented that the use of policies supporting elective caesarean delivery in this group should be weighed against the cost of maternal morbidity associated with caesarean delivery.

Thus, it will be seen that a broad spectrum of opinion exists regarding the use of prophylactic caesarean delivery in cases of ultrasonographically diagnosed fetal macrosomia. This practice may be considered pragmatic and controversial because a randomised trial has not been conducted to compare a policy of elective caesarean delivery for ultrasonographically diagnosed fetal macrosomia with a policy of standard obstetric management without ultrasonographic fetal weight prediction.

## EARLY INDUCTION OF LABOUR

It has been suggested that elective induction of labour before or near term may prevent macrosomia and its complications based on the knowledge that fetus continues to gain about 250 g per week after the 37th week.[77] One of the major concerns about this plan of management is that induction of labour in the presence of an unfavourable cervix (Bishop score < 5) may fail, resulting in an increased caesarean section rate.[53]

Current evidence does not support early induction of labour. Observational studies suggest that induction of labour at least doubles the risk of caesarean delivery without reducing the risk of shoulder dystocia or newborn morbidity.[50,65,78] There was no difference between expectant management and induction of labour in a group of women who subsequently experienced shoulder dystocia.[67] The authors reviewed 11 studies involving 1051 women who underwent induction of labour. Although the pooled analysis of the observational studies showed that women who were induced were less likely to achieve spontaneous vaginal delivery, analysis of randomised controlled trials showed no significant effect on the rate of spontaneous vaginal delivery. Both randomised controlled trials and observational studies showed no significant differences in the rates of operative vaginal delivery and of shoulder dystocia between groups of women who were managed expectantly and those whose labour was induced (8.9% versus 10.3%).

Hyperstimulation and hypertonus of uterine contractions are potential, but uncommon, complications during induction of labour either with prostaglandins or oxytocin. Accurate assessment of uterine contractions and adequate fetal heart rate monitoring are important whenever induction of labour is attempted. This becomes even more important when induction of labour is carried out for suspected fetal macrosomia in view of the increased risks of cephalopelvic disproportion and birth injury. The progress of labour should be closely monitored to detect arrest or delay.[79] Thus, the involvement of senior obstetricians in management decisions and the use of fetal electronic monitoring should be initiated as soon as is feasible.

## CONCLUSIONS

Although it is often suggested that the best plan of management should include an informed mother and a well-designed plan for obstetric emergencies, the literature regarding this topic is incomplete and often inconclusive. The major concern regarding the management of macrosomic fetuses is to reduce interventions in order to avoid complications. Most high birth-weight fetuses experience an excellent outcome, regardless of management.

The overall rate of significant birth injury among macrosomic infants is low. Antenatal diagnosis of macrosomia often results in an increase in operative deliveries. Reported neonatal mortality rates do not appear to differ significantly between different modes of delivery. However, small sample sizes and the relative rarity of neonatal deaths may preclude an accurate assessment of the mortality risk in this population.

It is difficult to ascertain the relative benefits of caesarean versus vaginal delivery among various birth-weight categories, as the effects of uncontrolled factors related to high birth-weight cannot be assessed. Furthermore, the lack of randomised trials comparing the risks and benefits associated with various methods of delivery hinders the formulation of a definitive answer to the question. At present, there seems to be little justification for wide-spread obstetric intervention in otherwise uncomplicated cases.

## Key points for clinical practice

- Fetal macrosomia complicates more than 10% of all pregnancies.
- The incidence of fetal macrosomia has increased in the last few decades, in both Europe and the USA.
- Birth weight is influenced by a variety of maternal, fetal, metabolic and genetic factors.
- Ultrasonography provides a more accurate means of obtaining an estimated fetal weight.
- The management of patients with fetal macrosomia is controversial.
- Expectant management reduces the rate of caesarean deliveries without compromising perinatal outcomes.
- It is important to have a good management plan for patients with fetal macrosomia, recognizing that there is currently no perfect solution.

### References

1. Boulet SL, Alexander GR, Salihu HM, Pass M. Macrosomic births in the United States: determinants, outcomes, and proposed grades of risk. *Am J Obstet Gynecol* 2003; **188**: 1372–1378.
2. Stotland NE, Caughey AB, Breed EM, Escobar GJ. Risk factors and obstetric complications associated with macrosomia. *Int J Gynaecol Obstet* 2004; **87**: 220–226.
3. Bonellie SR, Raab GM. Why are babies getting heavier? Comparison of Scottish births from 1980 to 1992. *BMJ* 1997; **315**: 1205.
4. Johar R, Rayburn W, Weir D, Eggert L. Birthweights in term infants. A 50-year perspective. *J Reprod Med* 1988; **33**: 813–816.
5. Orskou J, Kesmodel U, Henriksen TB, Secher NJ. An increasing proportion of infants weigh more than 4000 grams at birth. *Acta Obstet Gynecol Scand* 2001; **80**: 931–936.
6. Wollschlaeger K, Nieder J, Koppe I, Hartlein K. A study of fetal macrosomia. *Arch Gynecol Obstet* 1999; **263**: 51–55.
7. Surkan PJ, Hsieh CC, Johansson AL, Dickman PW, Cnattingius S. Reasons for increasing trends in large for gestational age births. *Obstet Gynecol* 2004; **104**: 720–726.
8. Okun N, Verma A, Mitchell BF, Flowerdew G. Relative importance of maternal constitutional factors and glucose intolerance of pregnancy in the development of newborn macrosomia. *J Matern Fetal Med* 1997; **6**: 285–290.
9. Ehrenberg HM, Durnwald CP, Catalano P, Mercer BM. The influence of obesity and diabetes on the risk of cesarean delivery. *Am J Obstet Gynecol* 2004; **191**: 969–974.
10. Jolly MC, Sebire NJ, Harris JP, Regan L, Robinson S. Risk factors for macrosomia and its clinical consequences: a study of 350,311 pregnancies. *Eur J Obstet Gynecol Reprod Biol* 2003; **111**: 9–14.
11. Orskou J, Henriksen TB, Kesmodel U, Secher NJ. Maternal characteristics and lifestyle factors and the risk of delivering high birthweight infants. *Obstet Gynecol* 2003; **102**: 115–120.
12. Dildy GA, Jackson GM, Fowers GK, Oshiro BT, Varner MW, Clark SL. Very advanced maternal age: pregnancy after age 45. *Am J Obstet Gynecol* 1996; **175**: 668–674.
13. Aldous MB, Edmonson MB. Maternal age at first childbirth and risk of low birthweight and preterm delivery in Washington State. *JAMA* 1993; **270**: 2574–2577.
14. Kerssen A, de Valk HW, Visser GH. Sibling birthweight as a predictor of macrosomia in

women with type 1 diabetes. *Diabetologia* 2005; **48**: 1743–1748.

15. Davis R, Woelk G, Mueller BA, Daling J. The role of previous birthweight on risk for macrosomia in a subsequent birth. *Epidemiology* 1995; **6**: 607–611.

16. Tanner JM, Lejarraga H, Healy MJ. Within-family standards for birth-weight. *Lancet* 1972; **2**: 1314–1315.

17. Spellacy WN, Miller S, Winegar A, Peterson PQ. Macrosomia – maternal characteristics and infant complications. *Obstet Gynecol* 1985; **66**: 158–161.

18. Ramos GA, Caughey AB. The interrelationship between ethnicity and obesity on obstetric outcomes. *Am J Obstet Gynecol* 2005; **193**: 1089–1093.

19. Steinfeld JD, Valentine S, Lerer T, Ingardia CJ, Wax JR, Curry SL. Obesity-related complications of pregnancy vary by race. *J Matern Fetal Med* 2000; **9**: 238–241.

20. Homko CJ, Sivan E, Nyirjesy P, Reece EA. The interrelationship between ethnicity and gestational diabetes in fetal macrosomia. *Diabetes Care* 1995; **18**: 1442–1445.

21. Gregory KD, Korst LM. Age and racial/ethnic differences in maternal, fetal, and placental conditions in laboring patients. *Am J Obstet Gynecol* 2003; **188**: 1602–1606, discussion 1606–1608.

22. Stotland NE, Cheng YW, Hopkins LM, Caughey AB. Gestational weight gain and adverse neonatal outcome among term infants. *Obstet Gynecol* 2006; **108**: 635–643.

23. Brown JE, Murtaugh MA, Jacobs Jr DR, Margellos HC. Variation in newborn size according to pregnancy weight change by trimester. *Am J Clin Nutr* 2002; **76**: 205–209.

24. Cogswell ME, Serdula MK, Hungerford DW, Yip R. Gestational weight gain among average-weight and overweight women – what is excessive? *Am J Obstet Gynecol* 1995; **172**: 705–712.

25. Dang K, Homko C, Reece EA. Factors associated with fetal macrosomia in offspring of gestational diabetic women. *J Matern Fetal Med* 2000; **9**: 114–117.

26. Langer O, Rodriguez DA, Xenakis EM, McFarland MB, Berkus MD, Arrendondo F. Intensified versus conventional management of gestational diabetes. *Am J Obstet Gynecol* 1994; **170**: 1036–1046, discussion 1046–1047.

27. Hawthorne G, Robson S, Ryall EA, Sen D, Roberts SH, Ward Platt MP. Prospective population based survey of outcome of pregnancy in diabetic women: results of the Northern Diabetic Pregnancy Audit, 1994. *BMJ* 1997; **315**: 279–281.

28. Langer O. Prevention of macrosomia. *Baillières Clin Obstet Gynaecol* 1991; **5**: 333–347.

29. Catalano PM, Drago NM, Amini SB. Longitudinal changes in pancreatic beta-cell function and metabolic clearance rate of insulin in pregnant women with normal and abnormal glucose tolerance. *Diabetes Care* 1998; **21**: 403–408.

30. Catalano PM, Huston L, Amini SB, Kalhan SC. Longitudinal changes in glucose metabolism during pregnancy in obese women with normal glucose tolerance and gestational diabetes mellitus. *Am J Obstet Gynecol* 1999; **180**: 903–916.

31. Boulet SL, Salihu HM, Alexander GR. Mode of delivery and birth outcomes of macrosomic infants. *J Obstet Gynaecol* 2004; **24**: 622–629.

32. Baskett TF, Allen AC. Perinatal implications of shoulder dystocia. *Obstet Gynecol* 1995; **86**: 14–17.

33. Anoon SS, Rizk DE, Ezimokhai M. Obstetric outcome of excessively overgrown fetuses (> or = 5000 g): a case-control study. *J Perinat Med* 2003; **31**: 295–301.

34. Zamorski MA, Biggs WS. Management of suspected fetal macrosomia. *Am Fam Phys* 2001; **63**: 302–306.

35. Acker DB, Sachs BP, Friedman EA. Risk factors for shoulder dystocia. *Obstet Gynecol* 1985; **66**: 762–768.

36. Ecker JL, Greenberg JA, Norwitz ER, Nadel AS, Repke JT. Birthweight as a predictor of brachial plexus injury. *Obstet Gynecol* 1997; **89**: 643–647.

37. Gross TL, Sokol RJ, Williams T, Thompson K. Shoulder dystocia: a fetal-physician risk. *Am J Obstet Gynecol* 1987; **156**: 1408–1418.

38. Gherman RB, Ouzounian JG, Goodwin TM. Obstetric maneuvers for shoulder dystocia and associated fetal morbidity. *Am J Obstet Gynecol* 1998; **178**: 1126–1130.

39. Nadas S, Reinberg O. Obstetric fractures. *Eur J Pediatr Surg* 1992; **2**: 165–168.

40. Gilbert A, Brockman R, Carlioz H. Surgical treatment of brachial plexus birth palsy. *Clin Orthop* 1991; **264**: 39–47.

41. Sandmire HF. Whither ultrasonic prediction of fetal macrosomia? *Obstet Gynecol* 1993;

**82**: 860–862.

42. Jennett RJ, Tarby TJ, Kreinick CJ. Brachial plexus palsy: an old problem revisited. *Am J Obstet Gynecol* 1992; **166**: 1673–1676, discussion 1676–1677.

43. Morrison JC, Sanders JR, Magann EF, Wiser WL. The diagnosis and management of dystocia of the shoulder. *Surg Gynecol Obstet* 1992; **175**: 515–522.

44. Rouse DJ, Owen J, Goldenberg RL, Cliver SP. The effectiveness and costs of elective cesarean delivery for fetal macrosomia diagnosed by ultrasound. *JAMA* 1996; **276**: 1480–1486.

45. Lipscomb KR, Gregory K, Shaw K. The outcome of macrosomic infants weighing at least 4500 grams: Los Angeles County + University of Southern California experience. *Obstet Gynecol* 1995; **85**: 558–564.

46. Chauhan SP, Lutton PM, Bailey KJ, Guerrieri JP, Morrison JC. Intrapartum clinical, sonographic, and parous patients' estimates of newborn birthweight. *Obstet Gynecol* 1992; **79**: 956–958.

47. Watson WJ, Soisson AP, Harlass FE. Estimated weight of the term fetus. Accuracy of ultrasound vs. clinical examination. *J Reprod Med* 1988; **33**: 369–371.

48. Gardosi J, Francis A. Controlled trial of fundal height measurement plotted on customised antenatal growth charts. *Br J Obstet Gynaecol* 1999; **106**: 309–317.

49. Chien PF, Owen P, Khan KS. Validity of ultrasound estimation of fetal weight. *Obstet Gynecol* 2000; **95**: 856–860.

50. Delpapa EH, Mueller-Heubach E. Pregnancy outcome following ultrasound diagnosis of macrosomia. *Obstet Gynecol* 1991; **78**: 340–343.

51. Altman DG, Chitty LS. Charts of fetal size: 1. Methodology. *Br J Obstet Gynaecol* 1994; **101**: 29–34.

52. Deter RL, Hadlock FP. Use of ultrasound in the detection of macrosomia: a review. *J Clin Ultrasound* 1985; **13**: 519–524.

53. Combs CA, Singh NB, Khoury JC. Elective induction versus spontaneous labor after sonographic diagnosis of fetal macrosomia. *Obstet Gynecol* 1993; **81**: 492–496.

54. Pollack RN, Hauer-Pollack G, Divon MY. Macrosomia in postdates pregnancies: the accuracy of routine ultrasonographic screening. *Am J Obstet Gynecol* 1992; **167**: 7–11.

55. Reece E, Friedman A, Copel J, Klienman C. Prenatal diagnosis and management of deviant fetal growth and congenital malformations. In: Reece E, Coustan D. (eds) *Diabetes Mellitus in Pregnancy*. New York: Churchill Livingstone, 1995; 222–226.

56. Landon MB, Mintz MC, Gabbe SG. Sonographic evaluation of fetal abdominal growth: predictor of the large-for-gestational-age infant in pregnancies complicated by diabetes mellitus. *Am J Obstet Gynecol* 1989; **160**: 115–121.

57. Sandmire HF, DeMott RK. The Green Bay cesarean section study. IV. The physician factor as a determinant of cesarean birth rates for the large fetus. *Am J Obstet Gynecol* 1996; **174**: 1557–1564.

58. Naylor CD, Sermer M, Chen E, Sykora K. Cesarean delivery in relation to birthweight and gestational glucose tolerance: pathophysiology or practice style? Toronto Trihospital Gestational Diabetes Investigators. *JAMA* 1996; **275**: 1165–1170.

59. Blackwell SC, Hassan SS, Wolfe HW, Michaelson J, Berry SM, Sorokin Y. Why are cesarean delivery rates so high in diabetic pregnancies? *J Perinat Med* 2000; **28**: 316–320.

60. Langer O, Berkus MD, Huff RW, Samueloff A. Shoulder dystocia: should the fetus weighing greater than or equal to 4000 grams be delivered by cesarean section? *Am J Obstet Gynecol* 1991; **165**: 831–837.

61. Nassar AH, Usta IM, Khalil AM, Melhem ZI, Nakad TI, Abu Musa AA. Fetal macrosomia (> or = 4500 g): perinatal outcome of 231 cases according to the mode of delivery. *J Perinatol* 2003; **23**: 136–141.

62. Diani F, Venanzi S, Zanconato G, Murari S, Moscatelli C, Turinetto A. Fetal macrosomia and management of delivery. *Clin Exp Obstet Gynecol* 1997; **24**: 212–214.

63. Kolderup LB, Laros Jr RK, Musci TJ. Incidence of persistent birth injury in macrosomic infants: association with mode of delivery. *Am J Obstet Gynecol* 1997; **177**: 37–41.

64. Gonen O, Rosen DJ, Dolfin Z, Tepper R, Markov S, Fejgin MD. Induction of labor versus expectant management in macrosomia: a randomized study. *Obstet Gynecol* 1997; **89**: 913–917.

65. Friesen CD, Miller AM, Rayburn WF. Influence of spontaneous or induced labor on

delivering the macrosomic fetus. *Am J Perinatol* 1995; **12**: 63–66.

66. Leaphart WL, Meyer MC, Capeless EL. Labor induction with a prenatal diagnosis of fetal macrosomia. *J Matern Fetal Med* 1997; **6**: 99–102.

67. Sanchez-Ramos L, Bernstein S, Kaunitz AM. Expectant management versus labor induction for suspected fetal macrosomia: a systematic review. *Obstet Gynecol* 2002; **100**: 997–1002.

68. El-Ghobashy A, Haw W, Tuffnell D. A Yorkshire medical staff survey on managing suspected fetal macrosomia during pregnancy. 2006; unpublished data.

69. Mulik V, Usha Kiran TS, Bethal J, Bhal PS. The outcome of macrosomic fetuses in a low risk primigravid population. *Int J Gynaecol Obstet* 2003; **80**: 15–22.

70. Mocanu EV, Greene RA, Byrne BM, Turner MJ. Obstetric and neonatal outcome of babies weighing more than 4.5 kg: an analysis by parity. *Eur J Obstet Gynecol Reprod Biol* 2000; **92**: 229–233.

71. Lim JH, Tan BC, Jammal AE, Symonds EM. Delivery of macrosomic babies: management and outcomes of 330 cases. *J Obstet Gynaecol* 2002; **22**: 370–374.

72. Gregory KD, Henry OA, Ramicone E, Chan LS, Platt LD. Maternal and infant complications in high and normal weight infants by method of delivery. *Obstet Gynecol* 1998; **92**: 507–513.

73. Conway DL. Delivery of the macrosomic infant: cesarean section versus vaginal delivery. *Semin Perinatol* 2002; **26**: 225–231.

74. Blickstein I, Ben-Arie A, Hagay ZJ. Antepartum risks of shoulder dystocia and brachial plexus injury for infants weighing 4,200 g or more. *Gynecol Obstet Invest* 1998; **45**: 77–80.

75. Gonen R, Bader D, Ajami M. Effects of a policy of elective cesarean delivery in cases of suspected fetal macrosomia on the incidence of brachial plexus injury and the rate of cesarean delivery. *Am J Obstet Gynecol* 2000; **183**: 1296–1300.

76. Conway DL, Langer O. Elective delivery of infants with macrosomia in diabetic women: reduced shoulder dystocia versus increased cesarean deliveries. *Am J Obstet Gynecol* 1998; **178**: 922–925.

77. Ott WJ. The diagnosis of altered fetal growth. *Obstet Gynecol Clin North Am* 1988; **15**: 237–263.

78. Weeks JW, Pitman T, Spinnato 2nd JA. Fetal macrosomia: does antenatal prediction affect delivery route and birth outcome? *Am J Obstet Gynecol* 1995; **173**: 1215–1219.

79. Oppenheim WL, Davis A, Growdon WA, Dorey FJ, Davlin LB. Clavicle fractures in the newborn. *Clin Orthop* 1990; 176–180.

*Jennifer Walsh  Deirdre J. Murphy*

6

# Operative vaginal delivery – a dying art?

The role of operative vaginal delivery has been controversial since its inception and the use of forceps, in particular, has been declining steadily in recent years.[1] Caesarean section in the second stage of labour, previously an uncommon phenomenon, is increasingly performed in preference to operative vaginal delivery or as a result of a failed attempt at operative vaginal delivery.[2] Despite recommendations from both the Royal College of Obstetricians and Gynaecologists (RCOG) and the American College of Obstetricians and Gynecologists (ACOG) to improve training in operative vaginal delivery in order to control ever-escalating rates of caesarean section, fear of litigation because of the morbidity associated with operative vaginal delivery has restricted the use of mid-cavity and rotational procedures and reduced the number of obstetricians sufficiently competent to teach trainees.[3,4] Safe and competent management of women in labour requires obstetricians to be confident in both forceps and vacuum delivery. If current trends continue, we will be lamenting the skills of operative vaginal delivery as a vanished art.

## HISTORICAL PERSPECTIVE

The history of forceps delivery dates back as far as 1500 BC, being originally used following fetal demise to save the mother's life.[5,6] The use of forceps has been debated since then. In 1752, William Smellie described the use of forceps in his *Treatise on the Theory and Practice of Midwifery* but, by the early 19th

**Jennifer Walsh** MRCOG MRCPI
Specialist Registrar in Obstetrics and Gynaecology, Coombe Women and Infants Hospital, Dolphin's Barn, Dublin 8, Republic of Ireland

**Deirdre J. Murphy** MD MRCOG (for correspondence)
Professor of Obstetrics, University Department of Obstetrics and Gynaecology, Trinity College Dublin & Coombe Women and Infants Hospital, Dolphin's Barn, Dublin 8, Republic of Ireland
E-mail: deirdre.j.murphy@tcd.ie

century, they had been almost completely abandoned due to neonatal and maternal morbidity associated with their use. This resulted in the infamous prolonged second stage of labour of Princess Charlotte of Great Britain in 1817. Her obstetrician, Sir Richard Croft, believed that forceps-assisted delivery should not be attempted until the fetal head had rested for 6 h on the perineum. Ultimately, the princess had a 24-h second stage of labour, resulting in a stillborn infant and her own untimely demise from post partum haemorrhage. Sir Richard himself committed suicide 6 weeks later. This tragedy sparked a revolution in the use of forceps to prevent such events from happening.

The use of forceps ultimately peaked to account for an extraordinary 70% of all deliveries by the late 1940s. Since then, their use has declined steadily in favour of unassisted delivery, vacuum extraction and caesarean section. The more recent decline in the use of forceps delivery is at odds with the overall increase in operative delivery rates in developed countries. In the UK, operative vaginal delivery rates are reasonably consistent at 10–15%. What has changed is the instrument of first choice, failure rates with the chosen instrument, sequential use of instruments and an increasing recourse to caesarean section in the second stage of labour. Historical swings in the approach to operative vaginal delivery have been dramatic and based largely on perceived risks and opinion leaders rather than a robust, evidence-based evaluation.

## TYPES OF OPERATIVE VAGINAL DELIVERY AND INDICATIONS FOR USE

There are numerous types of obstetric forceps, with more than 700 described.[7] However, they may be divided into three main groups – outlet, mid-cavity and rotational forceps – each of which are appropriate to specific situations and require differing levels of skill. The definitive metal vacuum extractor was first described by Malmström in 1954 and was modified by Bird in 1969. The first soft cups were available in the 1980s.[5] There is now a range of metal, sialastic and disposable vacuum extractors to choose from with specific devices for rotation and modifications that record the pressure exerted during the procedure.[8] Obstetricians vary greatly in their preferred use of instruments for specific circumstances.[9]

The indications for operative vaginal delivery have changed little over the years. They may be divided into maternal reasons and fetal reasons. Maternal indications include maternal exhaustion and maternal conditions in which pushing is contra-indicated, *e.g.* certain maternal cardiac disease or raised intracranial pressure. Fetal indications consist primarily of suspected fetal distress. Such situations call for careful evaluation by the obstetrician to determine whether abdominal or vaginal delivery is most appropriate and, if vaginal delivery is attempted, which choice of instrument will successfully complete the delivery with the least maternal and neonatal morbidity.

Importantly, however, there are certain situations in which forceps delivery is considered superior or where vacuum extraction is contra-indicated (Table 1). These include the delivery of the after-coming head of a breech, preterm assisted delivery, assisted delivery of a face presentation, operative vaginal

**Table 1** Indications for forceps delivery

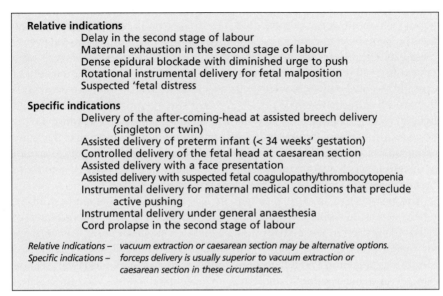

**Relative indications**
Delay in the second stage of labour
Maternal exhaustion in the second stage of labour
Dense epidural blockade with diminished urge to push
Rotational instrumental delivery for fetal malposition
Suspected 'fetal distress

**Specific indications**
Delivery of the after-coming-head at assisted breech delivery
(singleton or twin)
Assisted delivery of preterm infant (< 34 weeks' gestation)
Controlled delivery of the fetal head at caesarean section
Assisted delivery with a face presentation
Assisted delivery with suspected fetal coagulopathy/thrombocytopenia
Instrumental delivery for maternal medical conditions that preclude
active pushing
Instrumental delivery under general anaesthesia
Cord prolapse in the second stage of labour

*Relative indications – vacuum extraction or caesarean section may be alternative options.*
*Specific indications – forceps delivery is usually superior to vacuum extraction or*
*caesarean section in these circumstances.*

delivery with suspected coagulopathy or thrombocytopenia in the fetus or cord prolapse in the second stage of labour. These situations call for expedited delivery by forceps in trained hands and, therefore, emphasise the need for training in both types of instrument.

## EPIDEMIOLOGY

There has been a steady decrease in the proportion of women achieving spontaneous vaginal delivery in developed countries throughout the world.[10] This is reflected in a dramatic rise in rates of operative delivery and, specifically, of caesarean section. Data from the US suggest that the rate of caesarean section has increased to 27.6% following seven annual successive rises.[11] In contrast, rates of operative vaginal delivery are falling but remain highly variable with variations of 200–300% around a relatively low mean of 7% (SD ± 4%; range, 1–23%).[12] Such variation suggests a pattern of almost random decision-making perhaps reflecting a lack of reliable outcome-based data to guide clinical decisions. An evaluation of caesarean delivery by an ACOG task force reported that first-time mothers delivering a term singleton fetus with a cephalic presentation and women with a previous caesarean section account for two-thirds of all caesarean deliveries in the US.[4] Most of the dramatic variation in caesarean delivery rates occurred in these two groups. Improved training in operative vaginal delivery has been recommended and it has been suggested that safe use of these techniques may help to reduce the caesarean delivery rate. Current data suggest that this recommendation has not yet been widely implemented

The National Sentinel Caesarean Section audit provided detailed information on operative delivery rates for England, Wales and Northern Ireland.[10] The caesarean section rate in England was 21.3% with rates of 24.2%

and 23.9% in Wales and Northern Ireland, respectively. The primary caesarean section rate was 17% overall and, as the largest clinical group in the maternity population, these women contributed 70% to the overall caesarean section rate. Clearly, the management of a first labour will have a major impact on the overall caesarean section rate for any delivery unit. Operative vaginal delivery rates ranged from 10–12% and have remained fairly constant. Of note, the majority of operative vaginal deliveries were by forceps in 1980 but 60–70% were performed by vacuum extraction in 2000–2001.[10] A recent survey of practice in the UK and Ireland reports marked variation in instrument preference according to the position and station of the presenting part and, importantly, according to the grade of operator.[9] Current trainees are far more likely than consultants to prefer vacuum to forceps in all clinical circumstances and are more likely to proceed directly to caesarean section for mid-cavity or rotational procedures.

The perspective is very different in less and least developed countries where access to skilled care is the limiting factor. The observed rate of caesarean section in West Africa was 1.3% with a suggested range of 3.6–6.5% for maternal indications alone.[13] These estimates fall well below the World Health Organization (WHO) recommendation of a 10–15% caesarean section rate set to achieve optimal maternal and perinatal safety. Vacuum-assisted delivery has been shown to offer a safe alternative to caesarean section in Ecuador when introduced as a new skill for carefully selected deliveries (station no higher than +3).[14] However, a survey of 121 developing countries reported that 37% of respondents said the method was known but used by only a limited number of specialists who do not teach it and 15% admitted no knowledge of the procedure.[15] This is in settings where forceps delivery is not available and access to caesarean section may be limited. These reports suggest that there is restricted access to appropriate obstetric care in developing countries for maternal indications that are major determinants of serious maternal morbidity and mortality.

It is more difficult to establish rates of caesarean section in the second stage of labour. In a prospective cohort study of women in the South West of England, 4% of the total population were transferred to theatre for operative delivery in the second stage of labour and just over half of these women were delivered by caesarean section, the remainder by rotational or mid-cavity operative vaginal delivery.[16] A North American review of operative vaginal delivery in the year 2000 suggested that operative deliveries involving rotation of more than 45° were likely to be abandoned. This has been reflected in a survey of obstetric fellows of ACOG which showed that over half have abandoned mid-cavity assisted vaginal delivery in favour of caesarean section.[17] Clearly, there are concerns about maternal and infant safety in relation to operative vaginal delivery reinforced by limited opportunities to acquire the necessary skills to perform such deliveries competently. However, the complexity and consequences of caesarean section in the second stage of labour should not be overlooked.[2]

## ASSOCIATED MORBIDITY

For many women, operative vaginal delivery is not planned or even considered and is a particularly disappointing result when it is the outcome of a long and difficult labour. The complications that arise may have their origin in the indication for operative delivery (for example, prolonged second stage) or may result from the procedure itself. It is important to consider early and long-term complications both physical and psychological as well as the implications for future reproductive outcomes. Where operative vaginal delivery is appropriate, there is a choice to be made between forceps and vacuum delivery and for mid-cavity or rotational procedures a choice between attempted operative vaginal delivery and second-stage caesarean section.

## MATERNAL MORBIDITY

### Early morbidity

There is on-going debate on the relative merits and hazards of vacuum and forceps delivery (Table 2). A systematic review of several randomised controlled trials (RCTs) reported that use of the vacuum extractor was associated with significantly less maternal trauma (OR, 0.41; 95% CI, 0.33–0.50) and with more completed deliveries (OR, 1.69; 95% CI, 1.31–2.19) than forceps delivery.[18] However, this is potentially misleading as attempted vacuum delivery has a higher failure rate than forceps as a first-line instrument with failed vacuum deliveries frequently completed by forceps. Vacuum failure rates of 20–30% have been reported in two recent RCTs with higher failure rates for the hand-held vacuum device.[19,20] Failure of vacuum delivery is 3–4 times more likely with a fetal malposition and is associated with an increased

**Table 2** Advantages and disadvantages of forceps delivery

**Advantages of forceps delivery**

*Forceps versus vacuum extraction*
There is a lower failure rate with forceps
Forceps is faster where 'fetal distress' is present
Sequential use of instruments is less common with forceps
Cephalhaematoma and retinal haemorrhage is less common with forceps

*Forceps versus emergency caesarean section*
Major obstetric haemorrhage is less common following forceps
Length of hospital stay is shorter following forceps
Admission of the baby for intensive care is less common following forceps
Re-admission to hospital occurs less frequently following forceps
Subsequent spontaneous vaginal delivery is more likely following forceps

**Disadvantages of forceps delivery**

*Forceps versus vacuum extraction*
Forceps delivery requires a higher degree of maternal analgesia
Maternal perineal trauma is greater following forceps
Facial bruising and facial nerve palsy is more common following forceps
Forceps delivery requires greater clinical skill (this may also be an advantage)

*Forceps versus emergency caesarean section*
Trauma to the baby is less likely following immediate caesarean section
Maternal perineal trauma is less common following caesarean section
Dyspareunia is less common following caesarean section
Urinary and faecal incontinence is less common following caesarean section

risk of postpartum haemorrhage.[21,22] In a prospective cohort study of women transferred to theatre for arrested progress in the second stage of labour, attempted forceps was more likely to result in completed vaginal delivery than attempted vacuum (63% versus 48%; $P < 0.01$).[16] In a recent large retrospective study, vacuum extraction was associated with more shoulder dystocia and cephalhaematoma but fewer anal sphincter lacerations.[23]

Rotational delivery and mid-cavity arrest in the second stage of labour present the obstetrician with a choice between a potentially difficult operative vaginal delivery and caesarean section at full dilatation, each with inherent risks. In a retrospective review of the maternal and fetal outcome of failed operative vaginal delivery compared to proceeding directly to caesarean section in the second stage of labour, Revah et al.[24] found no increased morbidity for the mother in a setting where caesarean section could follow promptly. In a prospective cohort study of women transferred to theatre for second stage arrest, caesarean section was associated with an increased risk of major haemorrhage (adjusted OR, 2.8; 95% CI, 1.1–7.6) and prolonged hospital stay (OR 3.5, 95% CI 1.6-7.6).[16] However, caesarean delivery (OR, 0.63; 95% CI, 0.38–1.00) and major haemorrhage were less likely with an experienced obstetrician (OR, 0.5; 95% CI, 0.3–0.9). High rates of third and fourth degree tears are reported following operative vaginal delivery.[22,25] The comparable morbidity at caesarean section relates to extension of the uterine incision into the cervix, vagina or broad ligaments. Extension of the uterine incision at full dilatation has been reported in up to 35% of cases[26] and has been associated with an increased risk of caesarean hysterectomy and febrile morbidity. Long-term follow-up will determine whether this results in subsequent difficult deliveries or an increased risk of uterine rupture.

Clearly, choice of operative delivery in the second stage of labour presents a difficult risk/benefit dilemma. Caesarean section at full dilatation with anhydramnios and an engaged fetal head is a difficult procedure. This is reflected in high rates of major obstetric haemorrhage, extension of the uterine incision and prolonged hospital admission. These risks must be balanced with the potential for pelvic floor trauma following operative vaginal delivery.

## Pelvic floor morbidity

Operative vaginal delivery is associated with increased pelvic floor morbidity but comparisons between vacuum and forceps remain controversial. Forceps delivery incurred a higher risk of third-degree laceration than vacuum in two population-based studies (OR, 1.94; 95% CI, 1.30–2.89 and OR, 3.33; 95% CI 2.97–3.74, respectively).[27,28] In another study, vacuum delivery (OR, 2.30; 95% CI, 2.21–2.40) resulted in a greater risk of sphincter laceration than forceps delivery (OR, 1.45; 95% CI, 1.37–1.52).[29] In a recent randomised trial assessing anal sphincter function, symptoms of altered faecal continence were significantly more common following forceps delivery compared to vacuum.[30] More re-assuringly, there was no difference in rates of urinary and bowel dysfunction at 5-year follow-up of a previous randomised controlled study comparing forceps and vacuum delivery.[31] However, in the prospective cohort study of operative delivery in the second stage of labour there was a 3-fold increased risk of urinary incontinence at 1 and 3 years following operative vaginal delivery compared to second stage caesarean section.[32,33]

## Psychological morbidity

A previous delivery experience can have important implications for future pregnancies, not least whether a woman would contemplate another pregnancy. Fear of childbirth has been reported in up to 26% of women at 5 years following either operative vaginal delivery or caesarean section compared with 10% following spontaneous vaginal delivery.[34] In a second-stage prospective cohort study, women were far more likely to aim for a future vaginal delivery following operative vaginal delivery than caesarean section (79% versus 39%) although fear of childbirth was a frequently reported reason for avoiding a further pregnancy in both groups.[35,36] A randomised controlled trial was conducted in Australia to assess the effectiveness of a midwife-led debriefing session during the postpartum hospital stay in reducing maternal depression among women giving birth by caesarean section, forceps or ventouse extraction.[37] Midwife-led debriefing was ineffective in reducing maternal morbidity at 6 months postpartum and the authors commented that the possibility that debriefing contributed to emotional health problems for some women could not be excluded. Further research is required to establish an optimal approach to helping women come to terms with the fear, distress and depression that can result from operative delivery. Of note, a recent study suggests that elective caesarean section does not protect against postnatal depression and women should be counselled accordingly when making decisions about future mode of delivery.[38]

## Future delivery outcome

The mode of delivery for arrested progress in the second stage of labour may have important implications for the future mode of delivery. Women who have experienced a previous caesarean section at full dilatation generate anxiety in subsequent labours relating to the risk of further emergency caesarean section and potential uterine rupture. Mid-cavity and rotational operative vaginal deliveries have become unpopular in the US and are increasingly abandoned in favour of caesarean section. This may be a short-sighted view, however, if one fails to consider the outcome of future deliveries in the assessment of overall morbidity. In a follow-up study of primigravidae who required midcavity operative vaginal delivery, more than 75% achieved a spontaneous vaginal delivery with heavier babies in the second pregnancy and very low overall rates of birth trauma or asphyxia.[34] Women delivered by operative vaginal delivery compared to second-stage caesarean section were far more likely to aim for vaginal delivery and to achieve a vaginal delivery (78% versus 31%) at 3-year follow-up of the prospective cohort study.[36] Women's satisfaction with the subsequent delivery experience remains to be evaluated.

## NEONATAL MORBIDITY

The neonatal outcome is critical to the debate on the role of operative vaginal delivery in modern obstetric practice. The need for speed may compete with concerns about neonatal trauma particularly where there are features of potential fetal compromise. The operator's expertise may ultimately determine the preferred mode of delivery but each obstetrician should have the necessary skills to deliver the baby by the swiftest and safest means according to the individual circumstances.

## Condition at birth

The neonatal morbidity related to operative delivery needs to be evaluated where operative vaginal delivery is successfully achieved, where caesarean section is undertaken following a failed attempt at operative vaginal delivery and where delivery is by immediate caesarean section. In a systematic review of trials comparing vacuum extraction with forceps delivery, Johanson and Menon[18] reported that use of the vacuum extractor was associated with an increase in neonatal cephalhaematoma and retinal haemorrhages. Despite this finding, the vacuum extractor has become the instrument of choice in the interest of minimising maternal morbidity. If speed is of the essence, particularly in the presence of suspected fetal hypoxia, then delivery can be completed more quickly in the delivery room than the operating theatre with a higher chance of completed operative vaginal delivery with forceps than vacuum.[39,40]

To date, there has been inconsistency in the reported early neonatal morbidity when comparing operative vaginal delivery with caesarean section for mid-cavity arrest. Older retrospective studies found little difference in short-term neonatal morbidity and, re-assuringly, the study by Revah *et al*.[24] found no increase in neonatal morbidity among women who had a failed operative vaginal delivery in a setting where caesarean section could follow promptly. In a prospective cohort study of women transferred to theatre in the second stage of labour, delivery by caesarean section was associated with an increased risk of admission to the special care baby unit (SCBU) compared to operative vaginal delivery (OR, 2.6; 95% CI, 1.2–6.0).[16] Of note, there were equal rates of ominous fetal heart rate tracings in the two groups. The greater risk of admission to SCBU following caesarean section did not appear to be the result of a selective decision based on pre-existing fetal compromise but may reflect the decision to delivery interval, which is frequently longer for a caesarean section. However, neonatal trauma was significantly less common following caesarean delivery compared to operative vaginal delivery (OR, 0.4; 95% CI, 0.2–0.7). In the majority of cases, this represented facial and scalp bruising but there was one facial laceration in each group, and a fractured clavicle and six cases of brachial plexus injury in the operative vaginal delivery group. A low umbilical artery pH was more frequently recorded following failed operative vaginal delivery but there was no increase in admissions to SCBU. Trauma was significantly more likely following failed operative vaginal delivery than immediate caesarean section ($P = 0.03$) but was still less common than following completed operative vaginal delivery.[41] In a large North American, population-based study, the sequential use of vacuum and forceps was associated with an increased need for mechanical ventilation in the infant.[42] These findings suggest that neonatal complications could be reduced with careful selection of cases.

The safest, quickest mode of delivery needs to be the priority where there is evidence of fetal compromise and this may mean operative vaginal delivery in experienced hands. However, operative vaginal delivery is likely to incur an increased risk of birth trauma (usually transient) that may be avoided by immediate recourse to caesarean section.

## Developmental outcome

In situations where the baby is born in poor condition, fears about early morbidity are quickly replaced by concerns about survival and long-term neurological disability. This can occur following either operative vaginal delivery or caesarean section and may result from the indication for emergency operative delivery and/or the procedure itself. Badawi *et al.*[43] have reported an increased risk of neonatal encephalopathy following both operative vaginal delivery and emergency caesarean section in a large Australian population-based study (OR, 2.3; 95% CI, 1.2–4.7 and OR, 2.2; 95% CI, 1.0-4.6, respectively). Moderate and severe neonatal encephalopathy are strongly associated with cerebral palsy and death. The use of sequential instruments (particularly vacuum and forceps) has been associated with scalp trauma, intracranial haemorrhage and neonatal death.[44] Reassuringly, a 5-year follow-up of the second stage prospective cohort study reported low overall rates of neurodevelopmental morbidity, with comparable outcomes for each mode of delivery.[45]

Clearly, the choice and conduct of operative vaginal delivery in the second stage of labour may have far-reaching consequences. It is important that studies addressing morbidity evaluate long-term neurodevelopmental outcome as neurological, cognitive and social disability may not be apparent for some years.

## TRAINING

The vast majority of avoidable maternal and neonatal morbidity at operative vaginal delivery relates to inappropriate application of the instrument and operator inexperience.[41] Therefore, an essential prerequisite for operative vaginal delivery is a skilled operator. The obstetrician must be able to assess the bony pelvis and unequivocally determine the fetal position and station, as well as any degree of flexion, caput, moulding and asynclitism. The instrument must then be correctly placed and an appropriate amount of traction applied in the right direction. In such circumstances, successful operative vaginal delivery rates are high and morbidity low. But these skills are not easy to acquire, and certainly cannot be self-taught. In addition, the trainee obstetrician must know when to ask for help. Predictors of failed operative vaginal delivery include occipitoposterior position, high presenting part (station spines +0), inadequate analgesia and birthweight > 4 kg and these criteria should alert the obstetrician to be cautious and seek senior support.[16,46]

The RCOG has recommended that obstetricians be confident and competent in the use of both vacuum and forceps, and that operators should choose the instrument most appropriate to the clinical circumstances and their level of skill.[3] Clear and detailed guidelines are available and should be adapted within local practice-based protocols and followed up with regular audit and multidisciplinary review of adverse incidents. A UK study demonstrated substantial differences in the assessment of fetal position and station between consultants and specialist registrars and that a consultant was more likely to reverse a decision for caesarean section and to conduct an operative vaginal delivery safely.[47] A review of failed vacuum extractions reported suboptimal application in 40% of cases.[48] Clearly, appropriate supervision and the availability of skilled obstetricians on the labour ward at all times will be an essential component of training initiatives.

In the US in 1999, a survey of residency training directors reported that, although trainers taught outlet and low-cavity forceps deliveries, they did not expect proficiency in mid-forceps deliveries from their trainees.[49] A further study in 2007 examined chief residents' experience with vacuum and forceps deliveries and self-perceived competencies with the procedures.[50] Residents reported performing significantly fewer forceps than vacuum deliveries. Although virtually all residents wanted to learn how to perform both types of deliveries, only half felt competent to perform forceps deliveries. This clearly demonstrates that current training results in a substantial proportion of residents graduating who do not feel competent to perform forceps deliveries. Ultimately, this lack of adequate personnel comfortable with performing forceps deliveries will lead to a continuing downward trend, and escalation in the already worrying trend towards second-stage caesarean section. When subsequent pregnancies are taken into consideration, this trend will diminish the overall number of women who achieve a spontaneous vaginal delivery.

## CONCLUSIONS

Operative vaginal delivery continues to pose a challenge for the obstetrician. There is a balance to achieve between maternal and neonatal well-being and early and long-term morbidity. Obstetricians should aim to deliver by the safest and most appropriate mode within their expertise. A management approach that can only offer caesarean section for complications in the second stage of labour may prove limiting and short-sighted. We are gaining increasing knowledge about the long-term health implications of operative vaginal delivery for both mother and baby. The influence of obstetric management in such cases needs further evaluation in terms of maternal psychological morbidity, future fertility both voluntary and involuntary, and the delivery outcome of future pregnancies. Obstetric training needs to encompass the skills of clinical assessment, choice of instrument for specific circumstances, technical competence, judgement of when to abandon a procedure in favour of caesarean section and clear communication with the woman and within the multidisciplinary team. We need to be confident that, when we perform an operative vaginal delivery, the benefits outweigh the risks, taking account of the clinical circumstances, the woman's preferences and her overall reproductive outlook.

---

### Key points for clinical practice

- Currently, almost one in three first-time mothers in the UK experiences an operative vaginal delivery.

- The vacuum extractor is preferred to forceps delivery in the interest of minimising maternal perineal trauma but is associated with higher rates of neonatal trauma and a higher failure rate.

- An increasing proportion of deliveries for mid-cavity arrest and malrotation are undertaken by caesarean section with a loss of expertise in complex operative vaginal delivery.

- Caesarean section in the second stage of labour is associated with higher rates of major obstetric haemorrhage, prolonged maternal hospital admission and more frequent neonatal admission for special care than operative vaginal delivery.

**Key points for clinical practice** *(continued)*

- Operative vaginal delivery is associated with a greater risk of pelvic floor trauma and subsequent urinary and bowel incontinence than second-stage caesarean section.

- There is an increased risk of voluntary and involuntary sub-fertility following delivery by caesarean section.

- Operative vaginal delivery and particularly failed operative vaginal delivery are associated with higher rates of neonatal trauma than caesarean section. This is a particular problem with the use of sequential instruments.

- Adverse neurodevelopmental outcomes at 5 years are uncommon following mid-cavity operative vaginal delivery and usually occur as a result of the indication for delivery rather than the procedure itself. The outcomes are similar for operative vaginal delivery and caesarean section in the second stage of labour.

- Obstetricians should aim to deliver by the safest and most appropriate mode within their expertise balancing the risks of maternal and neonatal morbidity. This may be an indication for mid-cavity operative vaginal delivery in experienced hands.

- The current approach to obstetric training may limit the availability of expertise in mid-cavity and rotational operative vaginal delivery for women in the future.

### References

1. Patel RR, Murphy DJ. Forceps delivery in modern obstetric practice. *BMJ* 2004; **328**: 1302–1305.
2. Spencer, C, Murphy DJ, Bewley S. Caesarean section in the second stage of labour. *BMJ* 2006; **333**: 613–614.
3. Royal College of Obstetricians and Gynaecologists. *Operative vaginal delivery*. Green top Guideline No 26. London: RCOG, 2005.
4. American College of Obstetricians and Gynecologists. *Evaluation of Cesarean Delivery*. Washington, DC: ACOG, 2000.
5. Gilstrap LC, Cunningham GF, Vandorsten PJ. *Operative obstetrics*. New York: McGraw Hill, 1995.
6. Shute WB. History of obstetrical forceps from 1750 to the present era. *Acta Belg Hist Med* 1992; **5**: 65–69.
7. Gei AF, Belfort MA. Forceps-assisted vaginal delivery. *Obstet Gynecol Clin North Am* 1999; **26**: 345–370.
8. Vacca A. Vacuum-assisted delivery: an analysis of traction force and maternal and neonatal outcomes. *Aust NZ J Obstet Gynaecol* 2006; **46**: 124–127.
9. Macleod M, Murphy DJ. Operative vaginal delivery and the use of episiotomy – A survey of practice in the United Kingdom and Ireland. *Eur J Obstet Gynecol Reprod Biol* 2008; **136**: 178–183.
10. Thomas J, Paranjothy S, on behalf of Royal College of Obstetricians and Gynaecologists Clinical Effectiveness Support Unit. *National Sentinel Caesarean Section Audit Report*. London: RCOG, 2001.
11. Hamilton BE, Martin JA, Sutton PD. Births: preliminary data for 2003. *National Vital Statistical Reports* 2004; **53**: 1–18.

12. Clark SL, Belfort MA, Hankins GD, Meyers JA, Houser FM. Variation in the rates of operative delivery in the United States. *Am J Obstet Gynecol* 2007; **196**: 526.e1–e5.

13. Dumont A, de Bernis L, Bouvier-Colle M-H, Breart G, for the MOMA study group. Caesarean section rate for maternal indication in sub-Saharan Africa: a systematic review. *Lancet* 2001; **358**: 1328–1334.

14. Chang X, Chedraui P, Ross MG, Hidalgo L, Penafiel J. Vacuum assisted delivery in Ecuador for prolonged second stage of labor: maternal-neonatal outcome. *J Matern Fetal Neonatal Med* 2007; **20**: 381–384.

15. Fauveau V. Is vacuum extraction still known, taught and practiced? A worldwide KAP survey. *Int J Gynaecol Obstet* 2006; **94**: 185–189.

16. Murphy DJ, Liebling RE, Verity L, Swingler R, Patel R. Cohort study of the early maternal and neonatal morbidity associated with operative delivery in the second stage of labour. *Lancet* 2001; **358**: 1203–1207.

17. Bofill JA, Rust OA, Perry KG, Roberts WE, Martin RW, Morrison JC. Operative vaginal delivery: a survey of fellows of ACOG. *Obstet Gynecol* 1996; **88**: 1007–1010.

18. Johanson RB, Menon BK. Vacuum extraction versus forceps for assisted vaginal delivery. Cochrane Database Syst Rev 2000; (2): CD000224.

19. Attilakos G, Sibanda T, Winter C, Johnson N, Draycott T. A randomised controlled trial of a new handheld vacuum extraction device. *Br J Obstet Gynaecol* 2005; **112**: 1510–1515.

20. Groom KM, Jones BA, Miller N, Paterson-Brown S. A prospective randomised controlled trial of the Kiwi Omnicup versus conventional ventouse cups for vacuum-assisted vaginal delivery. *Br J Obstet Gynaecol* 2006; **113**: 183–189.

21. Bhide A, Guven M, Prefumo F, Vankalayapati P, Thilaganathan B. Maternal and neonatal outcome after failed ventouse delivery: comparison of forceps versus cesarean section. *J Matern Fetal Neonatal Med* 2007; **20**: 541–545.

22. Damron DP, Capeless EL. Operative vaginal delivery: a comparison of forceps and vacuum for success rate and risk of rectal sphincter injury. *Am J Obstet Gynecol* 2004; **191**: 907–910.

23. Caughey A, Sandberg PL, Zlatnik MG, Thiet MP, Parer JT, Laros Jr RK. Forceps compared with vacuum: rates of neonatal and maternal morbidity. *Obstet Gynecol* 2005; **106**: 908–912.

24. Revah A, Ezra Y, Farine D, Ritchie K. Failed trial of vacuum or forceps – maternal and fetal outcome. *Am J Obstet Gynecol* 1997; **176**: 200–204.

25. Kudish B, Blackwell S, Mcneeley SG *et al*. Operative vaginal delivery and midline episiotomy: a bad combination for the perineum. *Am J Obstet Gynecol* 2006; **195**: 749–754.

26. Rodriguez AI, Porter KB, O'Brien WF. Blunt versus sharp expansion of the uterine incision in low-segment transverse cesarean section. *Am J Obstet Gynecol* 1994; **171**: 1022–1025.

27. MacArthur C, Glazener CMA, Wilson PD *et al*. Obstetric practice and faecal incontinence three months after delivery. *Br J Obstet Gynaecol* 2001; **108**: 678–683.

28. De Leeuw JW, Struijk PC, Vierhout ME, Wallenburg HCS. Risk factors for third degree perineal ruptures during delivery. *Br J Obstet Gynaecol* 2001; **108**: 383–387.

29. Handa VL, Danielsen BH, Gilbert WM. Obstetric anal sphincter lacerations. *Obstet Gynecol* 2001; **98**: 225–230.

30. Fitzpatrick M, Behan M, O'Connell PR, O'Herlihy C. Randomised clinical trial to assess anal sphincter function following forceps or vacuum assisted vaginal delivery. *Br J Obstet Gynaecol* 2003; **110**: 424–429.

31. Johanson RB, Heycock E, Carter J, Sultan AH, Walklate K, Jones PW. Maternal and child health after assisted vaginal delivery: five-year follow up of a randomised controlled study comparing forceps and ventouse. *Br J Obstet Gynaecol* 1999; **106**: 544–549.

32. Liebling RE, Swingler R, Patel RR, Verity L, Soothill PW, Murphy DJ. Pelvic floor morbidity up to one year after difficult instrumental delivery and cesarean section in the second stage of labor: a cohort study. *Am J Obstet Gynecol* 2004; **191**: 4–10.

33. Bahl R, Strachan B, Murphy DJ. Pelvic floor morbidity at three years after instrumental delivery and caesarean section in the second stage of labor and the impact of a subsequent delivery. *Am J Obstet Gynecol* 2005; **192**: 789–794.

34. Jolly J, Walker J, Bhabra K. Subsequent obstetric performance related to primary mode of delivery. *Br J Obstet Gynaecol* 1999; **106**: 227–232.

35. Murphy DJ, Liebling R. Cohort study of maternal views on future mode of delivery following operative delivery in the second stage of labour. *Am J Obstet Gynecol* 2003; **188**: 542–548.

36. Bahl R, Strachan B, Murphy DJ. Outcome of subsequent pregnancy three years after previous operative delivery in the second stage of labour – cohort study. *BMJ* 2004; **328** : 311–314.

37. Small R, Lumley J, Donohue L, Potter A, Waldenstrom U. Randomised controlled trial of midwife led debriefing to reduce maternal depression after operative childbirth. *BMJ* 2000; **321**: 1043–1047.

38. Patel RR, Peters TJ, Murphy DJ, ALSPAC Study Team. Operative delivery and postnatal depression? A cohort study. *BMJ* 2005; **330**: 576–580.

39. Murphy DJ, Koh DK. Cohort study of decision to delivery interval and neonatal outcome for emergency operative vaginal delivery. *Am J Obstet Gynecol* 2007; **196**: 145.e1–e7.

40. Olagundoye V, MacKenzie IZ. The impact of instrumental delivery in theatre on neonatal outcome. *Br J Obstet Gynaecol* 2007; **114**: 603–608.

41. Murphy DJ, Liebling RE, Patel R, Verity L, Swingler R. Cohort study of operative delivery in the second stage of labour and standard of obstetric care. *Br J Obstet Gynaecol* 2003; **110**: 610–615.

42. Demissie K, Rhoads GG, Smulian JC *et al*. Operative vaginal delivery and neonatal and infant adverse outcomes: population based retrospective analysis. *BMJ* 2004; **329**: 24–29.

43. Badawi N, Kurinczuk JJ, Keogh JM *et al*. Intrapartum risk factors for newborn encephalopathy: the Western Australian case-control study. *BMJ* 1998; **317**: 1554–1558.

44. Towner D, Castro MA, Eby-Wilkens E, Gilbert WM. Effect of mode of delivery in nulliparaous women on neonatal intracranial injury. *N Engl J Med* 1999; **341**: 1709–1714.

45. Bahl R, Patel RR, Swingler R, Ellis N, Murphy DJ. Neurodevelopmental outcome at 5 years after operative delivery in the second stage of labor: a cohort study. *Am J Obstet Gynecol* 2007; **197**: 147.e1–e6.

46. Ben-Haroush A, Melamed N, Kaplan B, Yogev Y. Predictors of failed operative vaginal delivery: a single-center experience. *Am J Obstet Gynecol* 2007; **197**: 308.e5.

47. Olah KS. Reversal of the decision for caesarean section in the second stage of labour on the basis of consultant vaginal assessment. *J Obstet Gynecol* 2005; **25**: 115–116.

48. Sau A, Sau M, Ahmed H, Brown R. Vacuum extraction: is there any need to improve the current training in the UK? *Acta Obstet Gynecol Scand* 2004; **83**: 466–470.

49. Hankins GD, Uckan E, Rowe TF, Coller S. Forceps and vacuum delivery: expectations of residency and fellowship training program directors. *Am J Perinatol* 1999; **16**: 23

50. Powell JN, Gilo N, Foote M, Gil K, Lavin JP. Vacuum and forceps training in residency: experience and self reported competency. *J Perinatol* 2007; **27**: 343–346.

*Stergios K. Doumouchtsis*
*Sabaratnam Arulkumaran*

**7**

# Postpartum haemorrhage: changing practices

Maternal mortality globally is estimated at 529,000 deaths per year, a ratio of 400 maternal deaths per 100,000 live births. Postpartum haemorrhage (PPH) is the most common cause of maternal mortality and accounts for one-quarter of all maternal deaths world-wide.[1] In developing countries, PPH accounts for over one-third of all maternal deaths.[2] Fourteen million cases of PPH occur each year with a case-fatality rate of 1%.[3] In the UK, it accounts for 28% of all direct maternal deaths and, according to the Confidential Enquiry into Maternal and Child Health of 2000–2002, this makes it the second most common cause of maternal mortality.[4] In this report, seventeen maternal deaths were directly due to haemorrhage; and of these, ten were due to PPH. A striking increase in the numbers of deaths from PPH in the triennium was noted. Similar rates were noted in the most recent Confidential Enquiry (2004–2006) and the phenomenon of doing 'too little, too late' was highlighted.[56] The Scottish Confidential Audit of Severe Maternal Morbidity[5–7] showed that major obstetric haemorrhage is the commonest category of severe morbidity. In 2004, the incidence was 3.2 per 1000 births (range, 2.8–3.8 per 1000 births) and in 2005 4.5 per 1000 births (range, 3.9–5.1 per 1000 births). Severe obstetric morbidity may be a more sensitive measure of pregnancy outcome than mortality alone and Waterstone *et al.*[8] have shown that, of obstetric complications, the disease specific morbidity per 1000 deliveries is highest for haemorrhage. This study called for the development and evaluation of ways of reducing the risk of severe haemorrhage. Apart from the

**Stergios K. Doumouchtsis** PhD MRCOG (for correspondence)
Senior Specialist Registrar, Department of Obstetrics and Gynaecology, St George's Hospital,
University of London, Cranmer Terrace, London SW17 0RE, UK
E-mail: sdoum@yahoo.com

**Sabaratnam Arulkumaran** PhD FRCOG
Professor, Department of Obstetrics and Gynaecology, St George's Hospital, University of London,
Cranmer Terrace, London SW17 0RE, UK
E-mail: sarulkum@sgul.ac.uk

considerable suffering for women and their families, PPH also creates major demands on health systems.[3]

## DEFINITIONS

There is no single, satisfactory definition of PPH. An estimated blood loss in excess of 500 ml following a vaginal birth or a loss of greater than 1000 ml following caesarean birth often has been used for the diagnosis. The Scottish Confidential Audit of Severe Maternal Morbidity defines as major haemorrhage an estimated blood loss $\geq 2500$ ml, or the transfusion of 5 or more units of blood or treatment for coagulopathy (fresh frozen plasma, cryoprecipitate, platelets).[7] These definitions are somewhat arbitrary as clinical visual estimation of blood loss is not reliable[9] and the average volume of blood lost can approach amounts of 500 ml after otherwise uncomplicated vaginal delivery and 1000 ml after caesarean delivery.[10] Even with an accurate measurement method, the quantity of blood lost is often less important than the effect it has on the woman, which depends on her blood volume and any underlying health factors. For this reason, it has been suggested that a useful definition takes into account any blood loss that causes a major physiological change (*e.g.* a fall in blood pressure), as the risk of dying from PPH depends not only on the amount and rate of blood loss but also on the health of the woman.

PPH is classified as primary or secondary. Primary PPH occurs within the first 24 h after delivery, and secondary PPH occurs between 24 h and 6–12 weeks postpartum.[10]

## AETIOLOGY AND RISK FACTORS

PPH is commonly due to abnormalities of one or a combination of four basic processes, referred to in the '4Ts' mnemonic – tone (poor uterine contraction after delivery), tissue (retained products of conception or blood clots), trauma (to genital tract), or thrombin (coagulation abnormalities).

Common risk factors for PPH are related to an overdistended uterus due to multiple pregnancy, polyhydramnios or fetal macrosomia. Moreover, obesity, coagulation disorders, primigravidity, chorio-amnionitis, prolonged rupture of membranes, fibroid uterus, previous caesarean birth, antepartum haemorrhage, pre-eclampsia, induction of labour, prolonged labour, instrumental delivery and prior PPH[11] are clinically considered to be risk factors. It has become more common for women with risk factors for PPH to become pregnant in recent years. In the UK, there is an overall trend towards later child-bearing.[12] Increased maternal age at childbirth[13] with associated increased incidence of caesarean and instrumental deliveries as well as placenta previa,[14,15] an increasing number of women with complex medical disorders becoming pregnant and an increasing number of multiple pregnancies due to assisted reproduction can result in increased incidence of PPH. However, PPH can occur even in women without identifiable risk factors. Numerically, more women without risk factors have atonic PPH compared to those with risk factors.

# PATHOPHYSIOLOGY

The blood vessels that supply the placental bed pass through an interlacing network of muscle fibres (myometrium). The spiral arteriolar arrangement in the uterus might lower the arterial pressure with which the blood enters the uterus. Myometrial contraction is the main driving force for placental separation and constriction of the blood vessels. This haemostatic mechanism is known as 'physiological sutures' or 'living ligatures'. When the placenta separates, bleeding occurs from the placental bed. Uterine atony results in a failure of the living ligatures to stop the bleeding. The active management of the third stage of labour is associated with a reduction of the risk of PPH and less need for blood transfusion by enhancing this physiological process.[16]

Young and healthy women can compensate for considerable blood loss over lengthy periods without demonstrating any cardiovascular changes. Mild shock occurs when about 20% of the blood volume is lost, which results in decreased perfusion of non-vital organs and tissues (skin, fat, skeletal muscle, and bone), with pale, cool skin and a feeling of increasing coldness. When 20–40% of the blood volume is lost, moderate shock occurs with decreased perfusion of vital organs (liver, the gut, and kidneys), oliguria and/or anuria, a drop in blood pressure, and mottling of the skin in the extremities, especially the legs. When 40% or more of the blood volume is lost, severe shock occurs resulting in decreased perfusion to the heart and brain, restlessness, agitation, coma, electrocardiographic and electro-encephalographic abnormalities, and possibly cardiac arrest.

# PREVENTION

The prediction of PPH using antenatal risk assessment is poor: only 40% of women who develop PPH have an identified risk factor.[17] However PPH is often a predictable event. Women with identified risk factors should be transferred to centres with transfusion facilities and an intensive care unit (ICU) for delivery if these are not available locally. The Royal College of Obstetricians and Gynaecologists urges obstetric units to consider early or prophylactic interventional radiology for the prevention and management of PPH in high-risk cases and recommends the introduction of strategies for the management of unpredicted PPH.[18]

Prevention of PPH should include antenatal risk assessment and management that assures that anaemia or other health problems are treated and women are sufficiently healthy to withstand PPH, as well as appropriate management of labour and delivery. The International Confederation of Midwives (ICM) and the International Federation of Gynecology and Obstetrics (FIGO) have launched a world-wide initiative to promote active management of the third stage of labour for all women.[19] Active management consists of interventions designed to facilitate the delivery of the placenta by increasing uterine contractions and to prevent PPH by averting uterine atony. The usual components include administration of uterotonic agents, controlled cord traction and uterine massage after delivery of the placenta, as appropriate. This approach reduces the risks of PPH, post partum anaemia, blood transfusion requirements, prolonged third stage of labour and use of therapeutic drugs for PPH.[16] It is now recommended that active management should be routine for women in maternity hospitals. Furthermore, there is no evidence to suggest that this recommendation should not include births at home or in birth centres.[16]

Injectable oxytocin has been recommended for routine use in the active management of the third stage of labour. It is a synthetic nonapeptide that is routinely administered for prevention and treatment of PPH. Oxytocin is a first-line agent because it is effective 2–3 min after injection and, as it has minimal secondary effects, it can be used in all women. If oxytocin is not available, other uterotonics can be used, such as ergometrine maleate 500 μg i.m., ergometrine with oxytocin 5 IU/ml (Syntometrine®; Alliance Pharmaceuticals Ltd) or misoprostol.

Misoprostol (Cytotec®; Pfizer Ltd), a prostaglandin $E_1$ analogue, is more stable than oxytocin and has been administered by oral, sublingual and rectal routes;[20] however, there are concerns that misuse of misoprostol can lead to significant maternal morbidity and even death. The main side-effects are nausea, vomiting and diarrhoea. Shivering and elevated body temperature have also been reported with the use of misoprostol in the third stage of labour. The side-effects of oral, but not rectal, misoprostol are dose-related. Moreover, rectal misoprostol causes less pyrexia, and shivering than oral misoprostol. Oral administration of misoprostol should, therefore, be considered in low-resource settings where safe administration and/or appropriate storage conditions for injectable oxytocin and ergot alkaloids are not possible.[21] A recent Cochrane review on the use of prostaglandins for the prevention of PPH concluded that neither intramuscular prostaglandins nor misoprostol is preferable to conventional injectable uterotonics as part of the management of the third stage of labour especially for low-risk women.[22]

Carbetocin, a long-acting oxytocin agonist, has been used for the prevention of PPH. The potential advantage of intramuscular carbetocin over intramuscular oxytocin is its longer duration of action. In comparison to oxytocin, carbetocin induces a prolonged uterine response when administered postpartum, in terms of both amplitude and frequency of contractions, but there is insufficient evidence that intravenous carbetocin is as effective as oxytocin to prevent PPH. Nevertheless, carbetocin is associated with reduced need for additional uterotonic agents and uterine massage, and there are no significant differences in adverse effects between carbetocin and oxytocin.[23]

The active management of the third stage of labour originally included early cord clamping.[16] There is very little evidence to suggest that the timing of cord clamping has an impact on the incidence of PPH. One study reported no significant difference in PPH associated with timing of cord clamping.[24] However, immediate cord clamping may reduce the quantity of red blood cells a newborn receives, whereas delayed cord clamping is associated with less anaemia, intraventricular haemorrhage and late onset sepsis especially in preterm infants.[25,26] For these reasons, the collaborative ICM/FIGO group decided not to include early cord clamping in the active management protocol. The cord may be clamped at the time the baby is dried and wrapped and passed to the mother to breast-feed. The placenta usually separates by that time and it is appropriate to apply cord traction. Early clamping may be indicated in cases of fetal distress when immediate resuscitation is required.

FIGO now also advises that, if oxytocin or misoprostol are unavailable, skilled birth attendants should use physiological (or expectant) management of the third stage. This means that, to avoid maternal overexertion, they should not begin cord traction before the uterus has contracted and the expulsion of the placenta has begun, thus allowing the mother to expel the placenta without interference.[19]

The World Health Organization held a Technical Consultation on the Prevention of Postpartum Haemorrhage in 2006[27] and recommends that:

1. Active management of the third stage of labour should include administration of a uterotonic soon after birth of the baby, delayed cord clamping and delivery of the placenta by controlled cord traction, followed by uterine massage.

2. Active management of the third stage of labour should be offered by skilled attendants, as potential risks such as uterine inversion, may result from inappropriate cord traction.

3. Oxytocin should be offered for prevention of PPH in preference to oral, sublingual or rectal misoprostol.

4. In the absence of active management of the third stage of labour, a uterotonic drug (oxytocin or misoprostol) should be offered.

## TREATMENT

A systematic and step-wise management of PPH can be achieved with the use of the mnemonic 'HAEMOSTASIS' following each step in rapid succession (Table 1). The mnemonic is conveniently divided into two parts – medical and surgical.

**Table 1** HAEMOSTASIS algorithm

General medical management
    H – Ask for help
    A – Assess (vital parameters, blood loss) and resuscitate
    E – Establish aetiology, ecbolics, ensure availability of blood
            Establish aetiology: '4Ts' – tone, tissue, trauma, thrombin
            Ecbolics (syntometrine, ergometrine, bolus syntocinon)
            Ensure availability of blood and blood products
    M – Massage the uterus
    O – Oxytocin infusion, prostaglandins (intravenous, rectal, intramuscular, intramyometrial)

Specific surgical management
    S – Shift to operating theatre
         bimanual compression
         anti-shock garment, especially if transfer is required
    T – Tissue and trauma to be excluded and proceed to tamponade
         balloon, uterine packing
    A – Apply compression sutures
    S – Systematic pelvic devascularisation (uterine, ovarian, quadruple, internal iliac)
    I – Interventional radiology, uterine artery embolisation
    S – Subtotal or total abdominal hysterectomy

## MEDICAL (HAEMO-)

### H – Ask for help

Massive PPH should be managed appropriately with a multidisciplinary input. Senior obstetricians and anaesthetists, midwives and theatre staff, haematologists and the blood bank and hospital porters and the intensive care unit should be alerted.

### A – Assess (vital parameters, blood loss) and resuscitate

Early recognition, prompt resuscitation and rapid restoration of the circulating blood volume are the key components of the initial management of PPH. General resuscitation measures include assessment of the haemodynamic status by monitoring the patient's vital signs – level of consciousness, blood pressure, pulse and oxygen saturation. Meticulous estimation of the blood loss forewarns of impending haemorrhagic shock. Different methods of estimation have been evaluated[28] and guidelines to improve accuracy of the visual estimation of blood loss have been suggested.[29] Two large bore cannulae should be inserted and blood samples taken for full blood count, group and save or cross-match (depending on the severity of haemorrhage), coagulation screen and renal and liver profile.

Fluid resuscitation in PPH is often overly conservative because of underestimation of volume and rapidity of blood loss. It is important to remember that symptoms of hypovolaemia are often delayed due to compensatory mechanisms. Moreover, concerns that fluid overload will lead to pulmonary oedema, or failure, may be misleading. A loss of 1 litre of blood requires replacement with 4–5 litres of crystalloid (0.9% normal saline or lactated Ringer's solution) or colloids until cross-matched blood is available, as most of the infused fluid shifts from the intravascular to the interstitial space.[30]

### 'The golden hour'

Severe haemorrhage can lead to cardiovascular failure. As the severity depends on body weight, haemoglobin levels, and body metabolism, emergency measures should be initiated if the estimated blood loss is more than one-third of the woman's blood volume (blood volume [ml] = weight [kg] x 80) or more than 1000 ml or a change in haemodynamic status. As more time elapses between the onset of severe shock and resuscitation, the chances of survival decrease because metabolic acidosis sets in. The 'golden hour' is the time at which resuscitation must be commenced to ensure the best chance of survival. The probability of survival decreases sharply after the first hour if the patient is not effectively resuscitated.[19]

For the general acute management of PPH a 'rule of 30' has been proposed. If the patient's systolic blood pressure (SBP) falls by 30 mmHg, heart rate (HR) rises by 30 beats/min, respiratory rate (RR) increases to > 30 breaths/min and haemoglobin (Hb) or haematocrit (Hct) drop by 30%, and/or her urinary output is < 30 ml/h, then the patient is most likely to have lost at least 30% of her blood volume and is in moderate shock leading to severe shock.[31]

The use of 'Shock Index' (SI) may also be valuable in the monitoring and general management of women with PPH. It refers to heart rate (HR) divided by the systolic blood pressure (SBP). The normal value is 0.5–0.7; however, with significant haemorrhage, it increases to 0.9–1.1.[31] The change in SI of an individual patient appears to be a better correlate in identifying early acute blood loss than the HR, SBP, or DBP used in isolation.[32]

## E – Establish aetiology, ecbolics, ensure availability of blood

- establish aetiology – four Ts, tone, tissue, trauma and thrombin
- ecbolics (syntometrine, ergometrine, bolus syntocinon)
- ensure availability of blood and blood products.

A systematic assessment for identifying the cause of bleeding should be made using the '4Ts' mnemonic. Thorough assessment of the uterine size and tone should be followed by vigorous uterine massage and administration of therapeutic uterotonic agents if the uterus is atonic. Manual exploration of the uterine cavity, ideally under anaesthesia, is essential to exclude or remove retained placental tissues and membranes. If bleeding persists despite a well-contracted uterus, examination under anaesthesia should be performed to look for extended tears in the cervix or high in the vaginal vault, as these may extend into the uterus or the broad ligament or they may cause retroperitoneal haematomas. Pressure or packing over the repair may be useful to achieve haemostasis and prevent of formation of haematomas. If retained tissue or trauma is excluded and bleeding continues despite a well-contracted uterus, a defect in coagulation is a likely cause.

As uterine atony is the most common cause, medical management usually consists of oxytocin 10 units by slow intravenous injection, ergometrine 0.5 mg by slow intravenous injection, methergine 0.2 mg intramuscularly, oxytocin infusion, 15-methyl $PGF_{2\alpha}$ (Carboprost® or Haemabate®) intramuscularly or intramyometrially, dinoprostone vaginally or rectally, or misoprostol.[10,33]

Blood and blood product transfusion should be commenced if bleeding is continuing, if the estimated blood loss lost is over 30% of the blood volume or if the patient is haemodynamically unstable despite aggressive resuscitation. Group-specific or group O, Rh-negative blood should be transfused until cross-matched blood becomes available. Coagulopathy may be secondary to a number of factors: disseminated intravascular coagulation (DIC), depletion of clotting factors within blood clots ('washout phenomenon'), dilution of clotting factors with crystalloid fluid resuscitation, lack of clotting factors in stored blood, hypothermia and acidosis secondary to hypoxia.[31] Dilutional coagulopathy occurs when about 80% of the original blood volume has been replaced. One litre of fresh frozen plasma (FFP) should be administered (15 ml/kg) with every 6 units of blood transfused. Platelet concentration should be kept at more than $50 \times 10^9$ per litre or more than $80–100 \times 10^9$ per litre if surgical intervention is likely. Cryoprecipitate, which provides a more concentrated form of fibrinogen and other clotting factors (VIII, XIII, von Willebrand factor), may be required if there is DIC or if the fibrinogen level is less than 10 g/l.[30]

## M – Massage the uterus

Uterine massage, either manually (hand on the fundus) or bimanually (vaginal hand in the anterior fornix; abdominal hand on the posterior aspect of the fundus) is a simple and very effective first-line measure and reduces bleeding even if the uterus remains atonic, allowing resuscitation to take effect with a reduced blood loss. If uterine atony continues after oxytocics are given, bimanual compression is undertaken.

## O – Oxytocin infusion, prostaglandins

Oxytocin, can be administered as a slow i.v. bolus (10 units) or as an infusion (40 units in 500 ml of 0.9% normal saline, infused at a rate of 125 ml/h) in order to maintain uterine contraction. Although there are no absolute contra-indications, an antidiuretic effect with volume overload may develop with high cumulative doses. If the uterus remains atonic after initial oxytocic therapy, Syntometrine or ergometrine should be repeated.

Ergometrine is an ergot alkaloid and hypertension is a contra-indication to this agent due to the potential development of severe hypertension and myocardial ischaemia.

Carboprost (Haemabate®; Pfizer Ltd, Pharmacia & Upjohn Co, Kalamazoo, MI, USA) is a prostaglandin $F_2$ analogue which is administered intramuscularly or intra-myometrially. It is a second-line agent for uterine atony (0.25 mg repeated every 15 min to a maximum dose of 2 mg). This is 80–90% effective in stopping PPH in cases that are refractory to oxytocin and ergometrine. It has bronchoconstrictive properties and is, therefore, contra-indicated in asthma. Side-effects include diarrhoea, vomiting, fever, headache and flushing.

Dinoprostone (Prostin®) is a prostaglandin $E_2$ analogue which may be given vaginally (but note that it may get washed out with bleeding) or rectally. It has effects on hypothalamic thermoregulation and can cause temperature elevations. It must be stored in a freezer at –4°F and brought to room temperature before use. This is a major disadvantage in acute severe haemorrhage.

Misoprostol is a synthetic prostaglandin $E_1$ analogue which has been used in the management of PPH. Two placebo-controlled randomised trials compared misoprostol with placebo and showed that misoprostol use was not associated with any significant reduction of maternal mortality, hysterectomy, the additional use of uterotonics, blood transfusion, or evacuation of retained products. Misoprostol use was associated with a significant increase of maternal pyrexia and shivering.[34,35] However, an unblinded trial showed better clinical response to rectal misoprostol than a combination of syntometrine and oxytocin.[36] A recent Cochrane review concluded that there is insufficient evidence to show that the addition of misoprostol is superior to the combination of oxytocin and ergometrine alone for the treatment of primary PPH.[37] The pharmocodynamics of misoprostol and oxytocin may explain these inconsistencies. As the peak serum concentration of oxytocin is much shorter than oral misoprostol, which reaches its serum peak concentration at 20 min,[38] a combination of these two agents could provide a sustained uterotonic effect.

Recombinant activated factor VII (rFVIIa, NovoSeven; Novo Nordisk A/S, Bagsvaerd, Denmark) was originally used in treating haemorrhage in patients with haemophilia with inhibitors, acquired haemophilia or other inherited bleeding disorders. In recent years, it has also been used in non-haemophilic haemorrhage, including life-threatening obstetric haemorrhage. A number of case reports of empirical 'off-label' use of rFVIIa show that it may be an alternative haemostatic agent when the standard treatment is ineffective.[39]

## SURGICAL (-STASIS)

PPH often appears controlled but recurs. Repeated and prolonged attempts to control haemorrhage with oxytocics and compression of the uterus may lead to a waste of precious time and delay the decision to proceed to surgical measures. This delay may also be due to the reluctance to perform unnecessary difficult surgery with high morbidity and mortality. The Scottish Confidential Audit of Severe Maternal Morbidity recommends that, if conservative measures fail to control haemorrhage, surgical haemostasis should be commenced 'sooner rather than later'.[7] Recent reports recommend that obstetricians must consider all available interventions to stop haemorrhage including B-Lynch suture, embolisation of uterine arteries or radical surgery.[4] In addition, recommendations have been made that all hospitals with delivery units should aim to provide an emergency interventional radiology service as these have the potential to save lives of patients with catastrophic PPH.[18,40] The American College of Obstetricians and Gynecologists also suggests that uterine tamponade can be effective in decreasing haemorrhage secondary to uterine atony, and that procedures such as uterine artery ligation or B-Lynch suture may be used to obviate the need for hysterectomy. In patients with stable vital signs and persistent bleeding, arterial embolisation may be suitable, especially if the rate of loss is not excessive.[10]

### S – Shift to operating theatre (anti-shock garment, especially if transfer is required and bimanual compression)

In low-resource settings (home births, midwifery-led units or remote areas), transfer to a centre with facilities is indicated at this stage. A new type of non-pneumatic anti-shock garment (NASG) can reverse the effect of shock on the body's blood distribution by applying external counter pressure to the legs and abdomen and returning blood to the vital organs, thus stabilising women until a hospital can be reached. A pilot study showed that, compared with women in a control group, bleeding decreased by 50% in women experiencing various forms of obstetric haemorrhage (*e.g.* ruptured ectopic pregnancy, post-abortion complications, or PPH) in whom the NASG was used.[41] The use of this device could be critical to decrease maternal mortality in low-resource settings where reaching a health facility is time consuming.

### T – Tissue and trauma to be excluded and to proceed to tamponade with balloon or uterine packing

On-going bleeding indicates transfer and evaluation in the operating theatre. Examination with appropriate lighting, equipment, analgesia and assistance will permit re-assessment of the uterine tone and exclude retained tissue and trauma. Bimanual compression and direct pressure over lacerations may help control bleeding while monitoring and resuscitation continues and preparations are made for further intervention.

Uterine packing has long been considered safe, quick and effective for controlling PPH.[42] The use of uterine packing in the management of PPH fell into disfavour after the 1950s following concerns that it: (i) was a potentially traumatic and time-consuming procedure; (ii) might conceal on-going haemorrhage; (iii) might predispose to the development of infection; and (iv) represented a 'non-physiological approach'.[43] More recently, Maier[42] concluded that uterine packing is a safe, quick and effective procedure for controlling PPH.

Successful use of uterine balloon tamponade has been reported using a number of devices, including the Foley catheter, a condom, the Sengstaken–Blakemore

**Table 2** Uterine balloon tamponade

**How to do it**

- Exclude local trauma or retained tissue in the uterus under spinal, epidural, or general anaesthesia

- Secure the anterior lip of the cervix with a sponge forceps

- When the Sengstaken–Blakemore catheter is used, cut and remove the distal tube to facilitate insertion and retention in the uterine cavity

- Hold the balloon catheter with another sponge forceps and insert it into the uterine cavity

- Fill the balloon with warm sterile water or a warm saline solution until it becomes visible in the cervical canal. When the pressure exceeds that of the patient's blood pressure, no additional fluid needs to be added and the bleeding should stop

- If there is no bleeding through the cervix or through the drainage channel of the balloon catheter, the 'tamponade test' result is pronounced successful and no further fluid is added

- If the bleeding does not stop, the result is unsuccessful and laparotomy is indicated

- The uterine fundus is palpated abdominally and a mark is made with a pen as a reference line from which any uterine enlargement or distension would be noted

- Administer oxytocin infusion (40 IU in a litre of normal saline solution) to keep the uterus contracted

- Keep the patient under constant surveillance after insertion of the tamponade balloon catheter. Monitor pulse, blood pressure, uterine fundal height, and signs of any vaginal bleeding or bleeding through the lumen of the catheter every 30 min. Check temperature every 2 h and urinary output hourly via an in-dwelling Foley catheter with a urometer

- Give intravenous broad-spectrum antibiotics at the time of insertion and for up to 3 days

**Removal of the balloon**

- After 6–8 h, if the uterine fundus remains at the same level and there is no active bleeding through the cervix or the central lumen of the catheter, it is safe to remove the balloon provided that the woman is stable and adequate blood replacement has been provided

- Keep the patient fasting for 2 h after the balloon is removed in case surgery is needed under anaesthesia

- Deflate the balloon slowly, but do not remove it for 30 min

- Continue the oxytocin infusion even if there is no bleeding

- If there is still no bleeding after 30 min, discontinue the oxytocin infusion and remove the balloon catheter

- If bleeding starts when the balloon is deflated, inflate the balloon again

oesophageal catheter (SBOC), the Rusch urological hydrostatic balloon, and the Bakri balloon. The SBOC has been the most frequently reported device. Overall, the reported success rates vary between 70–100%.[44] Uterine tamponade with the SBOC has been described as a prognostic test in obstetric haemorrhage by Condous et al.[45] In their study, the 'tamponade test' had a positive result of > 87% for successful management of PPH. Furthermore, the use of balloon tamponade in the successful management of PPH secondary to extensive vaginal lacerations has recently been reported.[46]

The 'tamponade test' can arrest bleeding in the majority of women with severe PPH and allows the obstetrician to identify which women will require laparotomy. This method has the advantages that: (i) insertion is easy and rapid with minimal anaesthesia; (ii) it can be performed by relatively inexperienced personnel; (iii) removal is painless; and (iv) failed cases can be identified rapidly (Table 2). The early use of balloon tamponade may be expected to result in reduced total blood loss and haemorrhage-related maternal mortality. To date, no immediate problems (such as bleeding or sepsis) or long-term complications (such as menstrual problems or problems with conception) have been reported in women who have undergone uterine tamponade.

## A – Apply compression sutures

If the patient is stable and bimanual compression of the uterus successfully achieves haemostasis, then compression sutures may be of value. Various modifications have been reported to the original B-Lynch[47] suture technique.[48–50] The ease of application of such sutures is a major advantage, and fertility is preserved.[43] The obvious disadvantages are the need for laparotomy and, usually, hysterotomy (although some modified types have avoided this step of the procedure). Recognised complications include erosion through the uterine wall, pyometra and uterine necrosis.[44]

## S – Systematic pelvic devascularisation

Pelvic devascularisation requires laparotomy, and progressive, step-wise devascularisation,[51] whereby the uterine, ovarian and finally internal iliac arteries are ligated (Table 3). Vaginal ligation of the uterine arteries has also been described.[52] Internal iliac artery ligation is usually effective in arresting bleeding from all sources within the genital tract, but it can be time consuming, is technically challenging, and carries risks of injury to other structures. Prerequisites include a haemodynamically stable patient, substantial surgical expertise and a desire to preserve fertility. The reported success rates are between 40–100%.[44] When arterial ligation fails, hysterectomy is usually required and higher morbidity may be expected compared with those patients undergoing hysterectomy without previous attempted arterial ligation.[43]

## I – Interventional radiology with uterine artery embolisation

Arterial embolisation under fluoroscopic guidance was first described in 1979.[53] The success rates may be as high as 70–100% and the procedure has the potential to preserve fertility. Prophylactic embolisation may have a role in a planned caesarean section when the placenta is thought to be morbidly adherent.[54] Complications include haematoma formation, infection, contrast-related

**Table 3** The stepwise pelvic devascularisation technique

1   Absorbable sutures should be used for all ligatures

2   Bilateral uterine artery ligation at the level of the uterine border beside the upper part of the lower uterine segment is usually the first step

3   If bleeding continues and is likely to originate from the lower uterine segment:

  • The bladder should be reflected inferiorly

  • A second lower bilateral uterine vessel ligation should be performed at the lower part of the lower uterine segment, 3–5 cm below the upper ligatures. At this level, the uterine artery is ligated bilaterally at the reflection of the cervicovaginal branch. This ligature should obliterate most of the branches of the uterine artery to the lower uterine segment and a branch that extends to the upper portion of the cervix

  • The ligatures should include a significant amount of myometrium to avoid damage to the uterine vessels and to obliterate some of the arterial branches

4   Bilateral ovarian artery ligation. A suture is passed through the avascular area in the infundibulopelvic ligament to include the ovarian vessels

5   Bilateral internal iliac artery ligation. This step should be performed by surgeons with expertise in the anatomy of the pelvis

6   Concomitant blood and blood product transfusion (and resuscitation measures) should be provided according to the patient's haemodynamic status.

side-effects and ischaemia resulting in uterus and bladder necrosis.[44] The need for specialised equipment and an interventional radiologist with a high degree of expertise are limitations of this procedure.

We recently performed a systematic review of conservative management of PPH when medical measures fail. The success rates for arresting PPH were 84.0% for balloon tamponade, 90.7% for arterial embolisation, 91.7% for compression sutures, and 84.6% for pelvic devascularisation (including uterine or internal iliac artery ligation). There was no statistically significant difference in success rates among these procedures. This study failed to demonstrate that any one method for the conservative management of severe PPH was superior to any other (Table 4). Uterine balloon tamponade should, therefore, be considered as the first step in the management of intractable PPH which is not due to genital trauma or retained tissue, and which does not respond to medical treatment.[44] Nevertheless, the choice of any measure may depend on

**Table 4** Success rates of surgical and radiological measures in the management of PPH[44]

| Method | Cases (n) | Success rate (%) | 95% CI |
|---|---|---|---|
| B-Lynch/compression sutures | 108 | 91.7 | 84.9–95.5 |
| Arterial embolisation | 193 | 90.7 | 85.7–94.0 |
| Arterial ligation/pelvic devascularisation | 501 | 84.6 | 81.2–87.5 |
| Uterine balloon tamponade | 162 | 84.0 | 77.5–88.8 |

There was no statistically significant difference among the four groups ($P = 0.06$).

the availability of facilities and a number of rapidly changing parameters, such as the degree of on-going bleeding, the estimated blood loss and the haemodynamic status of the woman.

## S – Subtotal or total abdominal hysterectomy

Subtotal or total abdominal hysterectomy is usually the final option in the management of PPH and should not be delayed if the conservative measures have failed. A gravid uterus is vascular and urinary tract injuries are more common due to the anatomical changes in pregnancy. However, subtotal hysterectomy may not be effective when the source of the bleeding is in the lower segment, cervix, or vaginal fornices. Hysterectomy is associated with numerous postoperative complications, including urinary tract injury, fistula formation, bowel injury, vascular injury, pelvic haematoma and sepsis. The loss of child-bearing potential and the psychological consequences should also be considered.

All these surgical techniques (uterine tamponade, devascularisation, compression sutures, and hysterectomy) require the ready availability of specific instruments and equipment. For this purpose, an obstetric haemorrhage equipment tray in the labour ward will facilitate prompt surgical management of severe obstetric haemorrhage, and may reduce the need for blood transfusion and hysterectomy.[55]

## CONCLUSIONS

PPH is a leading cause of maternal morbidity and mortality. Although identification of risk factors antenatally and during labour may be useful in the prevention and management of PPH, severe life-threatening haemorrhage is often unpredictable. Prompt resuscitation of the patient with restoration of circulating blood volume and identification of the cause of bleeding should be performed by a multidisciplinary team approach. A rapid succession of treatment measures in a step-wise, systematic management of PPH can be facilitated using the algorithm 'HAEMOSTASIS' and assessment tools such as the 'rule of 30' and the 'shock index'. These indices, although currently in use, need to be scientifically validated. Protocols for the prevention and management of PPH should be in place in every maternity unit. Training in the management of this common obstetric emergency should include regular 'fire drills' involving all the members of staff.

---

### Key points for clinical practice

- 'Too little, too late' refers to delay in blood transfusion and surgery as well as inadequate transfusion and can result in severe morbidity and mortality. Interventions should be undertaken in a step-wise and rapid succession.

- A multidisciplinary team approach is essential in the management of postpartum haemorrhage and all the members of the team should be aware of the hospital protocol.

**Key points for clinical practice** (continued)

- The 'HAEMOSTASIS' algorithm is a step-wise and systematic mnemonic for the management of postpartum haemorrhage.

- Assessment tools such as the 'rule of 30' and the 'shock index' are helpful in the monitoring and the management of a patient with postpartum haemorrhage but need further evaluation.

- If medical measures fail to control haemorrhage, surgical haemostasis should be commenced sooner rather than later.

- Uterine balloon tamponade is easy to use and effective and allows the obstetrician to identify which women will require laparotomy.

- An obstetric haemorrhage equipment tray should be available in every labour ward as it facilitates prompt surgical management of severe obstetric haemorrhage, and may reduce the need for blood transfusion and hysterectomy.

- Regular 'fire drills' on the management of postpartum haemorrhage should be included in the educational programme of every maternity unit.

## References

1. World Health Organization. *The World Health Report 2005. Make every mother and child count.* Geneva: WHO, 2005.
2. Khan KS, Wojdyla D, Say L, Gulmezoglu AM, Van Look PF. WHO analysis of causes of maternal death: a systematic review. *Lancet* 2006; **367**: 1066–1074
3. Department of Reproductive Health and Research, World Health Organization. *Maternal Mortality in 2000: Estimates Developed by WHO, UNICEF, and UNFPA.* Geneva: WHO, 2004.
4. Royal College of Obstetricians and Gynaecologists. *Why Mothers Die 2000–2002. Confidential Enquiry into Maternal and Child Health.* London: RCOG Press, 2004.
5. Penney G, Brace V. *Scottish Confidential Audit of Severe Maternal Morbidity. 1st Annual Report 2003.* Edinburgh: Scottish Programme for Clinical Effectiveness in Reproductive Health, 2003.
6. Penney G, Adamson L, Kernaghan D. Scottish *Confidential Audit of Severe Maternal Morbidity. 2nd Annual Report 2004.* Edinburgh: Scottish Programme for Clinical Effectiveness in Reproductive Health, 2004.
7. Penney G, Kernaghan D, Adamson L. *Scottish Confidential Audit of Severe Maternal Morbidity. 3rd Annual Report 2005.* Edinburgh: Scottish Programme for Clinical Effectiveness in Reproductive Health, 2005.
8. Waterstone M, Bewley S, Wolfe C. Incidence and predictors of severe obstetric morbidity: case-control study. *BMJ* 2001; **322**: 1089–1093, discussion 1093–1094.
9. Razvi K, Chua S, Arulkumaran S, Ratnam SS. A comparison between visual estimation and laboratory determination of blood loss during the third stage of labour. *Aust NZ J Obstet Gynaecol* 1996; **36**: 152–154.
10. ACOG Practice Bulletin: Clinical Management Guidelines for Obstetrician-Gynecologists Number 76, October 2006: Postpartum Hemorrhage. *Obstet Gynecol* 2006; **108**: 1039–1047.
11. Kominiarek MA, Kilpatrick SJ. Postpartum hemorrhage: a recurring pregnancy complication. *Semin Perinatol* 2007; **31**: 159–166.
12. Office for National Statistics. *Average age of mother at childbirth: Social trends 33.* 2003 <www.statistics.gov.uk>.

13. Ohkuchi A, Onagawa T, Usui R *et al*. Effect of maternal age on blood loss during parturition: a retrospective multivariate analysis of 10,053 cases. *J Perinat Med* 2003; **31**: 209–215.

14. Cleary-Goldman J, Malone FD, Vidaver J *et al*. Impact of maternal age on obstetric outcome. *Obstet Gynecol* 2005; **105**: 983–990.

15. Oyelese Y, Smulian JC. Placenta previa, placenta accreta, and vasa previa. *Obstet Gynecol* 2006; **107**: 927–941.

16. Prendiville WJ, Elbourne D, McDonald S. Active versus expectant management in the third stage of labour. Cochrane Database Syst Rev 2000(3): CD000007.

17. Sherman SJ, Greenspoon JS, Nelson JM, Paul RH. Identifying the obstetric patient at high risk of multiple-unit blood transfusions. *J Reprod Med* 1992; **37**: 649–652.

18. Royal College of Obstetricians and Gynaecologists. *The Role of Emergency and Elective Interventional Radiology in Postpartum Haemorrhage. Good Practice Guidelines*. London: RCOG, 2007.

19. Lalonde A, Daviss BA, Acosta A, Herschderfer K. Postpartum hemorrhage today: ICM/FIGO initiative 2004–2006. *Int J Gynaecol Obstet* 2006; **94**: 243–253.

20. Hofmeyr GJ, Walraven G, Gulmezoglu AM, Maholwana B, Alfirevic Z, Villar J. Misoprostol to treat postpartum haemorrhage: a systematic review. *Br J Obstet Gynaecol* 2005; **112**: 547–553.

21. Derman RJ, Kodkany BS, Goudar SS *et al*. Oral misoprostol in preventing postpartum haemorrhage in resource-poor communities: a randomised controlled trial. *Lancet* 2006; **368**: 1248–1253.

22. Gulmezoglu A, Forna F, Villar J, Hofmeyr G. Prostaglandins for preventing postpartum haemorrhage. Cochrane Database Syst Rev 2007(3): CD000494.

23. Su L, Chong Y, Samuel M. Oxytocin agonists for preventing postpartum haemorrhage. Cochrane Database Syst Rev 2007(3): CD005457.

24. Ceriani Cernadas JM, Carroli G, Pellegrini L *et al*. The effect of timing of cord clamping on neonatal venous hematocrit values and clinical outcome at term: a randomized, controlled trial. *Pediatrics* 2006; **117**: e779–e786.

25. Rabe H, Reynolds G, Diaz-Rossello J. Early versus delayed umbilical cord clamping in preterm infants. Cochrane Database Syst Rev 2004(4): CD003248.

26. Mercer JS, Vohr BR, McGrath MM, Padbury JF, Wallach M, Oh W. Delayed cord clamping in very preterm infants reduces the incidence of intraventricular hemorrhage and late-onset sepsis: a randomized, controlled trial. *Pediatrics* 2006; **117**: 1235–1242.

27. Department of Making Pregnancy Safer, World Health Organization. *WHO Recommendations for the Prevention of Postpartum Haemorrhage*. Geneva: WHO, 2007.

28. Chua S, Ho LM, Vanaja K, Nordstrom L, Roy AC, Arulkumaran S. Validation of a laboratory method of measuring postpartum blood loss. *Gynecol Obstet Invest* 1998; **46**: 31–33.

29. Bose P, Regan F, Paterson-Brown S. Improving the accuracy of estimated blood loss at obstetric haemorrhage using clinical reconstructions. *Br J Obstet Gynaecol* 2006; **113**: 919–924.

30. Ramanathan G, Arulkumaran S. Postpartum hemorrhage. *J Obstet Gynaecol Can* 2006; **28**: 967–973.

31. Chandraharan E, Arulkumaran S. Massive postpartum haemorrhage and management of coagulopathy. *Obstet Gynaecol Reprod Med* 2007; **17**: 119–122.

32. Birkhahn RH, Gaeta TJ, Terry D, Bove JJ, Tloczkowski J. Shock index in diagnosing early acute hypovolemia. *Am J Emerg Med* 2005; **23**: 323–326.

33. The Management of Postpartum Haemorrhage. Scottish Obstetric Guidelines and Audit Project: SPCERH, 1998.

34. Hofmeyr GJ, Ferreira S, Nikodem VC *et al*. Misoprostol for treating postpartum haemorrhage: a randomized controlled trial [ISRCTN72263357]. *BMC Pregnancy Childbirth* 2004; **4**: 16.

35. Walraven G, Dampha Y, Bittaye B, Sowe M, Hofmeyr J. Misoprostol in the treatment of postpartum haemorrhage in addition to routine management: a placebo randomised controlled trial. *Br J Obstet Gynaecol* 2004; **111**: 1014–1017.

36. Lokugamage AU, Sullivan KR, Niculescu I *et al*. A randomized study comparing rectally administered misoprostol versus Syntometrine combined with an oxytocin infusion for

the cessation of primary post partum hemorrhage. *Acta Obstet Gynecol Scand* 2001; **80**: 835–839.

37. Mousa HA, Alfirevic Z. Treatment for primary postpartum haemorrhage. Cochrane Database Syst Rev 2007(1): CD003249.

38. Weeks A. Oral misoprostol for postpartum haemorrhage. *Lancet* 2006; **368**: 2123.

39. Franchini M, Lippi G, Franchi M. The use of recombinant activated factor VII in obstetric and gynaecological haemorrhage. *Br J Obstet Gynaecol* 2007; **114**: 8–15.

40. Investigation into 10 maternal deaths at, or following delivery at, Northwick Park Hospital, North West London Hospitals NHS Trust, between April 2002 and April 2005. London: Healthcare Commission, 2006.

41. Miller S, Hamza S, Bray EH *et al*. First aid for obstetric haemorrhage: the pilot study of the non-pneumatic anti-shock garment in Egypt. *Br J Obstet Gynaecol* 2006; **113**: 424–429.

42. Maier RC. Control of postpartum hemorrhage with uterine packing. *Am J Obstet Gynecol* 1993; **169**: 317–321, discussion 321–323.

43. Dildy 3rd GA. Postpartum hemorrhage: new management options. *Clin Obstet Gynecol* 2002; **45**: 330–344.

44. Doumouchtsis SK, Papageorghiou AT, Arulkumaran S. Systematic review of conservative management of postpartum hemorrhage: what to do when medical treatment fails. *Obstet Gynecol Surv* 2007; **62**: 540–547.

45. Condous GS, Arulkumaran S, Symonds I, Chapman R, Sinha A, Razvi K. The 'tamponade test' in the management of massive postpartum hemorrhage. *Obstet Gynecol* 2003; **101**: 767–772.

46. Tattersall M, Braithwaite W. Balloon tamponade for vaginal lacerations causing severe postpartum haemorrhage. *Br J Obstet Gynaecol* 2007; **114**: 647–648.

47. B-Lynch C, Coker A, Lawal AH, Abu J, Cowen MJ. The B-Lynch surgical technique for the control of massive postpartum haemorrhage: an alternative to hysterectomy? Five cases reported. *Br J Obstet Gynaecol* 1997; **104**: 372–375.

48. Cho JH, Jun HS, Lee CN. Hemostatic suturing technique for uterine bleeding during cesarean delivery. *Obstet Gynecol* 2000; **96**: 129–131.

49. Nelson GS, Birch C. Compression sutures for uterine atony and hemorrhage following cesarean delivery. *Int J Gynecol Obstet* 2006; **92**: 248–250.

50. Pereira A, Nunes F, Pedroso S, Saraiva J, Retto H, Meirinho M. Compressive uterine sutures to treat postpartum bleeding secondary to uterine atony. *Obstet Gynecol* 2005; **106**: 569–572.

51. AbdRabbo SA. Stepwise uterine devascularization: a novel technique for management of uncontrolled postpartum hemorrhage with preservation of the uterus. *Am J Obstet Gynecol* 1994; **171**: 694–700.

52. Hebisch G, Huch A. Vaginal uterine artery ligation avoids high blood loss and puerperal hysterectomy in postpartum hemorrhage. *Obstet Gynecol* 2002; **100**: 574–578.

53. Brown BJ, Heaston DK, Poulson AM, Gabert HA, Mineau DE, Miller Jr FJ. Uncontrollable postpartum bleeding: a new approach to hemostasis through angiographic arterial embolization. *Obstet Gynecol* 1979; **54**: 361–365.

54. Cheng YY, Hwang JI, Hung SW *et al*. Angiographic embolization for emergent and prophylactic management of obstetric hemorrhage: a four-year experience. *J Chin Med Assoc* 2003; **66**: 727–734.

55. Baskett TF. Surgical management of severe obstetric hemorrhage: experience with an obstetric hemorrhage equipment tray. *J Obstet Gynaecol Can* 2004; **26**: 805–808.

56. Saving mother's lives: Reviewing maternal deaths t make motherhood safer. 2003–2005. The Seventh Report of the Confidential Enquiries into Maternal Deaths in the United Kingdom. London:CEMACH, 2007.

*David Shepherd  Ophelia Ziwenga*

**8**

# The management of shock in obstetric patients

Shock is a critical condition and a life-threatening medical emergency. Shock results from acute, generalised, inadequate perfusion of the tissues below that needed to deliver the oxygen and nutrients for normal cell function. In obstetric cases, shock is most commonly due to either haemorrhage or sepsis.[1] Other causes are less common, but cause significant mortality and morbidity if inadequately managed. Substandard care is still an issue in the management of the shocked patient.[1] Prompt recognition and management can improve maternal and fetal outcome in shock.

## AETIOLOGY

The major classes of shock include: (i) hypovolaemic shock; (ii) septic shock; (iii) cardiogenic shock; and (iv) distributive shock. Table 1 summarises the important causes of each type of shock.

## PATHOPHYSIOLOGY

Untreated shock progresses through three stages as shown in Table 2. Inadequate management allows shock to progressively worsen passing through these stages until death occurs.

## DIAGNOSIS

There are no laboratory tests for shock. A high index of suspicion and physical signs of inadequate tissue perfusion and oxygenation are the basis for initiating prompt management. Initial management does not rely on knowledge of the underlying cause.

**David Shepherd** MB ChB FRCA (for correspondence)
Consultant Obstetric Anaesthetist, Department of Anaesthesia, Sheffield General Hospital, The Jessop Wing, Tree Root Walk, Sheffield S10 2SF, UK
E-mail: david.shepherd@shef.ac.uk

**Ophelia Ziwenga** MBChB(Hons) FRCA FCARSI
Currently Clinical Research Fellow in Regional Anaesthesia, University of Alberta, Canada

**Table 1** Aetiology of shock

| Type | Causes |
| --- | --- |
| **Hypovolaemic** | Haemorrhage (overt or occult)<br>Protracted vomiting (hyperemesis)<br>Diarrhoea<br>Diabetic ketoacidosis<br>Peritonitis<br>Burns |
| **Septic** | Sepsis, endotoxaemia |
| **Cardiogenic** | Massive pulmonary embolus |
|  | Cardiomyopathies – myocardial infarction, hypertrophic obstructive cardiomyopathy, cardiac amyloid, myocarditis |
|  | Obstructive non-structural – pulmonary embolism, cardiac tamponade, pulmonary hypertension, constrictive pericarditis |
|  | Obstructive structural – valvular aortic stenosis, valvular mitral stenosis, idiopathic hypertrophic subaortic stenosis (aka hypertrophic obstructive cardiomyopathy), coarctation of the aorta, left atrial myxoma |
|  | Dysrhythmias |
|  | Regurgitant lesions – mitral regurgitaion, aortic regurgitation, ventricular septal defect, left ventricular aneurysm, ventricular wall rupture |
|  | Blunt cardiac trauma – contusion |
| **Distributive** | Neurogenic – spinal injury, regional anaesthesia<br>Anaphylaxis |

## INITIAL MANAGEMENT

Successful management of the shocked patient requires teamwork. Maternity units should have established protocols for dealing with shock. Practice 'fire' drills allow deficiencies in the system to be identified and addressed without risk to patients.[2] Simulators, MOET and ALSO courses are helpful in training individuals and teams.

**Table 2** Stages of shock

**Stage 1 – Compensated**
- Changes in blood pressure and cardiac output compensated by adjustment of homeostatic mechanisms.
- In healthy patients this category of shock may not require fluid replacement if the cause is removed.

**Stage 2 – Decompensated**
- Maximal compensatory mechanisms are acting but tissue perfusion is reduced.
- Vital organ (cerebral, renal and myocardial) function becomes impaired.

**Stage 3 – Irreversible**
- Vital organ perfusion is impaired. Acute tubular necrosis, severe acidosis, decreased myocardial perfusion and decreased myocardial contractility occur.
- The profound decrease in perfusion leads to cellular damage and death.

Senior team members should be summoned early – anaesthetist, obstetrician, haematologist and midwife. Other support should be contacted as soon as practicable (e.g. neonatologist, radiologist, theatre team and a dedicated porter, *etc.*).

The management of shock should start as soon as the diagnosis is made, aiming for prompt restoration of tissue perfusion and oxygenation. The management of the underlying aetiology is secondary until resuscitation has been instituted.

All therapy is directed at optimising maternal condition. This is particularly important in the antenatal period as optimal maternal management improves intra-uterine conditions for the fetus. Delivery may need to be considered as part of the resuscitation in some forms of shock.

The resuscitation follows the familiar 'ABC' pattern common to all medical emergencies.

## AIRWAY

A patent airway should be assured and high flow oxygen (15 l/min) administered using a mask with reservoir bag. The airway should be protected by tracheal intubation if there is potential compromise.

## BREATHING

Ventilation (breathing) should be checked, and supported if inadequate.

## CIRCULATION (WITH CONTROL OF HAEMORRHAGE)

- Insert two wide-bore peripheral intravenous cannulas.

- Initial circulatory management aims to restore circulating volume and reverse hypotension with crystalloid. Blood may be required; therefore, as the first intravenous cannula is inserted, samples can be drawn for full blood count, coagulation screen, urea, electrolytes and cross matching. In shock management, the initial request should be for 6 units.

- Emergency O rhesus-negative blood or group-specific uncrossmatched blood may be needed in massive haemorrhage.

- Response to therapy can be monitored with simple clinical measurements – pulse, non-invasive blood pressure, pulse oximetry and urine output.

- Left lateral tilt, a wedge or manual displacement of uterus is required to avoid aortocaval compression which may further worsen hypotension.

After resuscitation has been initiated, the underlying cause of the shock should be identified and definitive treatment instituted.

Vasoactive drugs (inotropes and vasopressors) are considered if the cause of shock is thought to be due to myocardial depression or profound vasodilatation. They have no part in the management of hypovolaemic shock.

## SPECIFIC PROBLEMS

### Haemorrhage and hypovolaemic shock

Hypovolaemia is an absolute reduction of the intravascular volume. Cardiac output is reduced producing a low perfusion state. In addition, vasoconstriction diverts blood flow away from all but vital organs (heart, brain and kidneys).

Massive haemorrhage is the commonest cause of hypovolaemic shock seen in obstetric practice and remains a major cause of maternal mortality. Haemorrhage may be obvious, such as external bleeding or, occult such as blood loss in perineal haematoma or intra-abdominal bleeding.

Non-haemorrhagic causes of hypovolaemic shock are due to excessive extracellular fluid loss from protracted vomiting (hyperemesis) and diarrhoea, bowel obstruction, peritonitis or burn injury. Definitive management is not considered further.

### Haemodynamic considerations in pregnancy

Pregnancy produces a hyperdynamic, hypervolaemic maternal circulation. This serves to protect the mother against haemorrhage to some degree. Cardiac output increases by 50% and blood volume by about 45%, reaching a peak at 28–34 weeks of gestation. Correspondingly, greater fluid losses (> 30% of circulating volume) can occur before anything other than maternal tachycardia is seen. At this point, peripheral vasoconstriction and hypotension develop. Aortocaval compression aggravates the instability seen in haemorrhage.

In the antepartum period, uteroplacental hypoperfusion may occur before maternal signs are evident adversely affecting fetal well-being. This can be detected as abnormal fetal heart rate patterns on the cardiotocograph.

### Causes of haemorrhagic shock in pregnancy

Haemorrhagic shock can occur any time in pregnancy. Table 3 contains a list of causes. The major causes of death are postpartum haemorrhage, placenta praevia and placental abruption.[1]

**Table 3** Causes of haemorrhage in pregnancy

| |
|---|
| **Antenatal** |
|     Ruptured ectopic pregnancy |
|     Incomplete abortion |
|     Placenta praevia |
|     Placental abruption |
|     Uterine rupture |
| |
| **Postpartum** |
|     Uterine atony. Risk increased by: |
|         Retained products of conception |
|         Prolonged labour |
|         Precipitous labour (lasting less than 3 h) |
|         Oxytocin augmentation of labour |
|         Distended uterus (multiple gestations, polyhydramnios, fetal macrosomia) |
|         Grand multipara |
|         Halogenated anaesthetics |
|     Lacerations to genital tract (perineum, vagina and cervix) |
|     Chorio-amnionitis |
|     Large placental site (*e.g.* twins) |
|     Acute uterine inversion |
|     Uterine leiomyomata (fibroids) |
|     Puerperal sepsis |

# MANAGEMENT OF MASSIVE OBSTETRIC HAEMORRHAGE

The initial management of massive obstetric haemorrhage is aimed at maternal resuscitation and does not rely upon knowledge of the underlying cause. The diagnosis of the cause and definitive treatment is initiated once resuscitation is under way. Basic shock management, as outlined above, is always the first step. Specific conditions have special aspects in their definitive management.

## Management of uterine atony

Uterine atony accounts for the majority of cases of postpartum haemorrhage, occurring in about 5% of deliveries. Factors increasing the risk of this problem are also shown in Table 3. Special aspects in the management of uterine atony include:

1. **Optimise uterine tone** – bimanual massage of the uterus, oxytocin bolus followed by infusion, ergometrine bolus (care in hypertensive disease), and Carboprost (15-methyl prostaglandin $F_{2-\alpha}$).

2. **Surgery** – removal of retained products of conception, strategies to stop bleeding from placental bed by physical means (intra-uterine balloon tamponade, B-Lynch suture, hysterectomy), and arterial embolisation.

## Lacerations of genital tract

Lacerations of the cervix, vagina and perineum are the second commonest cause of post partum haemorrhage. Special aspects in the management of lacerations include surgery – repair of genital tract, vaginal pack.

## Uterine rupture

The incidence of uterine rupture is 0.05% of all pregnancies,[3] occurring between 1 in 140–300 of women with a pre-existing scar.[4] Uterine scarring occurs after caesarean section or other uterine surgery (*e.g.* myomectomy). The risk of rupture increases with the number of caesarean sections; two previous sections carry a 3–5-fold increased risk over one previous section.[5,6] Perinatal mortality is 10 times that of the maternal mortality.[3] Uterine rupture typically occurs in early labour, but can develop in late pregnancy.

Uterine rupture presents with acute fetal distress and cessation of uterine activity. Uterine or scar tenderness may suggest the diagnosis, but is not a constant feature. Vaginal bleeding may occur and examination may show that the baby is not as low in the birth canal earlier. Special aspects in the management of uterine rupture include:

1. Stop oxytocin infusion if running.

2. Continuous maternal and fetal monitoring.

3. Emergency laparotomy with rapid operative delivery.

4. Caesarean hysterectomy may need to be performed if haemorrhage is impossible to control.

## Uterine inversion

This is a rare complication of pregnancy that can be associated with massive haemorrhage. The estimated incidence varies widely from 1 in 1584 deliveries to 1 in 20,000 deliveries, nullipara being higher risk.[7,8]

**Table 4**  Factors predisposing to uterine inversion

- Short umbilical cord
- Excessive traction on the umbilical cord
- Excessive fundal pressure
- Fundal implantation of the placenta
- Retained placenta and abnormal adherence of the placenta
- Chronic endometritis
- Vaginal births after previous caesarean section
- Rapid or long labours
- Previous uterine inversion
- Certain drugs such as magnesium sulphate (drugs promoting tocolysis)

Part of the uterus indents towards the dilated cervix, eventually passing through into the vagina. Uterine relaxation is required to allow the initial indentation, followed by resumption of contractions in such a way that inversion results. Table 4 lists aetiological factors for uterine inversion.

Acute inversion presents as post partum haemorrhage, with a vaginal mass and cardiovascular collapse. Pain is extreme. Autonomic instability may aggravate this condition. The diagnosis is confirmed by inability to feel the uterine fundus abdominally. Obesity can make diagnosis more difficult. Chronic cases are uncommon and difficult to diagnose presenting with spotting, discharge and low back pain. Ultrasound may be required to confirm the diagnosis. Special aspects in the management of uterine inversion include:

1. Replacement of the uterus needs to be undertaken quickly as delay makes replacement more difficult.

2. Administer tocolytics (nitroglycerin, terbutaline, magnesium sulphate) to allow uterine relaxation.

3. Replacement is undertaken (with placenta if still attached) – manually by slowly and steadily pushing upwards, with hydrostatic pressure[9,10] or surgically.

4. Existing epidural or spinal anaesthesia can be used in the management of acute inversion provided the patient is cardiovascularly stable. In subacute or chronic cases, general anaesthesia is usually necessary (produces more uterine relaxation).

## DEVELOPMENTS IN MANAGEMENT OF HAEMORRHAGE

### CELL SALVAGE

Cell salvage is widely used in cardiac, vascular, trauma and other major surgery. Obstetric theatres have been slow to introduce this technique because of theoretical risks of amniotic fluid embolus and rhesus iso-immunisation. The former has never been documented and remains theoretical. The latter is preventable with adequate anti-D therapy, so Kleihauer testing should be performed as soon as practicable in rhesus-negative mothers with rhesus positive babies.

Autologous transfusion with salvaged red cells avoids the hazards of homologous blood transfusion. The technique is economically viable, the disposables costing less than a unit of red cells. Autologous transfusion has been used in over 400 reported obstetric cases, and many more that are unreported, without causing harm.[11]

Blood is removed from the operative site through heparinised suction tubing and a filter into a collecting reservoir and processed by washing and centrifugation to remove circulating debris and contaminants. The resulting red cells have a haematocrit of 55–80 and can be returned to the patient quickly. The cell saver only replaces red blood cells and will not correct coagulopathy.

The risk from transfusion of amniotic fluid is obviously a concern. The use of a separate suction for amniotic fluid and a leukocyte depletion filter during transfusion has been shown to be effective at removing fetal components from the salvaged blood.[12]

Other disadvantages with this technique are financial and logistic.

1. The units have capital and maintenance costs. The disposables appear relatively expensive.

2. Staff require training and regular exposure to the technology to retain their skills.

3. The unit can only be used for 'clean' blood, *i.e.* the technique is unsuitable for post partum haemorrhage on the labour ward due to faecal contamination.

Overall, the risk/benefit ratio, long-term financial savings and increasing difficulty with blood bank supplies outweigh the disadvantages and the balance is in favour of using cell salvage in obstetrics.

## RECOMBINANT ACTIVATED FACTOR VII

Activated recombinant factor VII (rFVIIa; NovoSeven, Novo Nordisk, Denmark) is a genetically engineered protein that promotes clot formation through its action at a number of points in the clotting cascade. The major activity occurs when factor VIIa forms a complex with exposed tissue factor at the site of endothelial damage. This complex is a key initiator in haemostasis, leading to production of small amounts of thrombin and activating factor V, factor VIII and platelets at the site of injury. Ultimately, there is conversion of fibrinogen to fibrin and the formation of a haemostatic clot. In addition, rFVIIa also activates factor IX that binds with factor VIIIa on the surface of activated platelets, generating more factor Xa and producing large-scale platelet surface thrombin generation and fibrin production

## PELVIC ARTERIAL EMBOLISATION

Some centres have access to radiological facilities to allow selective embolisation of pelvic vessels using interventional radiological techniques.[13] Success with this modality of treatment avoids the need for hysterectomy. The major problem is the transfer of the haemorrhaging, unstable patient from obstetric theatre to the angiography suite. Insertion of the intravascular catheters has been used in our unit with success in haemorrhage reduction, before procedures in women who might be expected to have major haemorrhage (placenta accreta undergoing elective caesarean section).

## BALLOON TAMPONADE

Tamponade techniques such as uterine packing and the use of hydrostatic balloon catheters have been shown to reduce the need for the more radical surgical options.[14] The balloon techniques have become popular in recent years. The hydrostatic urological Rusch balloon, gastric balloon, Foley's catheter, the Bakri balloon and a condom catheter have all been used. The Rusch balloon is used in our unit;[15] the technique involves the insertion of the balloon catheter into the uterine cavity, inflation with warm saline and then vaginal packing. Oxytocin infusion is used to maintain uterine tone. The balloon catheter remains *in situ* for 12–24 h. Fluid is removed gradually and the balloon catheter removed in a high-care area (high dependency unit or operating theatre). After balloon removal, the vaginal pack is removed.

## SEPTIC SHOCK

Septic shock is uncommon in pregnancy and maternal mortality from sepsis has reduced over the last century. It remains a significant cause of direct death in pregnancy. There were 13 deaths due to genital tract sepsis in the last *Confidential Enquiry into Maternal Deaths in the United Kingdom* report.[1] The obstetric patient is less likely to die of complications of septic shock than their general medical/surgical counterparts. Mortality rates with septic shock have been estimated to be about 3% in obstetric patients, compared with approximately 50% in non-obstetric patients.

Large-scale inflammatory response results in massive vasodilatation (decreased systemic vascular resistance), increased capillary permeability and cardiac depression leading to hypotension. Hypotension reduces tissue perfusion pressure and tissue hypoxia ensues. In addition to poor perfusion there is also impairment of oxygen utilisation by the tissues. These factors can lead to multiple organ failure and death.

### DEFINITIONS

There is a spectrum of sepsis-related pathologies.

#### Systemic inflammatory response syndrome

Systemic inflammatory response syndrome (SIRS) is a wide-spread inflammatory response to a variety of clinical insults. It is recognized by the presence of two or more of the following: (i) temperature $< 36°C$ or $> 38°C$; (ii) hart rate $> 90$ bpm; (iii) hyperventilation (respiratory rate) $> 20$ breaths/min or on blood gas $PaCO_2 < 4.3$ kPa (32 mmHg); (iv) white blood cell count $> 12,000$ cells/mm$^3$, or with $> 10\%$ immature neutrophils.

#### Sepsis

SIRS plus evidence of infection (suspected or known).

#### Septic shock

This is sepsis with hypotension despite adequate fluid resuscitation. To diagnose septic shock the following two criteria must be met: (i) evidence of infection, through a positive blood culture; and (ii) refractory hypotension –

hypotension despite adequate fluid resuscitation. Patients requiring vasopressor or inotropic therapy despite adequate fluid resuscitation are considered to be in septic shock.

### Sepsis with multi-organ dysfunction

Hypotension, hypoxaemia, oliguria, metabolic (with or without lactic acid) acidosis, thrombocytopenia, or depressed level of consciousness.

## PATHOPHYSIOLOGY OF SEPSIS

Better understanding of the pathogenesis of sepsis has contributed to the introduction of therapeutic agents that may improve outcome. Sepsis arises due to complex interactions within the body.

### Micro-organism and inflammatory response

There is convincing evidence that sepsis results from an exaggerated systemic inflammatory response induced by infecting organisms. The cell wall components of Gram-positive and Gram-negative bacteria induce a variety of pro-inflammatory mediators (cytokines) in host cells (macrophages/monocytes and neutrophils). These cytokines play a central role in initiating sepsis and shock. In Gram-negative bacteria, the most toxic component is the lipid A moiety of lipopolysaccharide and in Gram-positive bacteria, lipoteichoic acid. Some Gram-positive bacteria also produce superantigen cytotoxins leading to massive cytokine production.

### Coagulation

Inflammatory cytokines initiate coagulation by activation of tissue factor (TF), the principal trigger of coagulation. Thrombin production follows, cleaving fibrinogen to produce fibrin, leading to formation of microvascular thrombi.

Cytokines also disrupt the body's modulators of coagulation and inflammation (protein C, protein S, antithrombin III and tissue-factor-pathway inhibitor). This worsens the coagulopathy by decreasing fibrinolysis.

The imbalance among inflammation, coagulation, and fibrinolysis results in wide-spread microvascular thrombosis and suppressed fibrinolysis.

### Cardiovascular function in septic shock

Arterial vasodilatation occurs in septic shock and cardiac output rises. The low vascular resistance results from the dependency of blood pressure on cardiac output. Hypotension and shock occur if the rise in cardiac output is insufficient to compensate for this change. Early in septic shock, the rise in cardiac output often is limited by hypovolaemia and from fall in preload. When intravascular volume is augmented, the cardiac output is usually elevated. However, even though cardiac output increases, the performance of the heart is usually reduced by myocardial depressant substances, coronary blood flow abnormalities, pulmonary hypertension, various cytokines, nitric oxide, and β-receptor down-regulation.

### Peripheral circulation in septic shock

Peripheral blood flow abnormalities result from an altered balance between local regulation of arterial vascular tone and the activity of central mechanisms. Vasoactive substances (*e.g.* nitric oxide, prostacyclin and endothelin) also affect regional blood flow.

Oxygen delivery to the tissues is increased but the arteriovenous oxygen difference is usually reduced and the blood lactate level rises in sepsis. This implies reduced tissue oxygen extraction and anaerobic cellular metabolism.

If oxygen supply falls there is a redistribution of cardiac output, preferentially supplying vital organs, such as the heart and brain. This fact has obvious implications for the fetus *in utero*.

Systemic microvascular permeability increases, contributing to oedema of various organs, particularly the lung and acute respiratory distress syndrome (ARDS) commonly occurs.

Maldistribution of blood flow, disturbances in the microcirculation and peripheral shunting of oxygen are responsible for diminished oxygen extraction and uptake, pathological supply dependency of oxygen, and lactate acidaemia in patients experiencing septic shock.

## AETIOLOGY

Pyelonephritis is the most common cause of septic shock during pregnancy, followed by chorio-amnionitis and postpartum endometritis. Commonly isolated organisms include *Escherichia coli*, groups A and B *Streptococcus*, *Klebsiella* spp., and *Staphylococcus aureus*. Predisposing factors in obstetric patients are shown in Table 5. There are also all of the non-obstetric causes of sepsis that may occur fortuitously during pregnancy such as pneumonia and appendicitis.

## CLINICAL FEATURES OF SEPSIS

The onset of life-threatening sepsis in obstetrics can be insidious with rapid clinical deterioration. The Boxes 1 and 2 indicate the symptoms and signs of sepsis that will be found.

In addition, laboratory blood tests demonstrate abnormal white cell count, low platelet count, coagulopathy, raised urea and creatinine concentrations,

**Table 5** Predisposing factors for sepsis in obstetric patients

| |
|---|
| Post-caesarean delivery endometritis (15–85%) |
| Prolonged rupture of membranes |
| Retained products of conception |
| Cerclage in the presence of ruptured membranes |
| Septic abortion/retained products of conception (1–2%) |
| Post vaginal delivery endometritis (1–4%) |
| Intra-amniotic infection (1%) |
| Water birth (delivery in water) increases the of risk infection to both mother and baby due to faecal contamination |
| Emergency caesarean section |
| Pregnancy with a retained intra-uterine contraceptive device and instrumentation of the genito-uterine tract |
| Urinary tract infections (1–6%) |
| Toxic shock syndrome (< 1%) |
| Necrotising fasciitis (< 1%) |

| Box 1 Symptoms of sepsis | Box 2 Signs of sepsis |
|---|---|
| • Abdominal pain<br>• Vomiting<br>• Diarrhoea | • Signs of sepsis<br>• Sympathetic activation<br>• Tachycardia<br>• Hypertension<br>• Pallor<br>• Clamminess<br>• Peripheral shut down<br>• Systemic inflammation<br>• Fever or hypothermia<br>• Tachypnoea<br>• Organ hypoperfusion<br>• Cold peripheries<br>• Hypotension<br>• Confusion<br>• Oliguria<br>• Altered mental state |

deranged liver function tests, metabolic acidosis with high serum lactate and raised C-reactive protein.

## GENERAL MANAGEMENT OF SEPTIC SHOCK

The general management of septic shock includes basic shock management and circulatory management, which usually requires rapid volume expansion to correct absolute and relative hypovolaemia and maintain end-organ perfusion.

In pregnancy, optimal therapy for the mother remains the first priority. Fetal compromise in sepsis is directly attributable to maternal cardiovascular decompensation and decrease in the *in utero* placental blood flow. Improvements in maternal haemodynamic stability have positive effects on the fetus. Efforts to intervene on behalf of the fetus by caesarean delivery of an unstable mother may end in poor outcome for both mother and baby. If the fetal component is the source of sepsis, then delivery becomes an essential part of therapy while stabilizing the mother.

## SPECIAL ASPECTS IN MANAGEMENT OF SEPTIC SHOCK

These include:

1. Transfer to a higher level facility (high dependency or intensive care) is usually required.

2. Invasive monitoring will inevitably be necessary (direct arterial, central venous).

3 Obtain blood cultures as soon as possible and culture other sites such as wounds, urine sputum or other body fluids (*e.g.* amniotic fluid). Intravenous antibiotics should be started. Broad-spectrum antibiotics should be used initially.

4. Removal of infected tissue after initial resuscitation is critical for patient survival. In obstetrics this may include evacuation of the uterus, delivery (if sepsis is related to chorio-amnionitis with a viable fetus), drainage of abscesses and hysterectomy in case of myometrial micro-abscesses. Delivery may not necessarily be indicated if sepsis is not related to the uterus and will be based upon the gestational age and fetal condition. Radiological investigations should be performed early to identify infected tissue/collections where indicated.

5. Goal-directed therapy (see below).

## ADVANCES IN SEPSIS MANAGEMENT

### Early goal-directed therapy
Early goal-directed therapy involves modifying the components of treatment to achieve specific end-points (including mean arterial blood pressure ≥65 mmHg, urine output >0.5 ml/kg/h, CVP 8–12 nmmHg and normal mixed venous oxygen saturation), in an effort to reduce end-organ damage and death. Use of this approach has been demonstrated to improve outcome in septic patients.

### Insulin therapy
Aggressive control of blood sugar has been demonstrated to improve outcome in septic patients.[16] The impact of tight glycaemic control in the prevention of fetal complications such as macrosomia, still-birth, and neonatal hypoglycaemia is well documented. It remains to be seen whether tight glycaemic control will result in improved maternal outcomes in the critical care setting.

### Activated protein C (APC)
Patients with sepsis have decreased APC levels. APC administration in septic shock has been reported to decrease mortality[17] and reduce organ dysfunction.[18] Studies with APC have been confined to those septic patients with the highest risk of death (APACHE II score ≥ 25). During pregnancy there are significant changes in the coagulation cascade including elevated factor VIII. How this impacts on the responsiveness to APC is unknown. However, pregnancy is not a contra-indication to its use.

### Corticosteroids
Administration of corticosteroids in high doses does not improve survival in unselected septic patients and can worsen outcome because of secondary infection.

In critically ill, septic, patients there may be a 'relative' adrenal insufficiency. Physiological stresses normally cause marked increases in cortisol levels. In septic shock, the adrenal gland may not respond to adrenocorticotropic hormone appropriately and, while the levels of cortisol may be increased, the magnitude of this increase may be reduced.

One study[19] has reported improved survival in patients with septic shock who were treated with low-dose hydrocortisone and fludrocortisone. No studies have been done in pregnant women. The impact of adrenal suppression and the usefulness of low-dose steroids in patients with obstetric septic shock is unknown.

## CARDIOGENIC SHOCK

The failure of the heart to provide adequate output leads to tissue under-perfusion. In addition to under-perfusion, blood and tissue oxygenation can also be exacerbated because of the 'back pressure' on the lungs that leads to pulmonary oedema. Pregnancy puts progressive strain on the heart as gestation progresses. The peak cardiac demands are between 28– 32 weeks of gestation.

Pre-existing cardiac disease places the parturient at particular risk. Cardiac-related death in pregnancy is the second most common cause of death in pregnancy[1] and is commoner than the leading direct cause of maternal death, thrombo-embolism.

Less commonly, cardiogenic shock is a result, directly or indirectly, of cardiac trauma (*e.g.* cardiac contusion in sternal injuries) or as a result of an infective process such as myocarditis.

## ANAPHYLAXIS

An international consensus working definition of anaphylaxis has been proposed as:[20] 'A serious allergic reaction that is rapid in onset and may cause death'.

The incidence of anaphylaxis in the UK is unknown. It is a relatively uncommon event in pregnancy but has serious implications for both mother and fetus. There was one death from acute anaphylaxis in the last triennial *Confidential Enquiry into Maternal Deaths in the United Kingdom* report.[1]

Anaphylactic shock is usually drug related. Amniotic fluid embolism shares many of the features of anaphylactic shock (see below).

### PATHOPHYSIOLOGY

An anaphylactic reaction is an exaggerated immunological response to a substance (antigen) to which an individual has been previously sensitized. It is a type 1 hypersensitivity (IgE-mediated) response causing breakdown and degranulation of mast cells and basophils releasing mediators (histamine, serotonin, bradykinin, thromboxane, tryptase and leukotrienes) into the plasma. These substances cause increased mucous membrane secretions, increased capillary permeability and leakage, marked vasodilatation and bronchospasm.

### AETIOLOGY

Anaphylaxis can be caused by pharmacological agents, insect stings, foods, and latex (though true latex-induced anaphylaxis is very rare). In up to 5% of cases, the causative agent cannot be identified.

117

**Table 6**  Symptoms and signs of anaphylaxis

---

**Cutaneous** (around 80% patients)
    Flushing, pruritus, urticaria, rhinitis, conjunctival erythema, lacrymation

**Cardiovascular** (collapse most common CVS event)
    Cardiovascular collapse, hypotension, vasodialtation and erythema, pale,
    clammy cool skin, diaphoresis, nausea and vomiting

**Respiratory** (upper and lower airway oedema)
    Stridor, wheezing, dyspnoea, cough, chest/throat tightness, cyanosis,
    confusion (from hypoxia), increased airway pressures in artificially
    ventilated patients (*e.g.* anaesthesia)

**Gastrointestinal/pelvic**
    Nausea and vomiting, abdominal pain, pelvic pain (described as being
    like uterine contractions), vaginal discharge (late)

**Central nervous system**
    Hypotension causes: (i) collapse with/without unconsciousness; (ii)
    dizziness; and (iii) incontinence. Hypoxia causes confusion.
    Patients may complain of a throbbing headache.

---

## CLINICAL FEATURES

Anaphylaxis should be considered when two or more body systems are affected. It can occur with or without cardiovascular or airway involvement, but this is rare. Table 6 lists the features that may be seen.

Early signs and symptoms include urticaria, rhinitis, conjuctivis, abdominal pain, vomiting and diarrhoea. Flushing is common but pallor may also occur.

Hypotension is the commonest feature of cardiovascular compromise during anaphylaxis. It may be associated with clinically obvious vasodilatation (erythema) or a sudden onset of shock with peripheral circulatory failure.

## MANAGEMENT

Management includes: (i) basic shock management (ABC); and (ii) circulatory management.

## SPECIAL ASPECTS IN MANAGEMENT OF ANAPHYLACTIC SHOCK

In addition to the basic resuscitation, other considerations are immediate and late.

### Immediate

1. Stop administration of the suspected agent and call for help.
2. Airway – early intubation of the trachea should be considered because upper airway oedema makes this manoeuvre problematic.
3. Circulation – the supine or Trendelenburg position with legs elevated increases venous return.
4. Give epinephrine intramuscularly. Repeat every 5–15 min titrated to pulse and blood pressure until improvement occurs.

5. In severe hypotension, intravenous epinephrine titrated to blood pressure is an option.

6. Rapid intravascular volume expansion with crystalloid solution.

If cardiac arrest occurs, advanced life support (ALS) protocols should be followed. Obstetric patients suffering with anaphylaxis are often young, with healthy hearts and cardiovascular systems. Effective cardiopulmonary resuscitation may maintain sufficient oxygen delivery until the effects of anaphylactic reaction resolve.

## Secondary

1. If hypotension persists despite the primary management, intravenous epinephrine infusion can be considered. Alternative vasopressor agents can also be used by bolus or infusion (metaraminol, methoxamine, vasopressin).

2. Atropine may be necessary if there is significant bradycardia.

3. If bronchospasm persists give nebulised or intravenous $\beta_2$-agonist such as salbutamol. An intravenous infusion may be necessary. Inhaled Ipratroprium may be particularly useful for the treatment of bronchospasm in patients on β-blockers.

4. Antihistamines – intravenous Chlopheniramine.

5. Steroids – intravenous hydrocortisone can be used, but its effect is not immediate.

6. All patients with severe anaphylaxis shock should be referred to critical care.

## INVESTIGATIONS

### Immediate
Elevated serum tryptase indicates that the reaction was due to mast cell degranulation, but does not identify the causative agent. Three blood samples need to be taken. Samples are taken at 1 h, 3 h and 24 h following the suspected reaction.

### Late
The aim is to identify causative agent. Refer the patient to an immunologist/ allergist for investigation.

## AMNIOTIC FLUID EMBOLUS

Amniotic fluid embolism (AFE) is a rare, but devastating, condition. It is responsible for around 8% of the direct maternal deaths in the UK.[1] The incidence of this complication would appear to be somewhere between 1 in 80,000 to 1 in 120,000.[21] It is characterised by an abrupt cardiovascular collapse and coagulopathy during labour or in the immediate postpartum period.

## PATHOPHYSIOLOGY

The mechanism of AFE is poorly understood. Current data suggest that the process is more similar to anaphylaxis[23] than to embolism, and the term anaphylactoid syndrome of pregnancy has been suggested because fetal tissue or amniotic fluid components are not universally found in women who present with signs and symptoms attributable to AFE.[24]

Amniotic fluid within the pulmonary circulation produces intense pulmonary vasospasm and hypertension. When ventilation perfusion mismatch occurs, profound hypoxia ensues. Hypoxia may account for 50% of the mortality within the first hour following onset of symptoms. This initial haemodynamic response is resolved within 15–30 min (in animal models[22]) and may account for its infrequent documentation in the clinical situation.

Following the initial phase there is a phase of haemodynamic compromise caused by left heart failure accompanied by return of right heart parameters to almost normal. The mechanism of the left ventricular dysfunction is unclear.

## CLINICAL FEATURES

A woman in the late stages of labour who becomes acutely dyspnoeic with hypotension; seizures and cardiac arrest may quickly follow. Massive DIC-associated haemorrhage occurs in survivors of the initial event. Most patients die within an hour of onset.

In case reports, patients are described as developing acute shortness of breath, sometimes with a cough, followed by severe hypotension. The following signs and symptoms are indicative of possible AFE:

1. Hypotension.
2. Dyspnoea – laboured breathing and tachypnoea may occur.
3. Seizure – the patient may experience tonic-clonic seizures.
4. Cough – this is usually a manifestation of dyspnoea.
5. Cyanosis – as hypoxia/hypoxaemia progresses, circumoral and peripheral cyanosis and changes in mucous membranes may manifest.
6. Fetal bradycardia occurs as a consequence of the hypoxic insult. Pulmonary oedema identified on chest X-ray.
7. Uterine atony resulting in excessive bleeding after delivery. Failure of the uterus to become firm with bimanual massage is diagnostic.
8. Cardiac arrest.

## MANAGEMENT

### Basic shock management
The treatment is supportive. Initiate cardiopulmonary resuscitation if the patient arrests.

### Circulatory management
1. Treat hypotension with crystalloid and blood products. Use vasopressors as necessary.
2. Women who survive the initial event will require ICU admission. Left heart failure and DIC are common late occurrences.

3. Coagulopathy is treated with fresh frozen plasma (FFP), cryoprecipitate and platelets as directed by the coagulation studies. Activated recombinant factor VIIa has also been used.

### Surgery

Perform emergency caesarean delivery in arrested mothers who are unresponsive to resuscitation.

## DISTRIBUTIVE SHOCK

In distributive shock there is no loss in intravascular volume or cardiac function. The primary defect is a massive vasodilatation leading to relative hypovolaemia, reduced perfusion pressure and, therefore, poorer flow to the tissues.

### SPINAL INJURIES (NEUROGENIC SHOCK)

Spinal cord injuries may produce hypotension and shock as a result of sympathetic nervous system dysfunction. Loss of sympathetic tone causes wide-spread vasodilatation.

### SPECIAL ASPECTS IN MANAGEMENT OF NEUROGENIC SHOCK

Following initial fluid resuscitation, vasopressor drugs may be required to counteract vasodilatation. Atropine may be necessary in high lesions as bradycardia can occur due to unopposed vagal activity.

## ANAESTHESIA

Shock may occur during any form of anaesthesia or analgesia for labour or delivery. This section considers shock associated with regional anaesthesia techniques. Shock caused by general anaesthesia is usually due to adverse drug reaction (anaphylaxis) as discussed above.

### HIGH SPINAL BLOCK

This complication occurs when an absolute or relative overdose of local anaesthetic drug is administered into the epidural or subarachnoid spaces. Factors include:

1. Drug dose for subarachnoid anaesthesia in pregnancy is reduced. Use of 'standard' non-obstetric doses may lead to extensive block.

2. High spinal block may follow excessive spread of an intrathecal injection of an appropriate dose of local anaesthetic.

3. Extensive block may occur following accidental intrathecal injection of a local anaesthetic dose intended for the epidural space. This is particularly true with high concentration doses given for operative delivery. The underlying cause may be drug passing through an unrecognised dural

puncture or migration of the epidural catheter from the epidural space to the intrathecal space.

4. Hypotension can be aggravated by incorrect positioning, particularly absence of lateral tilt causing aortocaval compression.

## Clinical features

All regional anaesthesia techniques produce a degree of sympathetic blockade (causing vasodilatation) and motor blockade (causing weakness). This only becomes a problem when it is extensive. Signs of high block are:

1. Hypotension often preceded by complaint of nausea or generally 'not feeling well'.

2. Bradycardia occurring when the sympathetic blockade reaches the level of the cardio-acceleratory fibres (T1–T4). This leaves unopposed vagal tone.

3. Difficulty in breathing as the block progresses in the cephalad direction as first the intercostal muscles and then the diaphragm are progressively paralysed.

4. Upper limb neurological signs (C5–T1) such as tingling of fingers (C6–T1) and weakness.

## Management

Basic shock management (ABC).

## Special aspects in management of high block

1. Support of the cardiovascular system with vasopressor drugs and inotropes to maintain adequate blood pressure.

2. Sedative agents can be used to reduce the risk of awareness once the initial resuscitation has been effected.

## LOCAL ANAESTHETIC TOXICITY

Toxic side effects of local anaesthetics are related to high plasma drug concentrations. High plasma concentrations can be due to accidental intravenous injection, rapid absorption or absolute overdose. Inadvertent intravenous injection in obstetric anaesthesia may occur most commonly during subcutaneous infiltration or epidural top-up. However, there have been recent reports of inadvertent administration of epidural solutions into intravenous lines with severe consequences.

Infiltration anaesthesia may be used for paracervical or pudendal blocks by obstetricians, without the presence of the anaesthetist. The generous blood supply in this region encourages rapid absorption and increases the risk of toxicity.

## Clinical features

The primary symptoms and signs affect the central nervous system and cardiovascular system.

1. Central nervous system – light headedness, tinnitus, dizziness, circumoral numbness, metallic taste, anxiety, confusion, a feeling of impending doom,

generalised tonic-clonic seizures leading to loss of consciousness and coma and respiratory depression.

2. Cardiovascular system – hypertension and tachycardia may occur in conjunction with convulsions, hypotension and dysrhythmias, refractory cardiorespiratory arrest.

3. CNS toxicity typically precedes CVS toxicity. However, in bupivacaine toxicity, CVS toxicity may occur in the absence of CNS toxicity. Pregnant women appear to be more sensitive to bupivacaine, exhibiting signs of toxicity at lower levels.

### Management
Basic shock management (ABC).

### Special aspects in management of local anaesthetic toxicity

1. Circulation – advanced life support, with external cardiac massage and defibrillation. This may be prolonged as arrhythmias can be very resistant to conventional therapy.

2. Support of the cardiovascular system with vasopressor drugs and inotropes may be necessary to maintain adequate blood pressure.

3. Seizure management – anticonvulsant therapy (diazepam emulsion 5–10 mg can be used to try and control convulsions).

4. Other – LipidRescue™ is a recently reported intervention for the management of local anaesthesia toxicity.[25,26] The initial animal work now seems to have been translated into successful therapeutic use in humans.[27–29] The current treatment regimen is available from the LipidRescue™ website.[30]

5. Caesarean section may be considered as part of the resuscitation in order to salvage the baby.

6. Sedative agents can be used to reduce the risk of awareness once the initial resuscitation has been effected.

---

### Key points in shock management

- Shock results from acute, generalised, inadequate perfusion of the tissues.
- Substandard care is still an issue in the management of the shocked patient.
- Shock is most commonly due to either haemorrhage or sepsis in obstetric cases.
- Massive haemorrhage remains a significant cause of maternal mortality and morbidity.
- Signs of hypovolaemia occur relatively late because of physiological changes in pregnancy.

## Key points in shock management *(continued)*

- Successful management of the shocked patient requires teamwork.

- Obstetric units should have established protocols for dealing with shock and practice 'fire' drills regularly.

- Shock management should commence immediately diagnosis is made aiming for prompt restoration of tissue perfusion and oxygenation. The management of the underlying aetiology is secondary until resuscitation has been instituted.

- All therapy is directed at optimising maternal condition. This is particularly important in the antenatal period as this approach improves intra-uterine conditions for the fetus. Delivery may need to be considered as part of the resuscitation in some forms of shock.

- The resuscitation follows the familiar ABC pattern.

### References

1. Confidential Enquiry into Maternal Deaths in the United Kingdom. *Why Mothers Die 2000–2002.* London: Royal College of Obstetricians and Gynaecologists, 2004.
2. Confidential Enquiry into Maternal Deaths in the United Kingdom. *Why Mothers Die 1997–1999.* London: Royal College of Obstetricians and Gynaecologists, 2001.
3. Lynch JC. Uterine rupture and scar dehiscence. A five year survey. *Anaesth Intensive Care* 1996; **24**: 699–704.
4. CESDI 5th Annual Report published by the Maternal and Child Health Research Consortium in May 1998.
5. Miller D. Vaginal birth after cesarian: a 10 year experience. *Obstet Gynecol* 1994; **84**: 255–258.
6. Caughey AB. Rate of uterine rupture during a trial of labor in women with one or two prior cesarian sections. *Am J Obstet Gynecol* 1999; **181**: 872–876.
7. Hussain M, Jabeen T, Liaquat N *et al.* Acute puerperal uterine inversion. *J Coll Phys Surg Pakistan* 2004; 14: 215–217.
8. Shah-Hosseini R, Evrard JR. Puerperal uterine inversion. *Obstet Gynecol* 1989; **73**: 567–570.
9. O'Sullivan J. Acute inversion of the uterus. *BMJ* 1945; **2**: 282–283.
10. Ogueh O, Ayida G. Acute uterine inversion: a new technique of hydrostatic replacement. *Br J Obstet Gynaecol* 1997; **104**: 951–952.
11. Catling S. Blood conservation techniques in obstetrics: a UK perspective. *Int J Obstet Anesth* 2007; **16**: 241–249.
12. Waters JH, Biscotti MD, Potter PS, Phillipson E. Amniotic fluid removal during cell salvaged in the caesarean section patient. *Anesthesiology* 2000; **92**: 1531–1536.
13. Hansch E, Chitkara U, McAlpine J, El-Sayed Y, Dake MD, Razavi MK. Pelvic arterial embolization for control of obstetric haemorrhage: a five year experience. *Am J Obstet Gynecol* 1999; **180**: 1454–1460.
14. Johanson R, Kumar M, Obhrai M, Young P. Management of massive postpartum haemorrhage: use of a hydrostatic balloon catheter to avoid laparotomy. *Br J Obstet Gynaecol* 2001; **108**: 420–422.
15. Keriakos R, Mukhopadhyay A. The use of the Rusch balloon for management of severe postpartum haemorrhage. *J Obstet Gynaecol* 2006; **26**: 335–338.
16. van den Berghe G, Wouters P, Weekers F *et al.* Intensive insulin therapy in the critically

ill patients. *N Engl J Med* 2001; **345**: 1359–1367.

17. Bernard GR, Vincent JPL, Latherer PF *et al*. Efficacy and safety of recombinant activated protein C for sever sepsis. *N Engl J Med* 2001; **344**: 699–709.

18. Vincent JL, Angus DL, Artigas A *et al*. Effects of drotrecogin alpha activated on organ dysfunction in the PROWESS trial. *Crit Care Med* 2003; **31**: 834–840.

19. Annane D, Sebille V, Charpentier C *et al*. Effect of treatment with low doses of hydrocortisone and fludrocortisone on mortality in patients with septic shock. *JAMA* 2002; **288**: 862–871.

20. Sampson HA, Munoz-Furlong, A, Campbell RL *et al*. Second symposium on the management and definition of anaphylaxis: summary report – second National Institute of Allergy and Infectious Disease/Food allergy and anaphylaxis Network Symposium. *J Allergy Clin Immunol* 2006; **117**: 391–397.

21. Tuffnell DJ. United Kingdom Amniotic Fluid Embolism Register. *Br J Obstet Gynaecol* 2005; **112**: 1625–1629.

22. Hankins GD, Snyder RR, Clark SL, Schwartz L, Patterson WR, Butzin CA. Acute hemodynamic and respiratory effects of amniotic fluid embolism in the pregnant goat model. *Am J Obstet Gynecol* 1993; **168**: 1113–1129, discussion 1129–1130.

23. Farrar SC, Gherman RB: Serum tryptase analysis in a woman with amniotic fluid embolism. A case report. *J Reprod Med* 2001; **46**: 926–928.

24. Clark SL, Hankins GD, Dudley DA *et al*. Amniotic fluid embolism: analysis of the national registry. *Am J Obstet Gynecol* 1995; **172**: 1158–1167, discussion 1167–1169.

25. Picard J, Meek T. Lipid emulsion to treat overdose of local anaesthetic: the gift of the glob. *Anaesthesia* 2006; **61**: 107–109.

26. Weinberg G, Ripper R, Feinstein DL, Hoffman W. Lipid emulsion infusion rescues dogs from bupivacaine-induced cardiac toxicity. *Reg Anesth Pain Med* 2003; **28**: 198–202.

27. Litz RJ, Popp M, Stehr SN, Koch T. Successful resuscitation of a patient with ropivacaine-induced asystole after axillary plexus block using lipid infusion. *Anaesthesia* 2006; **61**: 800–801.

28. Rosenblatt MA, Abel M, Fischer GW *et al*. Successful use of a 20% lipid emulsion to resuscitate a patient after a presumed bupivacaine related cardiac arrest. *Anesthesiology* 2006; **105**: 217–218.

29. Foxall G, McCahon R, Lamb J, Hardman JG, Bedforth NM. Levobupivacaine-induced seizures and cardiovascular collapse treated with Intralipid. *Anaesthesia* 2007; **62**: 516–518.

30. Weinberg G. <www.lipidrescue.org> [Accessed 29 August 2007].

*Norbert Pateisky*

**9**

# Risk management in obstetrics and gynaecology

The publication of the book *To err is human* in 1999 changed the world of risk management in medicine forever.[1] After Brennan and Leape's *Harvard medical practice study* in 1991[2] (the first major publication where all aspects of preventable adverse events in medicine were discussed in detail), preventable errors in medicine started to become a focus of interest.

In summary, it turned out that preventable errors in medical practice were frequent, caused a much patient harm and cost a tremendous amount of money in all Western healthcare systems. Some of the most prominent problems in modern healthcare today include wrong-side surgery, retained foreign bodies, surgical site infections, burns during surgery, mismatched blood transfusion and medication errors. This is especially true for specialities like obstetrics, surgery and anaesthesia, where litigation is also common.

While the number of publications about medical risk management increased rapidly following publication of *To err is human*, success in the acceptance of effective methods in front-line practice has been only moderate. Despite all recommendations to use risk-management methods that have been implemented successfully for more than 30 years in so-called 'high-risk industries' like aviation, nuclear fuels, aircraft carriers, transportation, space travel or petrochemical processing, very few have started to adopt these strategies in clinical practice.

Because risk management is a very frequent problem, with solutions that are relevant to every medical discipline, it will be treated in a general way in this article. The practices that are useful for other specialities are often of importance in obstetrics and gynaecology.

**Norbert Pateisky** MD
Professor of Obstetrics and Gynaecology, Subdepartment of Clinical Risk Management, Department of Obstetrics and Gynecology, University of Vienna, Währinger Gürtel 18–20, A-1090 Vienna, Austria
E-mail: norbert.pateisky@meduniwien.a.at

## THE PROBLEM

'If you know the problem, the solution is quite clear'. Do we know the problem?

It is common knowledge today, that human error is involved in about 70% of all accidents in all industries, including healthcare.[3] While other industries such as military and civil aviation started to solve their problems some 30 years ago, healthcare systems have ignored the facts about human errors for a very long time. Robert Helmreich, a psychologist and pioneer in error management, wrote in one of his papers:[4] 'Error results from physiological and psychological limitations of humans. Causes of error include fatigue, workload, and fear as well as cognitive overload, poor interpersonal communications, imperfect information processing, and flawed decision making.' Effective error-management is based on understanding the nature and extent of human error. However, it is still the case that the consequences of errors in medicine often trigger the 'shame and blame' reaction towards the individuals involved in the case. The nurse or doctor at the end of the chain of events is found guilty for committing the error and for the adverse clinical outcome.

The best model to explain the real background to the great majority of accidents – in medicine and elsewhere – is James Reason's 'Swiss cheese theory'.[5]

In brief, the theory states, that no accident happens without a series of mishaps illustrated by the holes in slices of Swiss cheese. The slices of cheese represent the different stages in a process, while the holes in the cheese represent active and passive errors within each stage. The model thus demonstrates that the main reasons for errors are inherent in the system, rather than being caused by an individual person in the system. In the words of Don Berwick, Chief Executive Officer of the Institute of Health Care Improvement: 'Every system is perfectly designed to achieve exactly the results it gets'.

As long as this fact is ignored in favour of the 'shame and blame' culture, there is no hope for real improvement in risk reduction at the clinical front line. An appropriate or 'just' culture is the precondition to real patient safety and risk management. James Reason describes a 'just culture' as an atmosphere of trust in which people are encouraged (even rewarded) for providing essential safety-related information, but in which they are also clear about where the line must be drawn between acceptable and unacceptable behaviour.

Looking at the main reasons for catastrophes and complications in every industry including healthcare, the so called 'non-technical skills' (NOTECHS), also known as 'soft skills', represents 80% of all cases. Table 1 shows definitions, categorisation and elements of NOTECHS according to Flin *et al.*[6] In all dangerous clinical situations, where errors triggered by environmental and personal factors – high workload, time pressure, stress, insufficient orientation, lack of training, fatigue, illness, *etc.* – that lead to errors and sometimes patient harm, the lack of NOTECHS escalates the danger, as can be shown in aviation as well as in medicine.[7]

In summary, in order to reduce clinical risk successfully, it is necessary to solve the problems that arise because of the limitations of human performance, induced and enforced by environmental, personal and team factors.

These problems are neither addressed nor approached by the most prominent certification systems based on ISO-norms (International Standardisation Organisation) mainly used in European medicine. ISO-based QM-Systems are

**Table 1** Definition, main categories and elements of non-technical skills (NOTECHS)

> **Situational awareness**
> Developing and maintaining a dynamic awareness of the situation in theatre based on assembling data from the environment (patient, team, time, displays, equipment); understanding what they mean, and thinking ahead about what may happen next
> > Gathering information
> > Understanding information
> > Projecting and anticipating future state
>
> **Decision making**
> Skills for diagnosing the situation and reaching a judgement in order to choose an appropriate course of action
> > Considering options
> > Selecting and communicating option
> > Implementing and reviewing decisions
>
> **Communication and teamwork**
> Skills for working in a team context to ensure that the team has an acceptable shared picture of the situation and can complete tasks effectively
> > Exchanging information
> > Establishing a shared understanding
> > Co-ordinating team activities
>
> **Leadership**
> Leading the team and providing direction, demonstrating high standards of clinical practice and care, and being considerate about the needs of individual team members
> > Setting and maintaining standards
> > Supporting others
> > Coping with pressure
>
> Based on the classification of Flin et al.[6]

very effective in situations similar to assembly lines and also in blood banks, pharmacies, or laboratories, but have virtually no impact upon the emergency situations which arise frequently in clinical medicine, notably in obstetrics, emergency departments, surgery and anaesthesia.

In clinical practice, the definition of standard operation procedures (SOPs) such as PAP smear sampling, assisted delivery and many others, together with the necessary skills to perform them, are essential to provide a standardised routine service. SOPs have also been defined for clinical risk management (RM-SOP) but these are not widely known or accepted by healthcare workers at the front line. Examples of tools and RM-SOPs, including the skills required to use the tools in an effective way, are given in Tables 2 and 3.

High-risk industries can demonstrate that the acceptance of the value of tools and of RM-SOPs, including the need for 'non technical skills' in areas such as education, training and practice procedures, is an essential precondition for effective risk-management strategies. Again, the most important problems relate to poor communication and teamwork, important components of the NOTECHS system.

A number of different skills and tools (e.g. Reporting Systems, Root Cause Analysis, Failure Mode Effect Analysis, Outcome Monitoring, M&M Conferences, Improvement Strategies and Just Culture) are important in the field of clinical risk management. Unfortunately, without specific risk-management tools, such as RM-SOPs and NOTECHS, all of the aforementioned elements will have very little effect in reducing clinical risk at the front line. Therefore, the following sections will concentrate on this topic and will specifically address the question of how to implement risk management in the clinical situation.

## RISK MANAGEMENT TOOLS AND CORRESPONDING STANDARD OPERATING PROCEDURE

Acceptance and correct use of RM-SOPs is essential for effective risk reduction. The benefits and corresponding SOPs for the correct use of the most important tools are listed in Tables 2 and 3.

**Table 2** Tools of risk management

| |
|---|
| • Checklists |
| • Communication strategies (closed loop, read back, repeat back) |
| • Briefings |
| • Debriefings |

**Table 3** Standard operation procedures of risk management (RM-SOP)

| |
|---|
| • Correct use of checklists |
| • Skills of safe communication strategies |
| • Use of briefings |
| • Use of debriefings |

## CHECKLISTS

### Benefit

It is easily demonstrated that humans have very limited ability to remember more than five items at once. Activities such as going on vacation or visiting the supermarket encourage us to use checklists. Well-designed and complete checklists prevent us from forgetting things, even those that are not important – but only if we use them!

Checklists additionally free our minds for other more complex problems that cannot be managed successfully by such simple techniques.

### Clinical example

Treatment of an eclamptic seizure.

### How to perform the SOP

Checklists are only effective if they are used every time you perform the specific procedure, even when you are fully trained. When you are tired, when there is work overload or when there is some other operational problem, you will avoid problems if you are convinced of the value of a checklist and trained in its use.

## CLOSED LOOP COMMUNICATION

### Benefit

There are a number of situations in which we all use closed loop communication to ensure that information is correctly transmitted. The benefit is clear – there will be no misunderstandings.

### Clinical example

Ordering high-risk medications such as cytotoxic chemotherapy or anticoagulants.

### How to perform the SOP

Think about asking for a telephone number, or ordering food at McDonalds. The technique is:

1. Say it.

2. Ask the recipient to repeat it or write it down and read it.

3. Confirm it.

This is the best way to know whether the information has been understood correctly. The technique is valuable when ordering high-risk medications or medications that sound alike, such as Dioval/Diovan, Lasix/Luvox, Taxol/Taxotere and many others.

## BRIEFING

### Benefit

A briefing is a structured type of interaction used to achieve clear and effective communication in a timely manner. Each of us feels better as a team member if we know the plan of the team. It is evident that sports teams or orchestras will be more successful if all members are aware of the plan.

### Clinical example

Before starting an operation, confirm the following important information: (i) identification of the patient; (ii) correct procedure; (iii) correct site and side; (iv) possible allergies; and (v) previous drug reactions.

### How to perform the SOP

To make briefings successful, they must be clear, short and precise. Ideally there should also be the opportunity for questions from team members. Briefing should take place as a minimum: (i) at the start of the day; (ii) prior to a procedure; (iii) as the situation changes; and (iv) during hand-offs (*e.g.* breaks, shift change, *etc.*).

## DEBRIEFING

### Benefit

Whenever a team has completed an activity, there should be a short session including all team members to review the mission. This provides the greatest chance for individuals and teams to learn and thereby improve their future performance.

**Clinical example**

Following an obstetrical emergency

**How to perform the SOP**

The entire team meets and reviews the management which has taken place. Three questions should be answered: (i) what went well; (ii) what did not go so well; and (iii) what should we do next time?

## NON-TECHNICAL SKILLS (NOTECHS)

Technical skills are essential but are often not enough to get everything right – consider a perfect operation performed on the wrong side of the body. This type of risk may be minimised by using so-called 'non technical skills' (NOTECHS). The main categories and elements of NOTECHS are listed in Table 1 using the classification of Flin et al.[6]

When things have gone wrong in other industries, these skills have been found to have made a major contribution in up to 80% of cases. Examples include the loss of Challenger and the disasters at Chernobyl and Three Mile Island. The current education and training of surgeons focuses on knowledge, clinical expertise and technical skills. NOTECHS are often ignored completely.

A significant problem in dealing with NOTECHS was that they could not be measured objectively. However, this problem now seems to have been overcome. Professor Rhona Flin and her group at the University of Aberdeen have developed the NOTSS (Non-Technical Skills for Surgeons) rating scale for use in operating theatres.[8] The NOTSS system allows explicit rating and feedback to be given in relation to non-technical skills. It is, in effect, a behavioural marker system and may be used to structure training and evaluation of non-technical skills in surgery in a similar fashion to current practice in anaesthesia, civil aviation and the nuclear power industry.

## EFFECTIVE RISK MANAGEMENT IN CLINICAL MEDICINE

This section illustrates how RM-SOPs and NOTECHS can be used together.

The fact that certain catastrophes in medicine (e.g. wrong-side surgery and transfusion errors) happen over and over again is a clear indicator that we have not yet solved the problem of risk reduction at the front line.[9] In the words of Paul Watzlawick: 'If you have not found a solution for your problem, it is not the problem, but the solution you have to work on'. So what can we do to become as successful in risk and error reduction as high-risk industries have been for many years?

1. We have to accept that we, as humans, are limited in error-free performance by the so-called 'human performance limitations' mentioned above. To achieve this goal, it is necessary to have interactive classroom teaching involving all members of healthcare teams (nurses, doctors, midwives, secretaries and others). Didactic teaching without interactivity will not achieve the target. At the end, the trainees should be convinced that one needs the SOPs of risk management (Tables 1 and 2) to overcome the 'human factor'.

2. We have to teach and reinforce the RM-SOPs that protect us from committing errors and help us in critical situations to achieve the best possible outcomes, whether working alone or in teams. Even if you are convinced of the value of RM-SOPs and have been trained to perform them correctly, it is likely that you will fail in real life, if you ignore the use of NOTECHS. Lack of NOTECHS results in team and communication problems impairing good outcomes. One of the major problems in this context is the hierarchical structure of medical practice.[10]

3. Consequently, after education and training in RM-SOPs, one needs to be trained in NOTECHS to perform effective risk reduction in clinical medicine.

## CONCLUSIONS

The main reason for inadequate risk management in healthcare is the fact that most care-givers ignore effective strategies and the need for appropriate systemic implementation of risk management at the front line. Hierarchical working practices and the 'shame and blame' culture have to be eradicated in favour of a 'Just Culture' to overcome these problems. It has been demonstrated by other industries that effective risk reduction is only possible when the problems surrounding ethos, human performance limitations and non-technical skills are taken into account and treated seriously. Obstetricians and gynaecologists, a group of doctors who are frequently exposed to risky situations, should be among the first to implement these effective strategies.

## References

1. Corrigan J, Kohn LT, Corrigan J, Donaldson MS. (eds) *To Err Is Human: Building a Safer Health System*. Washington, DC: National Academy Press, 2000.
2. Brennan TA, Leape LL, Laird NM *et al*. Incidence of adverse events and negligence in hospitalized patients: results of the Harvard Medical Practice Study I. *N Engl J Med* 1991; **324**: 370–377.
3. Helmreich RL, Foushee HC. Why crew resource management? Empirical and theoretical bases of human factors training in aviation. In: Wiener E, Kanki B, Helmreich R. (eds) *Cockpit resource management*. San Diego, CA: Academic Press, 1993; 3–45.
4. Helmreich LH. On error management: lessons from aviation. *BMJ* 2000; 320: 781–785.
5. Reason J. The Swiss cheese model of defenses. In: Reason J. (ed) *Managing the risks of organizational accidents*. Aldershot: Ashgate, 1997; 9.
6. Flin R, Maran N. Identifying and training non-technical skills for teams in acute medicine. *Qual Safety Health Care* 2004; **13**: 80–88.
7. Leonard M, Graham S, Bonacum D. The human factor: the critical importance of effective teamwork and communication in providing safe care. *Qual Safety Health Care* 2004; **13**: 85–90.
8. University of Aberdeen. *NOTSS: Non-Technical Skills for Surgeons*. <www.abdn.ac.uk/iprc/notss> Last updated 9 March 2007.
9. Leape LL, Berwick DM. Five years after *To Err Is Human* – What have we learned? *JAMA* 2005; **293**: 2384–2390.
10. Walton MM. Hierarchies: the Berlin Wall of patient safety. *Qual Safety Health Care* 2006; **15**: 229–230.

*Jane Hook  Michael Seckl*

# 10

# Management of trophoblastic disease

Gestational trophoblastic disease (GTD) is an umbrella term for a group of pregnancy-related disorders arising from abnormal placental trophoblast cells. It encompasses two pre-malignant conditions – partial and complete hydatidiform moles (PHM, CHM) – and the malignant gestational trophoblastic neoplasias (GTN): invasive mole (IM), choriocarcinoma (CC) and the very rare placental site trophoblastic tumour (PSTT). All forms of GTD produce β-human chorionic gonadotrophin (β-hCG). The amount of β-hCG correlates with disease volume and so monitoring this hormone is an accurate biomarker for screening, diagnosis, therapeutic response and follow-up of women with GTD. Hydatidiform mole (HM), the commonest form of the disease, occurs in 1 in 714 pregnancies in the UK[1] and about 8% become malignant. GTN is a significant cause of morbidity, loss of fertility and, rarely, mortality in young women. However, it is now highly treatable due to its remarkable sensitivity to chemotherapy. The successful outcome for patients with GTD has been greatly facilitated by the establishment, in 1973, of a centralised registration and treatment system in the UK. Depending on geographical location, patients are registered in London (Charing Cross Hospital), Sheffield (Weston Park Hospital) or Dundee (Ninewells Hospital) for hCG surveillance, enabling early detection of GTN which is then treated either at Charing Cross or Sheffield. This has enabled the development of effective and safe management policies which are now used worldwide.

**Jane Hook** MBBChir MA(Cantab) MRCP
Specialist Registrar in Medical Oncology, St James' Institute of Oncology, St James' University Hospital, LeedsLS9 7TF, UK

**Michael Seckl** MBBS MD FRCP PhD (for correspondence)
Professor, Gestational Trophoblastic Disease Unit, Department of Medical Oncology, Charing Cross Hospital, Fulham Palace Road, London W6 8RF, UK
E-mail: m.seckl@imperial.ac.uk

Areas of on-going research and development in GTD include:

1. Understanding of the pathogenesis of gestational trophoblastic disease, particularly its genetic basis.

2. Improving the accuracy of diagnosis in early hydatidiform mole and identifying factors which predict transformation to gestational trophoblastic neoplasias.

3. Improving outcome for patients with relapsed or drug-resistant disease.

4. Improving the accuracy of human chorionic gonadotrophin monitoring.

This chapter describes recent advances in these areas and provides an overview of current evidence-based management of GTD based on our practice at Charing Cross Hospital.

## THE SPECTRUM OF GESTATIONAL TROPHOBLASTIC DISEASE

### PREMALIGNANT

Hydatidiform moles are abnormal conception events, which produce rapidly growing, highly vascular, placenta-like structures. They usually present with symptoms of early pregnancy failure and abnormal, but non-specific, appearance on ultrasound.[2] Untreated, they can result in life-threatening complications from local disease (vaginal bleeding and uterine rupture) and, uniquely for a premalignant lesion, spread to distant organs (respiratory failure from metastases or tumour emboli). Overall, 16% of CHM and 0.5% of PHM undergo malignant transformation and all cases are followed up for this by serial hCG monitoring (Figs 1 & 2).[3] It is now clear that PHM can give rise to all forms of GTN and must be followed up as closely as CHM.[3,4]

The incidence of CHM is 0.5–1 per 1000 pregnancies in Europe compared to 3 in 1000 for PHM.[2] Up to 90% of first trimester PHM may be misclassified as non molar abortion due to subtle pathological changes and the presence of

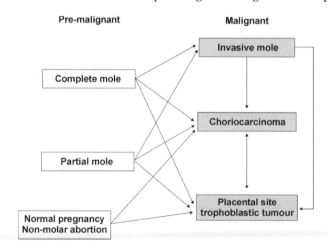

**Fig. 1** The spectrum of gestational trophoblastic disease. Normal pregnancy and pre-malignant molar pregnancy both give rise to gestational trophoblastic neoplasia.

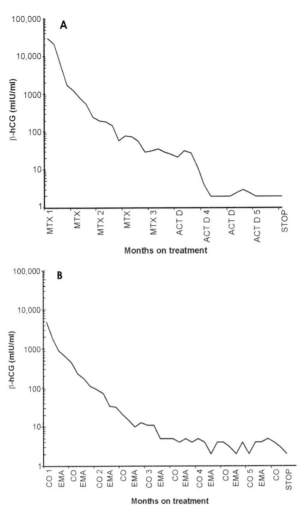

**Fig. 2** Monitoring response to chemotherapy by hCG levels. (A) Low-risk disease, developing methotrexate resistance; (B) high-risk disease successfully treated with EMA/CO chemotherapy.

some fetal material.[5] Risk factors for HM include maternal age (≤ 15 and ≥40 years old) and prior molar pregnancy. The risk of a second CHM is 1 in 76 and rises to 1 in 6.5 for a third.[6] There is ethnic variation in the incidence of HM with increased rates in Asian women.[1] The vast majority of cases are sporadic but an extremely rare familial syndrome of recurrent CHM has been described. These cases are of great interest in the search for the underlying genetic basis of HM. Rarely, a molar pregnancy may develop as a twin to a normal embryo. With careful monitoring and specialist obstetric care, 40% of these cases have continued into the third trimester and delivered live babies.[7]

Sporadic CHMs are androgenetic in origin. In most cases, a genetically empty ovum is fertilised by a single haploid sperm that then duplicates, forming a CHM with a homozygous 46XX karyotype. In a minority of cases, fertilisation is by two haploid sperm, producing a heterozygous 46XX or 46XY CHM. In contrast, PHMs are genetically biparental, usually with a triploid karyotype, and arise due to fertilisation of a normal egg by two sperm. Tetraploid PHMs have also been described. For a triploid embryo to give rise to a PHM pregnancy, at least two of the chromosome sets must be paternal.[8]

Cases were previously defined as PHM or CHM on the basis of classical pathological findings but, with most cases now presenting in the first trimester, these changes are increasingly of historical interest and new pathological techniques have been developed to differentiate the two.

## GESTATIONAL TROPHOBLASTIC NEOPLASIA

GTN arises when the normal regulatory mechanisms controlling the proliferation and invasiveness of trophoblastic tissue are lost.[9] The molecular changes underlying this transformation are not yet known.

IM and CC are neoplastic lesions arising from villous trophoblasts, whereas the cell of origin of PSTT is the intermediate trophoblast. Differentiating between IM and CC following a molar pregnancy is not clinically important: they tend to behave in the same way and respond to the same treatments. However, PSTT is important to recognise as it has distinct clinicopathological behaviour.

### Invasive mole

Invasive mole is a CHM or PHM that invades the myometrium. It is diagnosed on the basis of a persistent or rising hCG following evacuation of a HM, and radiological imaging suggesting the presence of molar tissue.

### Gestational choriocarcinoma

Gestational CC can follow any type of pregnancy and, although its incidence is greatest in the first year, the interval from the causative pregnancy can be highly variable. The longest interval on record at Charing Cross Hospital is 35 years. Rarely, the disease can also present during pregnancy. CHM is the most frequent antecedent pregnancy. The incidence of CC is hard to calculate as most cases are simply labelled as post-molar GTN but the incidence of CC following non-molar pregnancy is estimated at 1 in 50,000.

CC is extremely aggressive forming highly vascular lesions at any site in the body. Patients usually present with bleeding, which is most commonly vaginal but may also be from metastases. Around a third present with metastatic disease and this may be as a clinical emergency – for example: (i) respiratory failure from large volume lung disease; (ii) pulmonary haemorrhage or intra-abdominal haemorrhage; and (iii) neurological abnormalities due to cerebral metastases or haemorrhage. The diagnosis of CC should be considered in all women of reproductive age who present with one of these acute events as it can be easily confirmed by hCG testing, and the initiation of emergency chemotherapy is life-saving.

### Placental site trophoblastic tumour

PSTT is an extremely rare variant of GTN that most commonly follows a normal pregnancy but has been described following CHM, PHM and CC. There are just over 200 cases recorded in the literature. It arises at the placental implantation site and may be difficult to differentiate from benign placental site nodules. Review of suspected cases by specialist pathologists is essential.

It is usually slow growing and late to metastasise, spreading locally through the uterine wall and to pelvic lymph nodes as well as to the lungs, brain and elsewhere. The usual presentation is with irregular vaginal bleeding. An important clue to the diagnosis of PSTT versus CC is a low level of hCG relative to tumour burden. This is because hCG is produced in high levels by syncytiotrophoblasts, which are not present in PSTT, and only in low levels by intermediate trophoblasts. However, in our experience of over 60 cases, it is still an accurate biomarker. Unlike other forms of GTD, PSTT is relatively chemo-insensitive and surgery is the main-stay of treatment.[10]

### Epithelioid trophoblastic tumour

Recently, the existence of another distinct neoplasm arising from intermediate trophoblasts has been suggested. This has been termed epithelioid trophoblastic tumour.[11] Only a handful of cases have been described; so far, these have been managed in the same way as PSTT.

## STEPS TOWARDS ELUCIDATING THE GENETIC BASIS OF GTD

### HYDATIDIFORM MOLE

The theory of an underlying genetic cause of HM is based on two observations: (i) women who have had one mole have an excess risk of having another; and (ii) the discovery of an inherited syndrome of recurrent CHM pregnancies which has been identified in a handful of families globally. Familial CHM is diagnosed by the presence of more than one woman in a single family with ≥2 CHM and is inherited in an autosomal recessive pattern. These families are being extensively studied with the aim of identifying specific genetic abnormalities and their role in the pathogenesis of HM.

In sporadic cases, the HM phenotype is thought to be caused by an excess of paternal genes. However, all cases of familial CHM are genetically biparental with a normal complement of maternal and paternal chromosomes.[12] In these cases, there must be abnormal gene expression during embryogenesis that results in a paternal pattern of expression analogous to that found in androgenetic CHM. It has, therefore, been suggested that familial CHMs are caused by an inherited failure of maternal imprinting. Genetic imprinting is a process that occurs during gametogenesis and embryogenesis through epigenetic modification of the genome by methylation, and results in differential expression of the maternal and paternal alleles of the same gene. In support of this theory, underexpression of an imprinted gene has been demonstrated in cases of both familial and sporadic CHM,[13] and abnormal methylation patterns in another family.[14]

Extensive mapping studies have been performed on the families. These have demonstrated a defective locus at 19q13.4 in five families and this abnormality has, excitingly, been localised to a single gene – NALP7.[15] This is the first causative single gene defect identified in HM. NALP7 protein is a member of the CATERPILLER family, which is involved in inflammation and apoptosis. It is expressed in oocytes and endometrium and is a negative regulator of the pro-inflammatory cytokine IL-1β, which is involved in regulating trophoblast invasion during implantation. It is unclear how defects in *NALP7* result in HM formation but abnormal inflammation during embryogenesis is likely to be involved.

However, identification of *NALP7* is not the end of the story:

1. *NALP7* does not appear to be involved in the establishment of imprinting. Defects in *NALP7* may be a consequence of abnormal imprinting rather than its cause.

2. Further families have been identified that do not map to 19q13.4 proving that familial HM is genetically heterogeneous.[16]

3. Abnormal *NALP7* has not yet been demonstrated in sporadic cases.

The search for further gene defects and the molecular basis of HM is on-going.

## CHORIOCARCINOMA

Historically, cytogenetic studies of CC have demonstrated a diverse range of abnormalities. Recently, microsatellite studies have shown loss of heterozygosity at specific regions – deletions of 7p12-q11.2, amplification of 7q21-q31, and loss of 8p12-p21.[17] Abnormalities in the latter two are also found in some cases of ovarian and breast cancer and are postulated to encode novel tumour suppressor genes. Several groups have reproduced these findings in non-molar CC but results in post-molar CC have been inconsistent.[18] Only a minority of tumours showed loss of heterozygosity for all three regions suggesting that these defects are acquired late in the development of CC and not essential for malignant transformation. It was hoped that these loci would correspond to defects found in HM and be predictive of malignant transformation. This is a major goal in GTD research but no reliable genetic markers have yet been identified.

## IMPROVING DIAGNOSTIC ACCURACY IN EARLY HYDATIDIFORM MOLE

The mean age at evacuation of a HM is now 9.4 weeks. At this early stage, HM may be confused with non-molar abortion, and CHM can be morphologically similar to PHM. Ploidy analysis, by flow cytometry or digital image analysis, can differentiate between diploid and triploid lesions. It can, therefore, identify a PHM but cannot definitively diagnose a diploid lesion as CHM.

The most significant recent development in the pathological analysis of HM is the use of p57$^{kip2}$ immunostaining to make a definitive diagnosis of androgenetic CHM as opposed to a hydropic abortion or a PHM. *p57$^{kip2}$* is a paternally imprinted gene, which is maternally expressed. The absence of maternal genes in androgenetic CHM means that the gene cannot be expressed in CHM cytotrophoblasts so p57$^{kip2}$ staining is negative in contrast to PHM, hydropic abortion and normal placenta. This technique is well validated, easy and inexpensive to perform.[19]

Identification of cases of HM that will subsequently undergo malignant transformation is also a goal for the histopathologists. There is developing evidence that these HMs are more likely to show telomerase activity (*i.e.* have limitless replicative potential) and increased expression of the anti-apoptotic gene *Mcl-1*.[20] These findings need further prospective evaluation.

## MANAGEMENT OF GESTATIONAL TROPHOBLASTIC DISEASE

The management of most cases of GTD is well established, with the majority of patients being cured after one line of treatment. For this group, the focus is now on optimising treatment regimens and defining the period of follow-up needed. However, outcomes for patients with relapsed and resistant GTN can still be improved and there is no universally agreed standard of care. The management of PSTT is distinct and, unlike other forms of GTN, usually results in loss of fertility – fertility-sparing surgery is an area of on-going interest.

### HYDATIDIFORM MOLE

Initial treatment for a suspected HM is surgical; this will be curative in the majority of cases with spontaneous regression of any residual molar tissue at both intra-uterine and distant sites and return of hCG levels to normal. Only 1 in 10 cases go on to require chemotherapy. They should undergo suction evacuation only, as any other form of surgical intervention (including hysterectomy) or use of drugs to induce uterine contraction increases the likelihood of needing chemotherapy and the risk of trophoblastic embolism. Post-evacuation, all cases must be registered with a trophoblast screening centre for hCG surveillance to ensure early detection of post-molar GTN. Serum hCG levels are measured fortnightly until normalisation, and urine levels analysed monthly after this. The risk of developing GTN is greatest in the first 6 months following diagnosis – 98% of cases at Charing Cross Hospital present within this time-frame. Post-HM surveillance for all cases has, therefore, been reduced to 6 months after spontaneous hCG normalisation.[21] Women should avoid becoming pregnant during this period; the only extra monitoring recommended in subsequent pregnancies are hCG checks at 6 and 10 weeks post-delivery. The oral contraceptive pill should not be used until hCG levels have returned to normal (it may act as a growth factor for trophoblastic tissue) but is safe to use after this.

In patients with elevated hCG post evacuation and/or recurrent symptoms, it can be tempting to carry out a second evacuation. However, this is not routinely recommended, as most patients will still need chemotherapy. This is especially true for patients with high initial hCG levels; up to 80% of those with a pre-interventional hCG > 5000 IU/l undergoing a second evacuation subsequently receive chemotherapy.[22] Routine repeat evacuation exposes patients to the risk of a surgical procedure without the benefits of increased chance of cure. However, it may be useful for symptom control in selected patients with heavy bleeding, or curative if the recurrent molar tissue is confined to the uterine cavity, particularly in those with hCG levels < 1500 IU/l.[23] Cases where second evacuation is contemplated should be discussed with the trophoblast centre.

**Table 1** Indications for chemotherapy in GTD

- Histological evidence of choriocarcinoma
- Evidence of metastases in brain, liver or gastrointestinal tract, or radiological opacities > 2 cm on chest X-ray
- Pulmonary, vulval or vaginal metastases unless hCG falling
- Heavy vaginal bleeding or evidence of gastrointestinal or intraperitoneal haemorrhage
- Rising hCG after evacuation
- Serum hCG > 20,000 IU/l more than 4 weeks after evacuation, because of the risk of uterine perforation
- Elevated hCG 6 months after evacuation even if still falling

## GESTATIONAL TROPHOBLASTIC NEOPLASIA

The management of post-molar GTN and *de novo* CC is the same, and determined by FIGO prognostic score. Indications for assessment at a trophoblast centre and commencement of chemotherapy are listed in Table 1. During chemotherapy, response to treatment is monitored by intense hCG surveillance. In all cases, chemotherapy is given until normalisation of serum hCG and then continues for a consolidation phase of 6–8 weeks.

### Initial assessment

Initial assessment comprises history, examination, serum/urine hCG, chest X-ray and pelvic Doppler ultrasonography. Demonstration of a vascular mass (without evidence of fetal material) on ultrasonography in the context of an elevated hCG is highly suggestive of GTN.[2] The volume of the uterus should be measured; this correlates with tumour burden and is a prognostic indicator. Molar tissue has a low resistance circulation due to arteriovenous shunting.

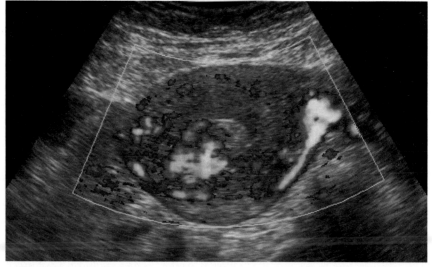

**Fig. 3** Large volume, highly vascular persistent molar tissue seen on Doppler ultrasonography of the uterus.

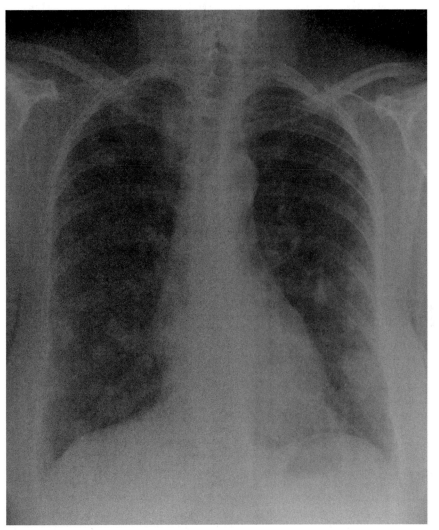

**Fig. 4** Extensive lung metastases visible on chest X-ray in a patient with an invasive mole.

The degree of shunting can be measured by Doppler studies calculating the pulsatility index (PI) of the uterine arteries. PI is an independent predictor of response to chemotherapy; low PI is an adverse prognostic factor.[24] It is being developed as a biomarker for monitoring response to treatment and is likely to be included in future prognostic scoring systems (Fig. 3). The presence of lung metastases on chest X-ray is predictive of CNS disease (Fig. 4); all patients with probable lung metastases should have a lumbar puncture and measurement of CSF hCG after CNS imaging confirms that it is safe to perform the procedure. A CSF:serum hCG ratio of > 1:60 is highly suggestive of the presence of CNS metastases. Further imaging for post-molar patients is only indicated in those with high-risk disease, or clinical features suggestive of metastases. Full staging is by computed tomography (CT) of the chest and abdomen, and magnetic resonance imaging (MRI) of the brain. Patients with CC and PSTT should also have an MRI of the pelvis.

**Table 2** FIGO anatomical staging

| | |
|---|---|
| Stage I | Disease confined to the uterus |
| Stage II | Disease outside of the uterus but limited to the genital structures |
| Stage III | Disease extends to the lungs with or without known genital tract involvement |
| Stage IV | All other metastatic sites |

**Table 3** FIGO prognostic score

| | 0 | 1 | 2 | 4 |
|---|---|---|---|---|
| Age (years) | ≤ 39 | >39 | | |
| Antecedent pregnancy | Hydatidiform mole | Abortion | Term pregnancy | |
| Interval from index pregnancy, months | < 4 | 4–6 | 7–12 | > 12 |
| Pretreatment hCG (mIU/ml) | < $10^3$ | $10^3$–$10^4$ | > $10^4$–$10^5$ | > $10^5$ |
| Largest tumour size, including uterus | 3–4 cm | 5 cm | | |
| Site of metastases | | Spleen, kidney | GI tract | Brain, liver |
| Previous failed chemotherapy | | | Single drug | Two or more drugs |

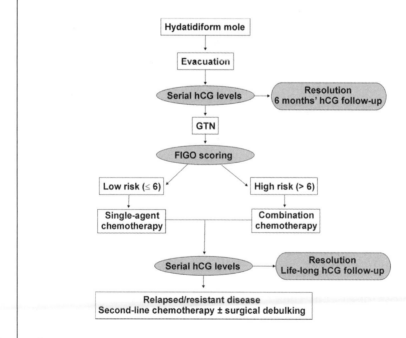

**Fig. 5** Management decisions in GTN.

## Prognostic score and staging

A single, universally accepted, anatomical staging and prognostic scoring system for GTN was developed by FIGO in 2000 (Tables 2 and 3).[25]

The prognostic score is central to the management of GTN (Fig. 5). It predicts the likelihood of a tumour developing resistance to single-agent chemotherapy and has been extensively validated. Patients are classified at diagnosis and divided into two categories – low-risk (score 0–6) and high-risk (score ≥7) to determine what chemotherapy regimen they receive. It is also predictive of the likelihood of cure: patients with low-risk disease have 5-year survival rates of nearly 100% which falls to 86% in high-risk disease.[26] Within the high-risk group, further adverse prognostic factors have been identified which include: (i) longer duration from antecedent pregnancy;[27] (ii) the presence of liver metastases; and (iii) combined liver and brain metastases. Long-term survival in patients with both liver and brain metastases is only 10%.[28]

## Treatment of low-risk patients

The aim of treatment in low-risk disease is to achieve cure without exposure to toxic chemotherapy. The majority of patients are cured with single agent chemotherapy, either methotrexate or actinomycin D. Neither agent has been shown to be superior but methotrexate with folinic acid rescue is most widely used due to its favourable safety/side-effect profile. A typical treatment regimen, and possible side-effects, is listed in Table 4. It is usually extremely well tolerated, there is no alopecia, myelosuppression is rare and there have been no reported cases of second malignancies.[29]

**Table 4** Low-risk treatment regimen

| | |
|---|---|
| Methotrexate/folinic acid | Cycle repeated every 14 days |
| Methotrexate | 50 mg by intramuscular injection repeated every 48 h for a total of 4 doses |
| Folinic acid | 15 mg orally 30 h after each injection of methotrexate |
| Typical side-effects | Stomatitis, conjunctivitis, abdominal and chest pain |

Methotrexate resistance is indicated by plateaued or rising hCG levels. Cure will no longer be achieved with methotrexate alone and alternative chemotherapy is needed – either single agent actinomycin D or combination chemotherapy depending on the hCG level (and thus likelihood of being cured with second-line single agent therapy). The cure rate for these patients remains nearly 100%, even for the rare cases who need three or more lines of treatment.[27]

## Treatment of high-risk patients

The likelihood of achieving cure with single agent chemotherapy in patients who fall into the high-risk category is low. Inadequate intensity of initial treatment and development of resistance in high-risk patients is associated with worse outcome. Therefore, these patients receive first-line combination chemotherapy. The most widely used regimen is EMA/CO (Table 5), which has remission rates of 80–95%,[26] but alternative regimens are in use. A recent

**Table 5** High-risk treatment regimen (EMA/CO)

| | |
|---|---|
| Week 1, days 1–2 | Etoposide/actinomycin D/methotrexate + folinic acid rescue |
| Week 2, day 8 | Vincristine/cyclophosphamide |
| Typical side-effects | Myelosuppression – granulocyte colony stimulating factor used to prevent neutropenia and maintain dose intensity |
| | Nausea/vomiting, mucositis, reversible alopecia, neuropathy |

meta-analysis failed to demonstrate the superiority of any regimen.[30] Short-term side-effects may be significant and, in the long term, there is a small excess risk of second malignancies, particularly acute myeloid leukaemia, breast and colon cancer.[29] Future fertility is not affected but age at menopause is lowered by an average of 3 years.[31]

At Charing Cross Hospital, all patients with lung metastases receive three doses of prophylactic intrathecal methotrexate. Those with proven CNS disease are treated with a modified EMA/CO containing higher doses of methotrexate plus fortnightly intrathecal methotrexate for the duration of their treatment.

## Management of residual post-treatment masses

After completing chemotherapy, patients are re-imaged. Pelvic ultrasound is repeated plus any investigations that were abnormal at diagnosis. The presence of a residual radiological abnormality can cause concern – does it still harbour active cancer cells and will it increase the risk of relapse?

Post-treatment Doppler ultrasonography may show the presence of uterine vascular malformations. These can haemorrhage and, in rare cases, cause massive vaginal or intraperitoneal bleeding. Intervention is not necessary unless there is active bleeding. If needed, uterine artery embolisation is a safe and effective treatment, avoiding the need for hysterectomy in the majority of cases. Patients with untreated vascular malformations and those post-embolisation have had successful pregnancies.[32]

At our centre, the recommended management of a residual metastatic mass depends on its anatomical site. Residual brain lesions are excised or treated with stereotactic radiotherapy. Chemotherapy penetration of the CNS may be reduced by the blood–brain barrier, increasing the likelihood of residual disease and making subsequent treatment with chemotherapy more difficult. Residual masses at other anatomical sites are generally not resected and follow-up is by standard hCG surveillance. Recent papers have demonstrated that patients with unresected residual lung masses are at no increased risk of relapse relative to similar patients who had a complete radiological response.[33,34] Complete serological response is necessary for cure but complete radiological response is not.

## Treatment of resistant and relapsed high-risk disease

GTN is one of a very small minority of malignant conditions where patients who progress on or after primary chemotherapy still have a good chance of cure (> 90% overall 5-year survival in a recent case series[27]). This is due to their exquisite chemotherapy sensitivity – the majority of patients who develop resistance to primary chemotherapy will still be cured after a second, or even third or fourth line of treatment. Relapsed, high-risk disease is defined by a rising hCG after complete serological response to EMA/CO chemotherapy (*i.e.* having at least 6 weeks of normal hCG values post-chemotherapy); resistant, or refractory, cases are those that have a rising, or plateaued, hCG while on EMA/CO.

Management of these patients is multidisciplinary, requiring careful radiological assessment to identify sites of potentially resectable disease and liaison with appropriate surgical teams. [18]FDG-PET may be used to locate sites of disease in cases showing serological relapse without visible abnormality on conventional imaging.[35] Treatment is usually with surgical resection plus postoperative chemotherapy or salvage chemotherapy alone. If no sites of disease are identified, a hysterectomy may be appropriate as the most likely site of relapse is uterine. The most effective second-line chemotherapy is EMA/EP, a weekly alternating regimen of EMA and etoposide plus cisplatin. This regimen is toxic but has reported remission rates of > 80%. An emerging, less toxic, alternative is a fortnightly regimen of Paclitaxel + Cisplatin alternating with Paclitaxel + Etoposide.[36]

Management beyond second line treatment is not clear and should be considered on an individual basis. Further surgery may be appropriate. A possible strategy is high-dose chemotherapy with peripheral blood stem cell rescue. There have been isolated case reports of patients with sustained remission following high-dose treatment, but a recent retrospective analysis of 11 patients undergoing this treatment at three trophoblast centres between 1993–2004 showed that only two patients achieved a transient response (lasting 4 and 12 months each).[37]

Developing evidence-based strategies for treating these patients is difficult due to their small numbers. Identifying prognostic factors for risk stratification and to guide treatment choice may be helpful. Recent analysis of patients undergoing second-line treatment at Charing Cross Hospital has shown different outcomes in patients with relapsed versus refractory disease. Five-year survival for patients with relapsed high-risk disease was 84% compared to 43% for those with refractory disease showing the need to identify effective treatments for this group of patients with chemoresistant disease.[27] Possibilities include the use of new chemotherapy agents (either alone or in combination with established drugs, *e.g.* the antimetabolite gemcitabine) or molecular-targeted therapies.

## Follow-up after chemotherapy

After successful treatment, patients are followed up by regular hCG surveillance (Table 6). The overall risk of relapse is 3% and is greatest in the first year. Currently, surveillance is life-long, as it remains unclear at what point it is safe to stop. Of treated patients, 83% have gone on to have successful pregnancies. Women are advised to avoid pregnancy for the first year as it may mask relapse and there is a theoretical risk of teratogenicity. Despite this advice, a number of women have become pregnant within 12 months without increased complications.[38] All patients who become pregnant should have an early ultrasound to check the normality of the pregnancy and should resume hCG surveillance at 6 weeks post delivery.

**Table 6** Schedule for hCG surveillance after chemotherapy

| | | hCG concentration Urine | Serum |
|---|---|---|---|
| Year 1 | Weeks 1–6 after chemotherapy | Weekly | Weekly |
| | Months 2–6 | 2-weekly | 2-weekly |
| | Months 7–12 | 2-weekly | – |
| Year 2 | | 4-weekly | – |
| Year 3 | | 8-weekly | – |
| Year 4 | | 3-monthly | – |
| Year 5 | | 4-monthly | – |
| Year 6 and above | Life-long monitoring | 6-monthly | – |

## PLACENTAL SITE TROPHOBLASTIC TUMOUR

PSTT is relatively chemoresistant and surgery, by specialist gynaecological surgeons, is the mainstay of treatment. Overall 5-year survival is 75%. The most important prognostic factor in PSTT is interval from the causative pregnancy. Those treated > 4 years post pregnancy have so far had 100% mortality; in contrast, at < 4 years there has been near 100% long-term survival for all stages of disease. Standard treatment for disease confined to the uterus is hysterectomy, with pelvic lymph node clearance and ovarian preservation. In metastatic disease, best results have so far been obtained using intensive chemotherapy (EMA/EP) with or without surgical resection. The majority of patients will need a hysterectomy to achieve cure.[10]

The major question in the management of PSTT, which frequently affects women of child-bearing age, is whether fertility-sparing surgery is safe in a minority of cases with good prognostic factors and disease localised to a single uterine site. There have been five reported cases of attempted fertility-sparing surgery using a variety of surgical techniques with and without postoperative chemotherapy, with mixed results. One case had a successful pregnancy, two achieved long-term remission but no term pregnancy, and two went on to need a hysterectomy for relapsed disease.[39–42] In one case at relapse, it was found post-hysterectomy that disease that appeared localised to a single uterine site on imaging, including [18]FDG PET, was in fact multifocal throughout the uterus. Any attempts at fertility-sparing surgery should be undertaken cautiously with pre-operative counselling of the patient and close follow up postoperatively.

## HUMAN CHORIONIC GONADOTROPHIN MONITORING – INCREASING COMPLEXITY WITH ACCURACY

Human chorionic gonadotrophin is a glycoprotein produced by trophoblasts and the pituitary. It is made up of two subunits – α which is common to hCG, TSH and LH and β which is specific to trophoblast-secreted hCG. It is now known that β-hCG exists in at least two intact forms – regular β-hCG which is produced in normal pregnancy and hCG-H a variant with double-sized oligosaccharide side chains that is produced by invasive cytotrophoblasts. Its presence is specific to the implantation phases of normal pregnancy and GTN. The differences between β-hCG and hCG-H are listed in Table 7. In GTN, fragmented β-hCG is also produced, *e.g.* free β-subunit, β-core, nicked free-β, and C-terminal fragments.

**Table 7** Differences between β-hCG and hCG-H

|  | β-hCG | hCG-H |
|---|---|---|
| Produced by | Syncytiotrophoblasts | Invasive cytotrophoblasts |
| Present in | Throughout normal pregnancy | Implantation phases of normal pregnancy |
|  | All forms of GTD | GTN only |
| Method of action | Endocrine | Autocrine |
| Role | Maintains progesterone production | Promotes trophoblast growth and invasion |

Accurate measurement of β-hCG is essential for the effective management of GTD. Complex decisions to initiate or stop chemotherapy, or proceed to irreversible surgical intervention (*e.g.* hysterectomy) are taken on the basis of hCG levels, so it is essential that the assays used in oncological hCG analysis are accurate and reliable. The increasing sensitivity of hCG assays and identification of β-hCG variants has led to the identification of a number of problems:

1. **False-negative results**. Unless an assay is able to detect all forms of β-hCG, it may result in failure to make the diagnosis of GTN or in inadequate treatment. This is a worry with many current commercially available hCG assays – assays used for hCG monitoring during pregnancy are not adequate for use in GTD.[43]

2. **False-positive results**. These occur due to cross-reactivity of the assay with circulating heterophile antibodies and can be eliminated by measuring urine hCG levels – the antibodies are too large to undergo glomerular filtration.

3. **Persistent low-level elevation of β-hCG without clinical or radiological evidence of active GTD**. This may occur in patients on hCG surveillance, or in healthy women who have had an incidental false-positive pregnancy test, and is a consequence of increasing assay sensitivity. Historically, women were often presumed to have GTN and treated with chemotherapy or even hysterectomy, but this did not result in hCG normalisation in the majority of cases. It is important to identify the cause of the elevation to target those who need treatment and avoid unnecessary intervention in the rest. It may be due to:

    i. *Quiescent GTN*, in patients with previous GTD. A minority of these patients will subsequently develop active disease and require chemotherapy. There is evidence that presence of an elevated hCG-H level can be used determine which cases in this group need chemotherapy.

ii *Pituitary-derived hCG*, which may be detectable in menopause or premature ovarian failure and is suggested by corresponding changes in LH/FSH levels.

iii *Non-gestational neoplasia* – germ cell and epithelial tumours with some trophoblast differentiation may produce hCG. Thorough investigation is needed to exclude this.[44]

iv *Physiological elevation* – some women may have an elevated baseline hCG.

New assays designed to detect specific hCG variants are in development and are leading to further increases in the specificity and sensitivity of hCG monitoring.

### hCG-H specific assays

An elevated hCG-H level has been shown to be specific to cases of HM that subsequently require chemotherapy; this elevation occurs earlier than rises in conventional hCG and before clinically apparent GTN develops. The routine use of hCG-H monitoring may allow earlier initiation of, or changes to, chemotherapy.[45]

### Diagnosis of PSTT by detection of free β-subunit

Currently, PSTT can be difficult to differentiate from CC or in other cases from benign placental site reactions. Recent work has shown that proportionately high levels of free β-fragments are produced in PSTT and that this is a highly sensitive test for discriminating cases of PSTT from CC.[46] Of note, it may also be elevated in some non-trophoblastic malignancies.

However, caution should be used when interpreting specific sub-type assays – is the tumour producing other forms of hCG which are not being identified?

Interesting research has recently been reported on the role of hCG-H in the development of GTN, particularly CC. hCG-H is secreted by invasive cytotrophoblasts and acts as an autocrine growth factor. An anti-hCG-H antibody has been developed that blocks tumourigenesis and progression of CC in mouse models. In the future, a human monoclonal antibody versus hCG-H could be a clinically useful targeted therapy in GTN. Alternatively, an anti-hCG-H vaccine could be used to promote endogenous antibody formation and prevent malignant transformation of HM.[47]

## CONCLUSIONS

Nearly all patients with GTD can now expect to be cured with their fertility intact and without long-term consequences. This success is creating new management problems: techniques for making accurate diagnosis of very early disease are being developed; the accuracy of hCG as a biomarker of disease activity is being improved; radiological techniques are being developed to improve prognostic scoring and accurate identification of sites of relapsed disease. Effective treatments for patients with chemotherapy-refractory disease still need to be developed. Advances are being made in identifying the genetic and molecular defects underlying the different forms of GTD. It is hoped that these will provide targets for treatment in the future and ultimately enable us to prevent the progression of HM to GTN.

# Key points for clinical practice

- All cases of hydatidiform mole should be registered for human chorionic gonadotrophin (hCG) surveillance: both partial and complete hydatidiform moles progress to gestational trophoblastic neoplasias.

- Initial treatment of suspected hydatidiform mole should be suction evacuation. Second evacuation increases the risk of subsequent chemotherapy and should be avoided.

- Gestational trophoblastic neoplasia post hydatidiform mole is diagnosed by rising hCG and abnormal radiology. Histological confirmation is not needed unless placental site trophoblastic tumour is a possible diagnosis. Placental site trophoblastic tumour is suggested by a relatively low hCG level for volume of radiological disease.

- The diagnosis of gestational trophoblastic neoplasia should be considered in all young women presenting as an emergency with unexplained respiratory failure or intracranial bleeding.

- Management of all cases of gestational trophoblastic neoplasia should be centralised.

- Type of chemotherapy given is determined by FIGO prognostic score; it should be calculated during the initial assessment.

- hCG assays used for monitoring must identify all forms of β-hCG. Pregnancy tests are not reliable for use in gestational trophoblastic neoplasia.

- Complete hCG response is necessary for successful treatment but complete radiological response is not. Intervention is not needed for residual post-treatment masses outside the central nervous system.

- Patients with relapsed disease still have a good chance of cure, even after multiple lines of treatment, and should be treated actively with a combination of chemotherapy and surgery.

- It is important to recognise cases of placental site trophoblastic tumour as management is primarily surgical.

## References

1. Tham BW, Everard JE, Tidy JA, Drew D, Hancock BW. Gestational trophoblastic disease in the Asian population of Northern England and North Wales. *Br J Obstet Gynaecol* 2003; **110**: 555–559.
2. Sebire NJ, Rees H, Paradinas F, Seckl M, Newlands E. The diagnostic implications of routine ultrasound examination in histologically confirmed early molar pregnancies. *Ultrasound Obstet Gynecol* 2001; **18**: 662–665.
3. Seckl MJ, Fisher RA, Salerno GA *et al.* Choriocarcinoma and partial hydatidiform moles. *Lancet* 2000; **356**: 36–39.
4. Palmieri C, Fisher RA, Sebire NJ *et al.* Placental site trophoblastic tumour arising from a partial hydatidiform mole. *Lancet* 2005; **366**: 688.
5. Newlands ES, Paradinas FJ, Fisher RA. Recent advances in gestational trophoblastic

disease. *Hematol Oncol Clin North Am* 1998; **13**: 225–244.
6. Bagshawe KD, Dent J, Webb J. Hydatidiform mole in the United Kingdom 1973–1983. *Lancet* 1986; **ii**: 673.
7. Sebire NJ, Foskett M, Paradinas FJ *et al*. Outcome of twin pregnancies with complete hydatidiform mole and healthy co-twin. *Lancet* 2002; **359**: 2165–2166.
8. Fisher RA. Genetic origins of hydatidiform moles. In: Hancock BW, Newlands ES, Berkowitz RS, Cole LA. (eds) *Gestational Trophoblastic Diseases*, 2nd edn. London: Chapman and Hall Medical, 2003; 6–38.
9. Hanahan D, Weinberg R. The hallmarks of cancer. *Cell* 2000; **100**: 57–70.
10. Papadopoulos AJ, Foskett M, Seckl MJ *et al*. Twenty-five years' clinical experience of placental site trophoblastic tumors. *J Reprod Med* 2002; **47**: 460–464.
11. Shih I, Kurman R. Epithelioid trophoblastic tumor: a neoplasm distinct from choriocarcinoma and placental site trophoblastic tumor simulating carcinoma. *Am J Surg Pathol* 1998; **22**: 1393–1403.
12. Helwani MN, Seoud M, Zahed L, Zaatari G, Khalil A, Slim R. A familial case of recurrent hydatidiform molar pregnancies with biparental genomic contribution. *Hum Genet* 1999; **105**: 112–115.
13. Fisher RA, Hodges MD, Rees H *et al*. The maternally transcribed gene *p57$^{KIP2}$* (CDNK1C) is abnormally expressed in both androgenetic and biparental complete hydatidiform moles. *Hum Mol Genet* 2002; **11**: 3267–3272.
14. Judson H, Hayward BE, Sheridan E, Bonthron DT. A global disorder of imprinting in the human female germ line. *Nature* 2002; **416**: 539–542.
15. Murdoch S, Djuric U, Mazhar B *et al*. Mutations in *NALP7* cause recurrent hydatidiform moles and reproductive wastage in humans. *Nat Genet* 2006; **38**: 300–302.
16. Zhao J, Moss J, Sebire NJ *et al*. Analysis of the chromosomal region 19q13.4 in two Chinese families with recurrent hydatidiform mole. *Hum Reprod* 2006; **21**: 536–541.
17. Matsuda T, Sasaki M, Kato H *et al*. Human chromosome 7 carries a putative tumor suppressor gene(s) involved in choriocarcinoma. *Oncogene* 1997; **15**: 2773–2781.
18. Burke B, Sebire NJ, Moss J *et al*. Evaluation of deletions in 7q11.2 and 8p12-p21 as prognostic indicators of tumour development following molar pregnancy. *Gynecol Oncol* 2006; **103**: 642–648.
19. Popiolek D, Herman Y, Mittal K *et al*. Multiplex short tandem repeat DNA analysis confirms the accuracy of p57$^{kip2}$ immonostaining in the diagnosis of complete hydatidiform mole. *Hum Pathol* 2006; **37**: 1426–1434.
20. Wells P. The pathology of gestational trophoblastic disease: recent advances. *Pathology* 2007; **39**: 88–96.
21. Sebire NJ, Foskett M, Short D *et al*. Shortened duration of human chorionic gonadotrophin surveillance following complete or partial hydatidiform mole: evidence for revised protocol of a UK regional trophoblastic disease unit. *Br J Obstet Gynaecol* 2007; **114**: 760–762.
22. Savage P, Seckl MJ. The role of repeat uterine evacuation in trophoblast disease. *Gynecol Oncol* 2005; **99**: 251–252, author reply 252–253.
23. Pezeshki M, Hancock BW, Silcocks P *et al*. The role of repeat uterine evacuation in the management of persistent gestational trophoblastic disease. *Gynecol Oncol* 2004; **95**: 423–429.
24. Agarwal R, Strickland S, McNeish IA *et al*. Doppler ultrasonography of the uterine artery and the response to chemotherapy in patients with gestational trophoblastic tumors. *Clin Cancer Res* 2002; **8**: 1142–1147.
25. Kohorn EI. The new FIGO 2000 staging and risk factor scoring system for gestational trophoblastic disease: description and critical assessment. *Int J Gynecol Cancer* 2001; **11**: 73–77.
26. Bower M, Newlands ES, Holden L *et al*. EMA/CO for high-risk gestational trophoblastic tumours: results from a cohort of 272 patients. *J Clin Oncol* 1997; **15**: 2636–2643.
27. Powles T, Savage P, Stebbing J *et al*. A comparison of patients with relapsed and chemo-refractory gestational trophoblastic neoplasia. *Br J Cancer* 2007; **96**: 732–737.
28. Newlands ES, Holden L, Seckl MJ, McNeish I, Strickland S, Rustin GJ. Management of brain metastases in patients with high-risk gestational trophoblastic tumors. *J Reprod Med* 2002; **47**: 465–471.

29. Rustin GJS, Newlands ES, Lutz J-M *et al*. Combination but not single agent methotrexate chemotherapy for gestational trophoblastic tumours (GTT) increases the incidence of second tumours. *J Clin Oncol* 1996; **14**: 2769–2773.

30. Xue Y, Zhang J, Wu TX, An RF. Combination chemotherapy for high-risk gestational trophoblastic tumour. Cochrane Database System Rev 2006; 3: CD005196.

31. Bower M, Rustin GJS, Newlands ES *et al*. Chemotherapy for gestational trophoblastic tumours hastens menopause by 3 years. *Eur J Cancer* 1998; **34**: 1204–1207.

32. Lim AKP, Agarwal R, Barrett N *et al*. Embolization of residual uterine vascular malformations in patients with gestational trophoblastic tumours. *Radiology* 2002; **222**: 640–644.

33. Powles T, Savage P, Short D, Young A, Pappin C, Seckl MJ. Residual lung lesions after completion of chemotherapy for gestational trophoblastic neoplasia: should we operate? *Br J Cancer* 2006; **94**: 51–54.

34. Yang J, Xiang Y, Wana X, Yanga X. The prognosis of a gestational trophoblastic neoplasia patient with residual lung tumor after completing treatment. *Gynecol Oncol* 2006; **103**: 479–482.

35. Dhillon T, Palmieri C, Sebire NJ *et al*. Value of whole body [18]FDG-PET to identify the active site of gestational trophoblastic neoplasia. *J Reprod Med* 2006; **51**: 879–887.

36. Newlands E. The management of recurrent and drug-resistant gestational trophoblastic neoplasias (GTN). *Best Pract Res Clin Obstet Gynaecol* 2003; **17**: 905–923.

37. El-Helw LM, Seckl MJ, Haynes R *et al*. High-dose chemotherapy and peripheral blood stem cell support in refractory gestational trophoblastic neoplasia. *Br J Cancer* 2005; **93**: 620–621.

38. Blagden SP, Foskett MA, Fisher RA *et al*. The effect of early pregnancy following chemotherapy on disease relapse and fetal outcome in women treated for gestational trophoblastic tumours. *Br J Cancer* 2002; **86**: 26–30.

39. Leiserowitz GS, Webb MJ. Treatment of placental site trophoblastic tumor with hysterotomy and uterine reconstruction. *Obstet Gynecol* 1996; **88**: 696–699.

40. Machtinger R, Gotlieb WH, Korach J *et al*. Placental site trophoblastic tumor: outcome of five cases including fertility preserving management. *Gynecol Oncol* 2005; **96**: 56–61.

41. Pfeffer P, Sebire NJ, Lindsay I, McIndoe A, Lim AKP, Seckl M. Fertility-sparing partial hysterectomy for placental-site trophoblastic tumour. *Lancet Oncol* 2007; **8**: 744–746.

42. Tsuji Y, Tsubamoto H, Hori M, Ogasawara T, Koyama K. Case of PSTT treated with chemotherapy followed by open uterine tumor resection to preserve fertility. *Gynecol Oncol* 2002; **87**: 303–307.

43. Mitchell H, Seckl M. Discrepancies between commercially available immunoassays in the detection of tumour-derived hCG. *Mol Cell Endocrinol* 2007; **262**: 310–313.

44. Palmieri C, Dhillon T, Fisher RA *et al*. Management and outcome of healthy women with a persistently elevated B-hCG. *Gynecol Oncol* 2007; **106**: 35–43.

45. Cole LA, Butler SA, Khanlian SA *et al*. Gestational trophoblastic diseases: 2. Hyperglycosylated hCG as a reliable marker of active neoplasia. *Gynecol Oncol* 2006; **102**: 151–159.

46. Cole LA, Khanlian SA, Muller CY, Giddings A, Kohorn E, Berkowitz RS. Gestational trophoblastic diseases: 3. Human chorionic gonadotrophin-free B-subunit, a reliable marker of placental site trophoblastic tumors. *Gynecol Oncol* 2006; **102**: 160–164.

47. Cole LA, Dai D, Butler SA, Leslie K, Kohorn E. Gestational trophoblastic diseases: 1. Pathophysiology of hyperglycosylated hCG. *Gynecol Oncol* 2006; **102**: 145–150.

*Malathy Appasamy  Shanthi Muttukrishna*

**11**

# Anti-Müllerian hormone: relevance in male and female infertility

Anti-Müllerian hormone (AMH) or Müllerian-inhibiting substance (MIS) is a glycoprotein hormone of the transforming growth factor beta (TGF-β) family with a molecular weight of 140 kDa. AMH is produced as a precursor and undergoes glycosylation or cleavage to form the mature molecule. Knowledge of recombinant AMH protein expression in the 1980s[1] resulted in successful antibody production against AMH that marked the beginning of a rapidly increasing knowledge of its biological effects and mechanism of action. In rats, AMH activity was localised to the immature Sertoli cells from the time of fetal sex differentiation to puberty in the testis[2] and to the granulosa cells of postnatal ovary to the end of ovarian activity.[3,4] The knowledge of the normal and pathological expression of AMH and the regulatory mechanisms involved encouraged scientists to study its clinical implications.

## ANTI-MÜLLERIAN HORMONE AND FEMALE INFERTILITY

### CIRCULATING AMH IN THE NORMAL MENSTRUAL CYCLE

Several studies have recently investigated the circulating levels of AMH throughout the menstrual cycle. Most studies[5-8] have reported that AMH levels do not alter significantly throughout the cycle whereas one recent study reports a significant rise in AMH in the late follicular phase compared to ovulation and early luteal phase of the cycle.[9] There is also some discrepancy

**Malathy Appasamy** MRCOG
Clinical Research Fellow, UCL Institute for Women's Health, University College London, 86–96 Chenies Mews, London WC1E 6HX, UK
E-mail: apmala01@yahoo.co.uk

**Shanthi Muttukrishna** PhD
Lecturer in Reproductive Science, UCL Institute for Women's Health, University College London, 86–96 Chenies Mews, London WC1E 6HX, UK
E-mail: s.muttukrishna@ucl.ac.uk

in the literature on the relationship between AMH and follicle stimulating hormone (FSH) during the menstrual cycle. Clearly defined studies with samples taken frequently with daily sample from days 7–21 of the cycle could confirm the levels of AMH during the menstrual cycle.

## OVARIAN RESERVE AND FERTILITY

Development of sensitive immunoassays for AMH has enabled investigators to study the role of AMH in women undergoing assisted reproduction. Fertility potential in a female is determined by the number and the quality of the primordial follicles remaining in the ovary, referred to as the ovarian reserve. Ovarian ageing (which essentially means decrease in ovarian reserve with time) is highly variable and results in depletion of primordial follicles in the ovary.[10,11] Although the underlying mechanism for reduction of ovarian reserve is poorly understood, predicting ovarian reserve can serve two purposes in a woman's reproductive life: (i) the diagnosis of premature menopause; and (ii) the determination of ovarian response to gonadotrophin stimulation in assisted reproductive treatment. Ovarian reserve testing (ORT) has been studied using static and dynamic biochemical markers (such as FSH, inhibin B, oestradiol [E2] and AMH) as well as biophysical markers (such as antral follicle count [AFC] and ovarian volume using transvaginal ultrasonography). However, the ideal ORT that may be useful clinically has yet to be ascertained.[12,13]

### AMH and ovarian reserve

AMH has received considerable attention in the field of reproductive medicine where its role as a marker of ovarian reserve has been increasingly explored. The reasons are clear: AMH is solely produced in the pre-antral and antral ovarian follicles and, therefore, may be representative of the quantity and quality of the ovarian follicle pool.[14] AMH activity starts to fade after the antral follicle stage and disappears in the pre-ovulatory follicles and corpora lutea. AMH plays a role in the recruitment of primordial follicles as suggested by the depletion of primordial follicle pool in AMH-deficient mice.[15] Furthermore, in the absence of AMH in mice, the pre-antral and antral follicles become more sensitive to the action of FSH.[15] Therefore, in mice, higher follicular phase AMH is likely to be associated with decreased number of FSH-sensitive large pre-antral and antral follicles that will be recruited into the follicular pool.[16,17] Hence, AMH inhibits initial recruitment of primordial follicles, thereby playing a role in preserving ovarian reserve as well as modulating cyclical follicular recruitment by decreasing the FSH sensitivity of the recruited primordial follicles. In turn, this keeps a check on the number of primordial follicles that will develop into pre-ovulatory follicles. This observation encouraged the study of AMH as a marker of ovarian reserve in women undergoing assisted reproduction technology (ART) as it could potentially determine the ovarian response to gonadotrophin stimulation in these women.[18]

### Role of ovarian reserve testing in ART

Anovulatory infertility accounts for 20–25% of couples undergoing ART. Anovulation could be the result of ovarian ageing, in other words, reduced ovarian reserve or result from polycystic ovarian syndrome. About 75% of the reserve has been shown to be exhausted in women between their early 30s and early 40s.[19] However, decreased ovarian reserve affects 5–10% of women under 30 years of age[20] and is associated with poor response to gonadotrophin stimulation. Assessment of ovarian reserve is useful before expensive IVF treatment is undertaken. This should help to identify both low and high responders prior to starting treatment thereby avoiding cancellation rate and side effects, the most serious of which is ovarian hyperstimulation syndrome (OHSS).This would also help physicians to evaluate and counsel patients before IVF stimulation and optimise stimulation protocols.

## Basal and dynamic hormonal markers of ovarian reserve

Screening for ovarian reserve as a prediction of IVF outcome started with measurement of basal hormonal markers in the follicular phase such as FSH[21] and inhibin B.[22] With FSH, there are problems of inter-cycle variability and its evaluation failed to prove useful in a meta-analysis.[23] Inhibin B levels rise progressively during the early follicular phase. Hence, testing for inhibin B in the early follicular phase when it peaks around day 5 of a cycle is a more reliable means of predicting ovarian reserve. However, published studies using inhibin B levels on day 3 to predict the number of oocytes retrieved are inconsistent.[24] Several dynamic tests of ovarian reserve have been developed that measure oestradiol, a product of granulosa cells, by pharmacological stimulation of the ovaries. These include the clomiphene citrate challenge test (CCCT),[25] the GnRH agonist stimulation test[26] and the FSH ovarian reserve (EFORT) test that analysed oestradiol and inhibin B on days 3–5 after FSH stimulation.[27] These dynamic tests appear more sensitive than basal FSH, inhibin B or chronological age. Dynamic inhibin B testing correlated well with the number of oocytes retrieved.[18] More recent studies have investigated AMH in dynamic ovarian reserve testing. In an ovarian stimulation test with gonadotrophin stimulation there was no significant change in AMH levels confirming that AMH levels are not altered by FSH in the cycle.[18]

## AMH as a basal marker of ovarian reserve

The role of AMH in follicular dynamics and prediction of ovarian response has received much recent attention. The observation that AMH was involved in inhibiting primordial follicular growth was further established by *in vitro* studies on cultured neonatal mouse ovary, where AMH was shown to appear immediately after the initiation of primordial follicle growth along with inhibin α-subunit. This initial increase was followed by inhibition of the recruitment of the remaining primordial follicle pool as shown by decrease in α-inhibin, used as a marker of early follicle development.[28] Therefore, AMH serves as an inhibitory growth factor in the early stages of folliculogenesis. In an *in vivo* study of 41 normo-ovulatory women, serum AMH showed a strong correlation with the number of antral follicles,[17] FSH and inhibin B levels. These findings were confirmed by other studies in patients undergoing IVF treatment.[18] Serum AMH strongly correlated with the antral follicle count, number of oocytes retrieved, age, FSH and inhibin B. Both antral follicle count and AMH served as equally important predictors of ovarian response in these studies.

## ROLE OF AMH AS A MARKER OF OVARIAN RESPONSE IN ART

Elevated concentrations of serum AMH, present in patients with polycystic ovaries,[29] associated with increased number of immature oocytes, suggesting that AMH could be used as a marker of successful oocyte retrieval during IVF treatment. All these early studies confirmed the role of AMH in the early follicular stage and its usefulness in predicting ovarian response. A further study by Fanchin *et al.*[30] looked at the dynamics of AMH secretion beyond the antral follicle stage by measuring AMH levels on days 3 (baseline), 6 and 8 after FSH treatment and on the day of hCG (pre-ovulatory phase) in patients undergoing controlled ovarian stimulation. These authors also studied the other serum markers (inhibin B, oestradiol, progesterone, testosterone and androstenedione) and established that serum AMH correlated positively with the number of small antral follicles and serum inhibin B throughout the cycle reflecting the same origin of these hormones from the small antral follicles,[31] but not with the other hormones. Serum AMH also showed a positive correlation with the number of oocytes retrieved and the strongest correlation was with baseline levels with a progressively declining still positive relationship with day 6, day 8 and pre-ovulatory levels. Therefore, serum AMH had a positive relationship with the number of mature oocytes retrieved, the weaker relationship is perhaps due to the decreased expression of AMH in the larger follicles. These authors also showed that day 3 serum AMH was more robustly correlated with the number of early antral follicles than inhibin B, E2, FSH and LH, suggesting that AMH may reflect ovarian follicular status better than the usual hormone markers.[32] AMH had a significantly higher inter-cycle reproducibility compared to inhibin B, FSH and early antral follicle count by transvaginal ultrasonography and reached satisfactory reliability with a single measurement.[33] More recent prospective studies have suggested

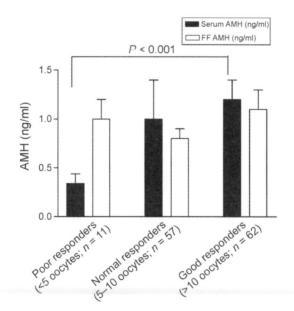

**Fig. 1** Pre-ovulatory serum and follicular fluid (FF) AMH (ng/ml) in patients undergoing controlled ovarian stimulation and its relationship to ovarian response.

an association between AMH and oocyte yield and support the concept of using AMH as a reliable predictor of ovarian reserve (Fig. 1).[29] Thus, AMH can serve as a cost-effective, reliable marker of ovarian fertility potential.

## AMH as a predictor of poor response and cycle cancellation in ART

In a prospective study of patients undergoing IVF treatment and who were likely to be poor responders based on their elevated day 3 FSH levels, serum AMH was identified to be the single best marker in determining the ovarian response.[34] In this study, serum FSH, inhibin B and AMH were measured and the results were analysed in relation to the number of oocytes retrieved in a group of clinically defined poor responders. About 75% of patients who had cancelled IVF treatment cycle had AMH levels below the detection limit, while FSH levels were significantly higher and inhibin B were 50-fold lower compared to the patients who completed treatment. On the other hand, AMH levels were undetectable in 12% of the patients who completed successful treatment. Therefore, it was clear that AMH measurement alone is insufficient to predict IVF cycle cancellation reliably. This observation led to study of the use of combined basal hormonal markers in predicting the success of an IVF treatment cycle. A cumulative score obtained by a using a panel of markers such as age, AFC, basal FSH, AMH, delta E2 and inhibin B may be useful in predicting ovarian response.[18] According to this study, a cumulative score of 12 could correctly identify 87% of poor responders and 80% of good responders (Fig. 2). A further study evaluated the role of an ultrasound marker (AFC) and dynamic basal and luteal phase hormonal markers (FSH, inhibin B, AMH and oestradiol) to predict outcome.[35] This study confirmed that poor responders had lower luteal AMH levels and good responders had higher AFC, AMH and luteal stimulated inhibin B and oestradiol compared to normal responders. Their multivariate regression analysis showed that the best models for predicting oocyte number included AFC, follicular phase AMH and stimulated inhibin B. Follicular phase and luteal phase AMH were predictive of

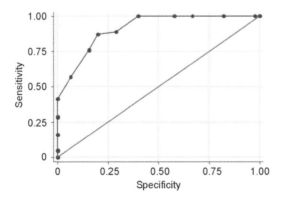

**Fig. 2** Receiver operating curve (ROC) for the identification of cut-off score for the cumulative score model to predict poor response to ovarian stimulation. The area under the curve was 0.91. ROC analysis is used to quantify the accuracy of the diagnostic tests. The area under the ROC curve commonly summarises the global performance of a diagnostic test. This area is interpreted as the probability that the result of a diagnostic test would be correct.

pregnancy outcome. A recent study evaluating the role of multiple endocrine markers and biophysical ovarian markers in predicting IVF outcomes in poor responders confirmed that day 3 inhibin B, AMH and mean ovarian volume are best predictors of successful ovarian response and cycle cancellations with AMH showing the least inter-cycle variability.[36]

The general consensus from prospective clinical studies so far is that AMH is a promising tool in the assessment of ovarian response and prediction of cycle cancellations in ART. However, whether it would serve as a useful tool to predict pregnancy outcome, in other words oocyte quality, is still controversial. While some studies have not seen an association with embryo quality and pregnancy outcome,[37] other studies claim a predictive value in live-birth rates.[38] Therefore, large-scale studies testing various patient populations are awaited before a consensus on pregnancy outcome can be achieved. Use of AMH as a marker for ovarian reserve in predicting the success of ART cycles has started to reach clinical application in several reproductive medicine units. However, its role in predicting oocyte quality remains to be ascertained.

## AMH IN MALE INFERTILITY

Development of the male reproductive system is dependent on genetic and hormonal factors. AMH is secreted from the Sertoli cells of the testis from the onset of testicular differentiation that is responsible for the regression of Müllerian ducts. Testosterone, secreted from the Leydig cells virilises the Wolffian duct and the development of external genitalia is dependent on 5-α-reductase, an enzyme that converts testosterone to the active form, dihydrotestosterone. The differentiation of the male reproductive system is complete by the 12th week of intra-uterine life followed by the descent of the testes from their position by the kidneys to the adult position in the scrotum. It is well established that testicular function is regulated by the hypothalamic–pituitary–ovarian axis, with the pituitary gonadotropins, FSH and LH, playing an important role in the initiation and maintenance of spermatogenesis. LH stimulates the synthesis of testosterone that maintains spermatogenesis. Both FSH and testosterone promote spermatogenesis by acting on the Sertoli cells. Sertoli cells produce several factors involved in sperm maturation. Sertoli cells produce an androgen-binding protein under the stimulus of FSH and testosterone that helps to maintain high concentrations of androgens in the seminiferous tubules in close proximity to the developing spermatocytes.

## ROLE OF AMH AS A MARKER OF SPERMATOGENESIS

Circulating levels of AMH remain high until puberty, when they progressively decrease to basal levels due to high testicular secretion of testosterone.[39] AMH has no role to play in gonadal determination and does not affect meiosis. However, high levels of AMH block Leydig cell differentiation from the mesenchymal cells and inhibit testosterone synthesis, acting through Leydig cell receptors thereby indirectly affecting spermatogenesis.[40] This triggered interest in studying its role in the adult male and its potential value as a marker of spermatogenesis in infertility.

After puberty, AMH is secreted preferentially by the apical pole of the Sertoli cell, towards the lumen of seminiferous tubules resulting in high concentrations in seminal plasma compared to serum. However, AMH is detectable in serum and serum levels reflect the seminal plasma levels and could be used as a non-invasive marker in the evaluation of male infertility.[41] Serum AMH was also positively correlated with sperm concentration and semen volume as well as serum inhibin B in a cohort of sub-fertile patients suggesting the value of serum AMH as a potential marker of spermatogenesis.[42] It was suggested that seminal plasma AMH could be subjected to the influence of seminal proteases and measurement of serum levels may be more representative of the actual levels.[43]

## AMH LOCALISATION IN THE TESTIS

The role of AMH in the post-pubertal male and its clinical relevance is still uncertain. AMH concentration in the seminal plasma was significantly lower in infertile oligospermic men compared to healthy volunteers and correlated with sperm concentration and mean testicular volume.[44] It was speculated that AMH may play a role in spermatogenesis. However, it could not be ascertained that lower AMH concentration in these men was due to a primary alteration in Sertoli cell function that also led to spermatogenic arrest.[45] In infertile obstructive azoospermia patients, seminal plasma AMH was undetectable, suggesting the testicular origin of AMH.[44] In the same study, infertile men with non-obstructive azoospermia had lower levels of AMH compared to fertile donors. Histological studies for AMH expression in testicular biopsy specimens from these men showed lack of AMH expression in men who had no spermatozoa and presence of AMH expression in those who had spermatozoa. Therefore, measurement of seminal plasma AMH is suggested as a non-invasive marker of normal spermatogenesis and for identifying infertile azoospermic men with the presence of testicular spermatozoa and successful sperm retrieval. Testicular biopsy specimens from oligospermic infertile patients showed AMH immunoactivity in the Sertoli cells of the seminiferous tubules that had spermatogenic arrest at the level of spermatogonia. Similar expression of AMH has been detected in prepubertal testis. However, AMH immunoactivity was absent in adult testis with normal spermatogenesis.[46] This suggests expression of AMH is associated with a population of Sertoli cells showing a prepubertal stage of development. Similarly, germ cell maturation has an effect on AMH expression from the Sertoli cells such that germ cells that have initiated meiosis cease to produce AMH earlier than their neighbouring germ cells that are still immature. Collectively, these findings reflect that testicular androgens and a synergistic effect of meiotic germ cells are potent inhibitors of AMH expression in pubertal testis. This was supported by the absence of AMH suppression and high AMH levels in patients with androgen insensitivity syndrome.

## ROLE OF AMH IN THE EVALUATION OF AZOOSPERMIA

In a recent study, we have shown that serum AMH levels are lower in men with obstructive azoospermia compared to non-obstructive azoospermia and controls suggesting that serum AMH levels may be potential markers of obstructive azoospermia in men with azoospermia.[47] A study on the measurement of seminal plasma AMH in different subgroups of male infertility patients supports the previous studies in that AMH levels were undetectable in patients with obstructive azoospermia but were detected in lower levels in the non-obstructive azoospermia compared to fertile controls.[48] There was also a positive correlation between seminal plasma AMH and testicular volume, sperm concentration and motility and a negative correlation with abnormal sperm morphology. Thus AMH can be a useful marker of normal spermatogenesis. However, AMH levels were not significantly different in the two groups whether they had successful sperm retrieval or not.

## CONCLUSIONS

AMH signals the existence of functional testicular tissue and allows the distinction between gonadal dysgenesis and tubulo-interstitial dysfunction in men with infertility or sexual dysfunction. This knowledge has expanded its clinical application from the evaluation of children with non-palpable gonads with or without ambiguous genitalia to the evaluation of adolescent males with precocious puberty, hypogonadotrophic hypogonadism and sex-cord stromal cell tumours. In adult men with infertility, AMH is a promising non-invasive marker for evaluating the underlying cause of spermatogenic defects. Its role in the evaluation of successful sperm retrieval in infertile men with non-obstructive azoospermia remains to be ascertained.

### Key points for clinical practice

- Serum anti-Müllerian hormone (AMH) is predictive of ovarian reserve.

- AMH is a marker of antral follicle count in the early follicular phase

- AMH levels are predictive of ovarian response to gonadotrophin stimulation in assisted reproductive therapy.

- AMH levels are predictive of cycle cancellation in poor responders in assisted reproductive therapy.

- AMH levels are higher in women with polycystic ovaries.

- In males, serum AMH could be a potential marker of obstructive azoospermia.

### References

1. Picard JY, Goulut C, Bourrillon R, Josso N. Biochemical analysis of bovine testicular anti-Müllerian hormone. *FEBS Lett* 1986; **195**: 73–76.
2. Donahoe PK, Ito Y, Marfatia S, Hendren III WH. The production of Müllerian inhibiting substance by the fetal, neonatal and adult rat. *Biol Reprod* 1976; **15**: 329–334.
3. Vigier B, Picard JY, Tran D, Legeai L, Josso N. Production of anti-Müllerian hormone:

another homology between Sertoli and granulosa cells. *Endocrinology* 1984; **114**: 1315–1320.

4. Rajpert-De ME, Jorgensen N, Graem N, Muller J, Cate RL, Skakkebaek NE. Expression of anti-Müllerian hormone during normal and pathological gonadal development: association with differentiation of Sertoli and granulosa cells. *J Clin Endocrinol Metab* 1999; **84**: 3836–3844.

5. La Marca A, Stabile G, Artensio AC, Volpe A. Serum anti Müllerian hormone throughout the human menstrual cycle. *Hum Reprod* 2006; **21**: 3103–3107.

6. Hehenkamp WJ, Looman CW, Themmen AP, de Jong FH, te Velde ER, Broekmans FJ. Anti Müllerian hormone levels in the spontaneous menstrual cycle do not show substantial fluctuation. *J Clin Endocrinol Metab* 2006; **91**: 4057–4063.

7. Streuli I, Fraisse T, Pillet C, Ibecheole V, Bischof P, de Ziegler D. Serum antimüllerian hormone levels remain stable throughout the menstrual cycle and after oral or vaginal administration of synthetic sex steroids. *Fertil Steril* 2007; Oct 3; [Epub ahead of print] PMID: 17919608 [PubMed – as supplied by publisher].

8. Tsepelidis S, Devreker F, Demeestere I, Flahaut A, Gervy CH, Englert Y. Stable serum levels of anti Müllerian hormone during the menstrual cycle: a prospective study in normo-ovulatory women. *Hum Reprod* 2007; **22**: 1837–1840.

9. Wunder DM, Bersinger NA, Yared M, Kretschmer R, Birkhauser MH. Statistically significant changes of antiMüllerian hormone and inhibin levels during the physiologic menstrual cycle in reproductive age women. *Fertil Steril* 2007; Jun 29; [Epub ahead of print]. PMID: 17603052 [PubMed – as supplied by publisher]

10. Richardson SJ, Senikas V, Nelson JF. Follicular depletion during the menopausal transition: evidence for accelerated loss and ultimate exhaustion. *J Clin Endocrinol Metab* 1987; **65**: 1231–1237.

11. Faddy MJ, Gosden RG. A model confirming the decline in follicle numbers to the age of menopause in women. *Hum Reprod* 1996; **11**: 1484–1486.

12. Lutchman SK, Davies M, Chatterjee R. Fertility in female cancer survivors: pathophysiology, preservation and the role of ovarian reserve testing. *Hum Reprod Update* 2005; **11**: 69–89.

13. Broekmans FJ, Kwee J, Hendriks DJ, Mol BW, Lambalk CB. A systematic review of tests predicting ovarian reserve and IVF outcome. *Hum Reprod Update* 2006; **12**: 685–718.

14. Durlinger AL, Visser JA, Themmen AP. Regulation of ovarian function: the role of anti-Müllerian hormone. *Reproduction* 2002; **124**: 601–609.

15. Durlinger AL, Kramer P, Karels B *et al*. Control of primordial follicle recruitment by anti-Müllerian hormone in the mouse ovary. *Endocrinology* 1999; **140**: 5789–5796.

16. Durlinger AL, Gruijters MJ, Kramer P *et al*. Anti-Müllerian hormone attenuates the effects of FSH on follicle development in the mouse ovary. *Endocrinology* 2001; **142**: 4891–4895.

17. Gruijters MJ, Visser JA, Durlinger AL, Themmen AP. Anti-Müllerian hormone and its role in ovarian function. *Mol Cell Endocrinol* 2003; **211**: 85–90.

18. Muttukrishna S, McGarrigle H, Wakim R, Khadum I, Ranieri DM, Serhal P. Antral follicle count, anti-Müllerian hormone and inhibin B: predictors of ovarian response in assisted reproductive technology? *Br J Obstet Gynaecol* 2005; **112**: 1384–1390.

19. Block E. Quantitative morphological investigations of the follicular system in women; variations at different ages. *Acta Anat (Basel)* 1952; **14**: 108–123.

20. Hofmann GE, Sosnowski J, Scott RT, Thie J. Efficacy of selection criteria for ovarian reserve screening using the clomiphene citrate challenge test in a tertiary fertility center population. *Fertil Steril* 1996; **66**: 49–53.

21. Chuang CC, Chen CD, Chao KH, Chen SU, Ho HN, Yang YS. Age is a better predictor of pregnancy potential than basal follicle-stimulating hormone levels in women undergoing *in vitro* fertilization. *Fertil Steril* 2003; **79**: 63–68.

22. Hall JE, Welt CK, Cramer DW. Inhibin A and inhibin B reflect ovarian function in assisted reproduction but are less useful at predicting outcome. *Hum Reprod* 1999; **14**: 409–415.

23. Bancsi LF, Broekmans FJ, Mol BW, Habbema JD, te Velde ER. Performance of basal follicle-stimulating hormone in the prediction of poor ovarian response and failure to become pregnant after *in vitro* fertilization: a meta-analysis. *Fertil Steril* 2003; **79**:

1091–1100.

24. Dumesic DA, Damario MA, Session DR *et al*. Ovarian morphology and serum hormone markers as predictors of ovarian follicle recruitment by gonadotropins for *in vitro* fertilization. *J Clin Endocrinol Metab* 2001; **86**: 2538–2543.

25. Navot D, Rosenwaks Z, Margalioth EJ. Prognostic assessment of female fecundity. *Lancet* 1987; **2**: 645–647.

26. Ranieri DM, Quinn F, Makhlouf A *et al*. Simultaneous evaluation of basal follicle-stimulating hormone and 17 beta-estradiol response to gonadotropin-releasing hormone analogue stimulation: an improved predictor of ovarian reserve. *Fertil Steril* 1998; **70**: 227–233.

27. Dzik A, Lambert-Messerlian G, Izzo VM, Soares JB, Pinotti JA, Seifer DB. Inhibin B response to EFORT is associated with the outcome of oocyte retrieval in the subsequent *in vitro* fertilization cycle. *Fertil Steril* 2000; **74**: 1114–1117.

28. Durlinger AL, Gruijters MJ, Kramer P *et al*. Anti-Müllerian hormone inhibits initiation of primordial follicle growth in the mouse ovary. *Endocrinology* 2002; **143**: 1076–1084.

29. Appasamy M, Jauniaux E, Serhal P, Al-Qahtani A, Groome NP, Muttukrishna S. Evaluation of the relationship between follicular fluid oxidative stress, ovarian hormones, and response to gonadotropin stimulation. *Fertil Steril* 2007; Aug 4: [Epub ahead of print]. PMID: 17681319 [PubMed – as supplied by publisher].

30. Fanchin R, Schonauer LM, Righini C, Frydman N, Frydman R, Taieb J. Serum anti-Müllerian hormone dynamics during controlled ovarian hyperstimulation. *Hum Reprod* 2003; **18**: 328–332.

31. Groome NP, Illingworth PJ, O'Brien M *et al*. Measurement of dimeric inhibin B throughout the human menstrual cycle. *J Clin Endocrinol Metab* 1996; **81**: 1401–1405.

32. Fanchin R, Schonauer LM, Righini C, Guibourdenche J, Frydman R, Taieb J. Serum anti-Müllerian hormone is more strongly related to ovarian follicular status than serum inhibin B, estradiol, FSH and LH on day 3. *Hum Reprod* 2003; **18**: 323–327.

33. Fanchin R, Taieb J, Lozano DH, Ducot B, Frydman R, Bouyer J. High reproducibility of serum anti-Müllerian hormone measurements suggests a multi-staged follicular secretion and strengthens its role in the assessment of ovarian follicular status. *Hum Reprod* 2005; **20**: 923–927.

34. Muttukrishna S, Suharjono H, McGarrigle H, Sathanandan M. Inhibin B and anti-Müllerian hormone: markers of ovarian response in IVF/ICSI patients? *Br J Obstet Gynaecol* 2004; **111**: 1248–1253.

35. Eldar-Geva T, Ben-Chetrit A, Spitz IM *et al*. Dynamic assays of inhibin B, anti-Müllerian hormone and estradiol following FSH stimulation and ovarian ultrasonography as predictors of IVF outcome. *Hum Reprod* 2005; **20**: 3178–3183.

36. McIlveen M, Skull JD, Ledger WL. Evaluation of the utility of multiple endocrine and ultrasound measures of ovarian reserve in the prediction of cycle cancellation in a high-risk IVF population. *Hum Reprod* 2007; **22**: 778–785.

37. Smeenk JM, Sweep FC, Zielhuis GA, Kremer JA, Thomas CM, Braat DD. Antimüllerian hormone predicts ovarian responsiveness, but not embryo quality or pregnancy, after *in vitro* fertilization or intracytoplasmic sperm injection. *Fertil Steril* 2007; **87**: 223–226.

38. Nelson SM, Yates RW, Fleming R. Serum anti-Müllerian hormone and FSH: prediction of live birth and extremes of response in stimulated cycles implications for individualization of therapy. *Hum Reprod* 2007; **22**: 2414–2421.

39. Rey R. Assessment of seminiferous tubule function (anti-Müllerian hormone). *Baillières Best Pract Res Clin Endocrinol Metab* 2000; **14**: 399–408.

40. Racine C, Rey R, Forest MG *et al*. Receptors for anti-Müllerian hormone on Leydig cells are responsible for its effects on steroidogenesis and cell differentiation. *Proc Natl Acad Sci USA* 1998; **95**: 594–599.

41. Al-Qahtani A, Muttukrishna S, Appasamy M *et al*. Development of a sensitive enzyme immunoassay for anti-Müllerian hormone and the evaluation of potential clinical applications in males and females. *Clin Endocrinol (Oxf)* 2005; **63**: 267–273.

42. Appasamy M, Muttukrishna S, Pizzey AR *et al*. Relationship between male reproductive hormones, sperm DNA damage and markers of oxidative stress in infertility. *Reprod Biomed Online* 2007; **14**: 159–165.

43. Isikoglu M, Ozgur K, Oehninger S, Ozdem S, Seleker M. Serum anti-Müllerian hormone

levels do not predict the efficiency of testicular sperm retrieval in men with non-obstructive azoospermia. *Gynecol Endocrinol* 2006; **22**: 256–260.

44. Fujisawa M, Yamasaki T, Okada H, Kamidono S. The significance of anti-Müllerian hormone concentration in seminal plasma for spermatogenesis. *Hum Reprod* 2002; **17**: 968–970.

45. Fenichel P, Rey R, Poggioli S, Donzeau M, Chevallier D, Pointis G. Anti-Müllerian hormone as a seminal marker for spermatogenesis in non-obstructive azoospermia. *Hum Reprod* 1999; **14**: 2020–2024.

46. Steger K, Rey R, Kliesch S, Louis F, Schleicher G, Bergmann M. Immunohistochemical detection of immature Sertoli cell markers in testicular tissue of infertile adult men: a preliminary study. *Int J Androl* 1996; **19**: 122–128.

47. Muttukrishna S, Yussoff H, Naidu M, *et al*. Serum anti Müllerian hormone and inhibin B in disorders of spermatogenesis, *Fertil Steril* 2007; **88**: 516–518.

48. Mustafa T, Amer MK, bdel-Malak G *et al*. Seminal plasma anti-Müllerian hormone level correlates with semen parameters but does not predict success of testicular sperm extraction (TESE). *Asian J Androl* 2007; **9**: 265–270.

*Sue Zaher  Lesley Regan*

**12**

# Magnetic resonance guided thermal ablation therapy for uterine fibroids

Uterine fibroids are the most common solid pelvic tumours in women during the reproductive years. They are estimated to be present in 20–50% of women over the age of 30 years, they increase with age, and the prevalence is higher in Afro-Caribbean women.[1] Fibroids are a significant cause of personal, social and financial distress for women of child-bearing age, with up to 25% of those women diagnosed requiring therapy.[2]

Symptoms typically fall into three groups: (i) heavy and/or prolonged menses; (ii) pressure symptoms due to the pelvic mass, leading to abdominal distension and pain, urinary frequency and nocturia; and (iii) reproductive dysfunction, including sub-fertility, miscarriage and pre-term delivery.[3]

The pathophysiology of uterine fibroids is not well understood. However, genetic predisposition as well as steroid hormone concentrations play a role in the formation and growth of these tumours, as do fibrotic and angiogenetic growth factors.[4]

Considerable debate exists regarding the optimal management of fibroids. Historically, the mainstay of treatment for uterine fibroids has been surgical, either myomectomy or hysterectomy.[5] However, recent changes in cultural attitudes together with an increase in maternal age at child-birth have resulted in women becoming increasingly reluctant to undergo open pelvic surgery. During the last decade, these societal changes have led to a decline in hysterectomy rates and an increased uptake of non-surgical interventions, such as the Mirena Intra Uterine System (IUS) and uterine artery embolisation (UAE). However, many women find the unpredictable bleeding pattern

**Sue Zaher** MBChB
Gynaecology Research Fellow, Department of Radiology, Imperial Healthcare NHS Trust at St Mary's Hospital, South Wharf Road, London W2 1NY, UK

**Lesley Regan** MD FRCOG
Professor and Head, Department of Obstetrics and Gynaecology, Imperial Healthcare NHS Trust at St Mary's Hospital, Mint Wing, South Wharf Road, London W2 1NY, UK
E-mail: l.regan@imperial.ac.uk

associated with the Mirena coil to be unacceptable and the safety of uterine artery embolisation in women wishing to preserve their fertility is debatable.[6]

## THERMAL ABLATION TECHNIQUES

The principles of thermal ablation are that the application of heat leads to a localised tissue destruction. Since the resulting cell necrosis is a coagulative rather than an ischaemic process, the painful infarction syndrome which is recognised after UAE is avoided.[7]

First generation thermal ablation was delivered via the laparoscopic approach.[8] Although this procedure achieved good symptom relief, concerns were raised regarding the high rate of dense pelvic adhesions following the introduction of the live laser fibres into the fibroid at laparoscopy.[9] Damage to the uterine serosa was frequently noted due to lack of thermal monitoring. The operator had to rely on a change in the external appearance of the fibroid as the only means of assessment that sufficient heat had been applied.

Reports of uterine rupture prior to the onset of labour did little to improve confidence in this technique; indeed, it was later suggested that laparoscopic myolysis be reserved for women who have completed their families.[10,11]

Second generation thermal ablation techniques relied on the superiority of magnetic resonance (MR) as an imaging modality and its unique ability to create thermal mapping using phase shift imaging. This gives the operator real-time, colour-map feedback on the temperature levels achieved, together with re-assurance that heating is occurring only in the target tissue, thus ensuring both the safety and efficacy of the treatment.[12]

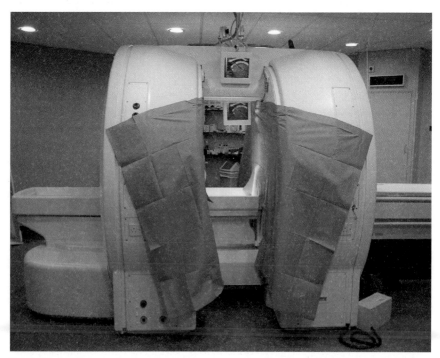

**Fig. 1** Open MRI scanner.

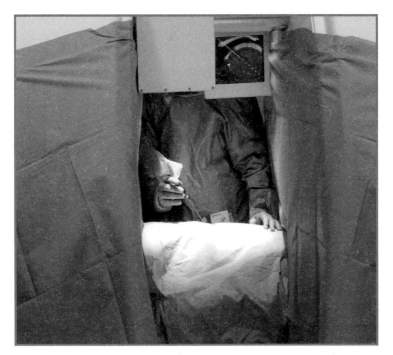

**Fig. 2** MR-guided laser ablation.

The technique of MR-guided laser ablation was made possible by the design of an open magnet (Fig. 1) which allows the operator direct access to the patient. The open scanner is composed of two magnet rings, 'the double doughnut', through the centre of which is placed the patient on the MR table. The scanner allows access to the patient in the vertical plane between the two magnet rings. The operator can stand beside the patient and insert four double-bore needles percutaneously through the abdominal wall and into the uterine fibroids (Fig. 2). The protective inner sheath is then pulled back and the live laser fibres are threaded through and inserted into the fibroids. The procedure is carried out under real-time MR imaging guidance ensuring that the bladder and bowel can be avoided. The thermal ablation begins distant from the serosal surface and, therefore, serosal tissue damage is limited to the puncture wounds.

In a previous publication from our group,[13] we followed a total of 66 patients with symptomatic uterine fibroids wishing to avoid surgery, who were treated with MR-guided laser ablation. MR thermal mapping ensured that maximal doses of energy were applied. Fibroid volume was measured at 3 and 12 months post laser ablation, menstrual blood loss was quantified before and after treatment and a menorrhagia outcomes questionnaire (MOQ) used to assess patient symptoms and satisfaction. There was a reduction in mean fibroid volume of 31% at 3 months and 41% at 1 year. Quality-of-life satisfaction scores were similar to those seen in women undergoing hysterectomy. In summary, 80% of patients said they would recommend the procedure to a friend. In direct contrast to laparoscopic laser ablation, there were no cases of pelvic adhesions. Approximately 150 women have now been treated with MR-guided percutaneous laser ablation with consistently good outcomes.

## FOCUSED ULTRASOUND SURGERY

The ability of ultrasound energy to interact with biological tissues has been recognised for many years. In fact, the earliest medical uses of ultrasound were therapeutic rather than diagnostic, and the ability of ultrasound energy to cause a rise in tissue temperature was recognised as long ago as 1927.[14] Limitations of accuracy and temperature monitoring hampered clinical development of this technique until the recent introduction of modern image guidance. The feasibility of an MRI guided system was first described in 1995.[15] High intensity ultrasound can be focused into a small volume to

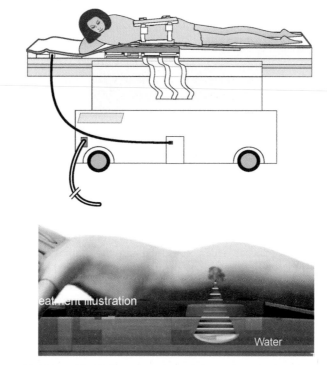

**Fig. 3** MR-guided focused ultrasound. Patient positioned on the MR table. Ultrasound beam focused at a specific target within the fibroid.

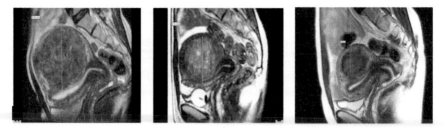

**Fig. 4** Before and after treatment images. MRI sagittal views of a fibroid, pretreatment, after GnRH, and 12 months following MRgFUS treatment.

produce a rise in tissue temperature sufficient to cause lethal cell damage to the target at depth within the body.[16] Concurrent MRI allows accurate tissue targeting and real-time temperature feedback, thereby achieving controlled, localised, thermal ablation without causing damage to surrounding tissues. Focused ultrasound energy is not just minimally invasive, but a completely non-invasive, low-risk therapy for treating uterine fibroids. Using this technique, complete areas of tissue within solid organs can be destroyed without invasion of the skin barrier (Fig. 3).

The fibroid centre at St Mary's Hospital, London was one of the first in the world to be involved in the clinical development of a focused ultrasound surgery system. The Exablate 2000™ (Insightec, Haifa, Israel) fully integrates with our standard closed 1.5 tesla MRI system. A specially integrated patient bed containing an ultrasound transducer is used, upon which the patient is positioned supine. An ultrasound beam is generated from the phased array transducer. The beam travels through a gel pad and a water bath, which help to create acoustic coupling (Fig. 4). The ultrasound energy travels easily through the skin and propagates through the tissue, focusing at a specific target within the body. Very quickly, the tissue at the focus reaches temperatures sufficient to cause cell coagulation. It is important to remember that there is no damage to adjacent tissue and only the target tissue undergoes necrosis.

Concurrent MR imaging allows:

1.   Three-dimensional anatomical information for exact tumour targeting.

2.   Beam path visualisation for safe treatment.

3.   Real-time MR thermometry to achieve planned outcome.

4.   Post-treatment contrast imaging for evaluating treatment outcome.

This closed-loop therapy design provides the operator with immediate feedback, an ability to react to that feedback and appreciate in real time the outcome of therapy, thereby providing the physician with total control of the procedure, in addition to ensuring safety and efficacy.


## RESEARCH STUDY OUTCOMES

To date, over 400 women have taken part in formal research trials and, since US FDA approval was granted for commercial treatments in 2004, more than 3000 women have been treated world-wide.[17] The FDA approved the system based on a review of clinical studies of safety and effectiveness conducted by the manufacturer and on the recommendation of a panel of outside experts convened by the agency to review the device. A total of 109 women with uterine fibroids were treated at seven medical centres around the world, including the unit at St Mary's Hospital. The original goal of the first study was to ensure safety of the treatments while investigating the level of efficacy possible. As such, restrictions were placed on the volume of fibroid tissue that could be treated in any patient. This study compared the results of 109 women who underwent MR-guided focused ultrasound surgery (MRgFUS) with those of 82 women who had a hysterectomy. Only 9 adverse events were reported, including pre-existing medical conditions and continued heavy menses. There was only one device-related adverse incident, with a patient experiencing leg numbness which resolved spontaneously. When the MRgFUS-treated women were reviewed 6 months later, 79.3% reported successful reduction in fibroid-related problems. The mean reduction in fibroid volume was 13.5%.[18]

Having established the safety of the device and the fibroid ablation procedure, the FDA expanded the allowable treatment volume. The Continued Access Study followed 160 women – 96 were treated under the original restricted treatment guidelines, and 64 women were treated under the expanded treatment guidelines. Of this latter group, 84.6% experienced significant symptomatic improvement at 24 months' post-treatment versus 76.2% in women treated under the original guidelines. The conclusions were that results following MRgFUS were constant and reproducible. Furthermore, the expanded treatment guidelines indicated that the greater the volume of tissue treated, the greater the symptomatic improvement.[19] Published results show that with non-perfused volumes of 60% and over, only 11% of patients will require alternative treatments at 24 months.[19]

## ADJUVANT GONADOTROPHIN-RELEASING HORMONE THERAPY

Initial research exclusion criteria dictated a maximum fibroid diameter of 10 cm because the time required to perform the procedure is volume-dependent. This limitation had important clinical implications since fibroids may be asymptomatic until this size threshold has been crossed, particularly amongst black women in whom presentation at a younger age with larger fibroids is common.[20] Hence, we designed and carried out the gonadotrophin-releasing hormone (GnRH) large fibroid study at St Mary's Hospital, London. We postulated that, by administering GnRH agonists to effect a temporary shrinkage in fibroid volume prior to carrying out MRgFUS, we could extend this innovative treatment to a much wider patient group. This was a prospective study, with a 12-month follow-up. Women received a 3-month course of GnRH agonist treatment followed by MRgFUS treatment. The primary outcome measurement was a reported change in Symptom Severity Score (SSS) as judged by the Uterine Fibroid Symptoms and Quality of Life Questionnaire (UFS-QOL). Comparison was made at enrolment, treatment, and at 3- and 6- and 12-months' post-treatment. A secondary outcome was the measured change in target fibroid volume. Fifty women were enrolled in the study. There was a 50% reduction in mean SSS at 6 months and 48% at 12 months post-treatment with 83% of women achieving at least a 10-point reduction in symptom scoring ($P < 0.001$). There was an average reduction in target fibroid volume of 21% overall at 6 months ($P < 0.01$) and 37% at 12 months (Fig. 4). No serious infective complications or emergency operative interventions were recorded.[20]

The initial FDA recommendation was that only women who had completed their families should be treated with MRgFUS. However, with the advantage of consistently good safety and efficacy results being reported, multicentre fertility studies were commenced and are on-going. These studies are recruiting women with symptomatic uterine fibroids, who wish to become pregnant. The non-invasive nature of the ExAblate system, whereby only the uterine fibroids undergo thermal ablation (with no damage to healthy surrounding tissue) suggests that MRgFUS should be a safe approach for women who want to preserve their fertility. The initial results have been very promising and evidence has been accumulating to show that women are able to conceive promptly and successfully deliver children after undergoing MRgFUS treatment for their uterine fibroids.[21,22] To date, 13 women have delivered healthy infants at term without complications and further pregnancies are on-going. Eight women delivered vaginally and five by caesarean section. Most importantly, there were no cases of uterine rupture, pre-term labour, placental abruption, abnormal placentation or fetal growth restriction, with a mean birth weight of 3.4 kg. MRgFUS has the potential to deliver safe and effective treatment for uterine fibroid symptoms without damaging patient fertility or creating additional pregnancy-related risks. Accordingly, the Conformitée Européene (CE) marking for the ExAblate system has been changed to include patients wishing to preserve their fertility.

## FUTURE RESEARCH INTO MRGFUS FOR ADENOMYOSIS

Adenomyosis is a common, benign, gynaecological disorder affecting premenopausal women, which is characterised by the growth of ectopic endometrial glands and stroma deep within the myometrium.[23] The 'benign invasion of endometrium into myometrium' that occurs in adenomyosis can lead to enlargement of the uterus with reactive hyperplasia and hypertrophy of the neighbouring myometrium.[24] The prevalence of adenomyosis in hysterectomy specimens can be found in up to 30% of cases.[25]

Symptoms of adenomyosis include menorrhagia, dysmenorrhoea, and diffuse uterine enlargement, sometimes leading to pelvic pressure and frequent urination. The severity of symptoms correlates roughly with extent of disease.[26] Adenomyosis is difficult to distinguish clinically from uterine leiomyoma, since many symptoms for these two conditions are similar. Further, adenomyosis and leiomyoma are not easily distinguishable on ultrasound and MRI is currently regarded as the best imaging tool for the differential diagnosis.[27]

Due to the accuracy and precision of this technique, we hypothesise that MRgFUS can also treat adenomyosis successfully without deleterious effects on the surrounding myometrium and on subsequent fertility. This hypothesis is also based on past experience in some patients with combined disease, in whom we have successfully ablated both leiomyomatic and adenomyotic lesions.

## CONCLUSIONS

MR-guided focused ultrasound treatment of uterine fibroids has been shown in phase I, II and III clinical trials to be a safe treatment option. Efficacy, in terms of sustained symptomatic relief, improves with more complete fibroid ablation and this should secure its place as a valid alternative to current therapies. Recent trials with the pre-treatment of adjuvant GnRH analogues have demonstrated efficacy in patients with larger fibroids, thus increasing the eligible patient population.

The non-invasive nature of MRgFUS holds particular attraction for candidates who intend subsequent conception without potential impairment of fertility. Current fertility data are encouraging and several published case-studies demonstrate that pregnancy following MRgFUS is safe, and does not increase maternal or fetal morbidity. Further experience with this technique is needed to counsel patients effectively. The UK National Institute for Health and Clinical Excellence (NICE) has recently published guidelines, recognising MRgFUS as a treatment alternative for symptomatic fibroids, and has encouraged our continuing research programme.

## References

1. Kjerulff K, Guzinski G, Langenberg P. Uterine leiomyomas: racial differences in severity, symptoms and age at diagnosis. *J Reprod Med* 1996; **41**: 483–490.
2. Veasy B, Reiter RC. Uterine leiomyomata: etiology, symtomatology and management. *Fertil Steril* 1981; **36**: 433–445.
3. Stewart EA. Uterine fibroids, seminar. *Lancet* 2001; **357**: 293–298.
4. Bosens IA, Lunenefeld B, Donnez J. (eds) Pathogenesis and Medical Management of Uterine Fibroids. London: Parthenon, 1999.
5. Carlson KJ, Miller BA, Fowler Jr FJ. The Maine Women's Health Study: I, Outcomes of hysterectomy. Obstet Gynecol 1994; **83**: 556–565.
6. Hehenkamp WJ, Volkers NA, Broekmans FJ et al. Loss of ovarian reserve after uterine artery embolization: a randomized comparison with hysterectomy. Hum Reprod 2007; **22**: 1996–2005.
7. Gupta JK, Sinha AS, Lumsden MA, Hickey M. Uterine artery embolization for symptomatic uterine fibroids. Cochrane Database Syst Rev 2006; (1): CD005073.
8. Goldfarb HA. Neodymium-yttrium aluminum garnet (YAG) laser laparoscopic coagulation of symptomatic myomas. J Reprod Med 1992; **37**: 636–638.
9. Donnez J, Squifflet J, Polet R, Nisolle M. Laparoscopic myolysis. Hum Reprod Update 2000; **6**: 609–613.
10. Arcangeli S, Pasquarette M. Gravid uterine rupture after myolysis. Obstet Gynecol 1997; **89**: 857.
11. Vilos G, Daly L, Tse B. Pregnancy outcome after laparoscopic electromyolysis. J Am Assoc Gynecol Laparosc 1998; **5**: 289–292.
12. Law PA, Gedroyc WM, Regan L. Magnetic resonance guided percutaneous laser ablation of uterine fibroids. Lancet 1999; **354**: 2049–2050.
13. Hindley JT, Law PA, Hickey M et al. Clinical outcomes following percutaneous magnetic resonance image guided laser ablation of symptomatic uterine fibroids. Hum Reprod 2002; **17**: 2737–2741.
14. ter Haar G. Wood and Loomis: the physical and biological effects of high frequency sound waves of great intensity. Philos Mag 1927; **4**: 7–14.
15. Cline HE, Hynynen K, Watkins RD *et al.* Focused US system for MR imaging-guided tumor ablation. *Radiology* 1995; **194**: 731–737.
16. Lynn J, Zwemer R, Chick A, Miller A. A new method for the generation and use of focused ultrasound in experimental biology. *J Gen Physiol* 1942; **26**: 179–193.
17. Insightec. Exablate 2000 for the treatment of uterine fibroids. Summary of semi annual report to FDA. 2006.
18. Hindley J, Gedroyc WM, Regan L *et al.* MRI guidance of focused ultrasound therapy of uterine fibroids: early results. *AJR Am J Roentgenol* 2004; **183**: 1713–1719.
19. Stewart EA, Gostout B, Rabinovici J, Kim HS, Regan L, Tempany CM; for the Magnetic Resonance Imaging Guided Focused Ultrasound for Uterine Fibroid Group. Sustained relief of leiomyoma symptoms by using focused ultrasound surgery. *Obstet Gynecol* 2007; **110**: 279–287.
20. Smart OC, Hindley JT, Regan L, Gedroyc W. Gonadotrophin-releasing hormone and magnetic resonance-guided focused ultrasound surgery for uterine leiomyomata. *Obstet Gynecol* 2006; **108**: 49–54.

21. Gavrilova-Jordan LP, Rose CH, Traynor KD, Brost BC, Gostout BS. Successful term pregnancy following MR-guided focused ultrasound treatment of uterine leiomyoma. *J Perinatol* 2007; **27**: 59–61.
22. Morita Y, Ito N, Ohashi H. Pregnancy following MR-guided focused ultrasound surgery for a uterine fibroid. *Int J Gynaecol Obstet* 2007; **99**: 56–57.
23. Arnold LL, Ascher SM, Schruefer JJ, Simon JA. Limitations of transvaginal sonography for the diagnosis of adenomyosis, with histopathological correlation. *Obstet Gynecol* 1995; **86**: 461–465.
24. Benson RC, Sneeden VD. Adenomyosis: a reappraisal of symptomatology. *Am J Obstet Gynecol* 1958; **76**: 1044–1057, discussion 1057–1061.
25. Bird CC, McElin TW, Manalo-Estrella P. The elusive adenomyosis of the uterus revisited. *Am J Obstet Gynecol* 1972; **112**: 583–593.
26. Bergholt T, Eriksen L, Berendt N, Jacobsen M, Hertz JB. Adenomyosis. *Hum Reprod* 2001; **16**: 2418–2421.
27. Ascher SM, Jha RC, Reinhold C. Benign myometrial conditions: leiomyomas and adenomyosis. *Top Magn Reson Imaging* 2003; **14**: 281–304.

*Francesco Fiorentino   Marina Baldi*

**13**

# Pre-implantation genetic diagnosis: current status and future prospects*

Couples who are carriers of genetic disorders, including recessive or dominant single-gene defects, sex-linked conditions, or chromosome re-arrangements, face a reproductive risk: affected pregnancies may result in miscarriage or in the birth of a child with significant phenotypic abnormality, sometimes resulting in early death. Such couples have the option of undergoing prenatal diagnosis once a pregnancy is established, either by amniocentesis or chorionic villus sampling (CVS), to allow the detection of the genetic disorder in the fetus. However, if the fetus is found to be carrying a genetic abnormality, the only options available to couples are to have a child with a genetic disease or to terminate the affected pregnancy. This is a difficult and often traumatic decision, as termination, especially in advanced pregnancies, can have substantial psychological and even physical morbidity. Some couples may also experience repeated pregnancy terminations in attempts to conceive a healthy child and might feel unable to accept further affected pregnancies. The prospect of repeating the process of pregnancy and termination one or more times in an attempt to achieve an unaffected pregnancy will be unacceptable to many. Other couples may not contemplate termination because of religious or moral principles.

Such couples have other reproductive choices such as gamete donation or adoption, or to remain childless, but each of these alternatives carries drawbacks.

Pre-implantation genetic diagnosis (PGD) has been introduced as an alternative to prenatal diagnosis in order to increase the options available for

* List of abbreviations at end

**Francesco Fiorentino** PhD
CEO and Lab Director, GENOMA – Molecular Genetics Laboratory, EmbryoGen, Centre for Pre-implantation Genetic Diagnosis, via Po 102, 00198 Rome, Italy
E-mail: fiorentino@laboratoriogenoma.it

**Marina Baldi** PhD (for correspondence)
GENOMA – Molecular Genetics Laboratory, EmbryoGen, Centre for Pre-implantation Genetic Diagnosis, via Po 102, 00198 Rome, Italy
E-mail: marinabaldi@laboratoriogenoma.it

fertile couples who have a known genetically transmittable disease. PGD is a very early form of prenatal diagnosis. Its intended goal is to reduce significantly a couple's risk of transmitting a genetic disorder by diagnosing a specific genetic disease in oocytes or early human embryos that have been cultured *in vitro*, before a clinical pregnancy has been established. After diagnosis, only embryos diagnosed as unaffected are selected for transfer to the woman's uterus.[1,2] The great advantage of PGD over prenatal diagnosis is that a potential termination of pregnancy is avoided. This gives couples the opportunity to start a pregnancy with the knowledge that their child will be unaffected by the genetic disorder. Consequently, PGD does not require a decision regarding possible pregnancy termination.

Following its first application in 1990,[3] PGD has become an important complement to the presently available approaches for prevention of genetic disorders and an established clinical option in reproductive medicine. The number of centres performing PGD has risen steadily, along with the number of diseases that can be tested,[4] and new applications and methodologies are introduced regularly. The range of genetic defects which can be diagnosed includes structural chromosomal abnormalities, such as reciprocal or Robertsonian translocations, in which it has proven to decrease the number of spontaneous abortions while preventing the conception of affected babies,[5] and most of the common single gene disorders (SGDs).[6–8] The scope of PGD has also been extended to improve IVF success for infertile couples, by screening embryos for common or age-related chromosomal aneuploidies in patients at increased risk, including advanced maternal age and repeated miscarriage.[9,10]

More recently, PGD has been used not only to diagnose and avoid genetic disorders, but also to screen out embryos carrying a mutation predisposing to cancer or to a late-onset disease, or to select for certain characteristics, such as matching for tissue type with the aim of recovering compatible stem cells from cord blood at birth for transplantation to an existing sick child.[11–14]

There are several stages during pre-implantation development at which genetic testing can be performed. PGD is usually performed by testing single blastomeres removed from cleavage stage embryos (6–8 cells). An alternative approach is represented by testing the first polar body (1PB) before oocyte fertilisation (so-called 'pre-conception genetic diagnosis', PCGD)[15] or sequential analysis of both first and second (2PB) polar bodies,[16] which are by-products of female meiosis as oocytes undergo maturation and fertilisation. In women who are carriers for a genetic disease, genetic analysis of 1PB and 2PB allows the identification of oocytes that contain the maternal unaffected gene. Analysis of PBs might be considered an ethically preferable way to perform PGD for couples with moral objections to any micromanipulation and potential discarding of abnormal embryos (so-called 'pre-embryonic genetic diagnosis').[17] It may also be an acceptable alternative in those countries where genetic testing of the embryos is prohibited.[15,18] Polar body analysis may be also preferred to blastomere biopsy as it is minimally invasive and damaging since the integrity of the embryo is not compromised. However, this technique is labour intensive, because all oocytes must be tested despite the fact that a significant number will not fertilise or will fail to form normal embryos suitable for IVF. Furthermore, it cannot be used for conditions where the male partner carries the genetic disorder, because only the maternal genetic contribution can be studied.

Single cells for genetic analysis may also be obtained from the embryo at blastocyst stage, on day 5 or 6 after fertilisation.[19] Biopsy at this stage has the advantage of allowing more cells to be sampled (5–10 cells), making genetic tests more robust. It also removes trophectoderm cells, leaving the integrity of the inner cell mass intact. However, due to the difficulty in extended culturing of human embryos, together with the fact that same day testing is required, blastocyst biopsy is currently used routinely in only a few centres.

## MAIN INDICATIONS

Currently, there are mainly three groups of patients who may benefit from PGD.

The first group consists of couples having a reproductive risk, *i.e.* risk of conceiving a child with a genetic disease. This can be a monogenic disorder (autosomal recessive, autosomal dominant or X-linked disorders) or a chromosomal structural aberration (such as a balanced translocation).

The second group consists of couples that undergo IVF treatment and whose embryos are screened for chromosome aneuploidies to increase the chances of an on-going pregnancy. The main indications for pre-implantation genetic screening (PGS) are an advanced maternal age, a history of recurrent miscarriages or repeated unsuccessful implantation. It has also been proposed for patients with obstructive azoospermia (OA) and non-obstructive azoospermia (NOA), in cases of unexplained infertility, or for patients with a previous child or pregnancy with a chromosomal abnormality.

A third group of indications can be defined that include ethically difficult cases. These include situations such as HLA typing of the embryo, so that the child born out of this treatment could be a cord-blood, stem-cell donor for a sick sibling, or PGD to diagnose late-onset diseases and cancer predisposition syndromes.

## SINGLE GENE DISORDERS

Many genetic disorders are a consequence of mutations in single genes. PGD is then indicated for couples at risk for transmitting a monogenic disease to their offspring.

Although it is more than a decade since the first PGD for a SGD was performed,[20] the complexity of the approach has so far limited its clinical application. PGD is a multidisciplinary procedure that requires combined expertise in reproductive medicine and molecular genetics. Additionally, genetic diagnosis of single cells is technically demanding, and protocols have to be stringently standardised before clinical application.

Thus, only a few centres world-wide are offering PGD for SGDs as a clinical service. Nowadays, PGD is available for a large number of monogenic disorders. It is estimated that PGD has been applied for more than 60 different SGDs in over 1800 cycles, resulting in the birth of more than 300 unaffected children.[4] The monogenic diseases for which PGD protocols have been developed generally reflect those for which prenatal diagnosis is already offered and includes a continuously growing list of autosomal recessive, dominant, and X-linked diseases. The most frequently diagnosed autosomal recessive disorders are cystic fibrosis, β-thalassemia, sickle cell disease and

**Table 1** Summary of the common monogenic disorders for which a PGD protocol has been established

| Indication | Gene | OMIM disease | OMIM gene |
|---|---|---|---|
| **PGD for monogenic disorders** | | | |
| Adrenoleukodystrophy (ALD) | ABCD1 | 300100 | *300371 |
| Agammaglobulinaemia non-Bruton type | IGHM | #601495 | *147020 |
| Alport syndrome | COL4A5 | #301050 | *303630 |
| Amyloid neuropathy – Andrade disease | TTR | #105210 | 176300 |
| Angioneurotic oedema | C1NH | #106100 | *606860 |
| Bartter syndrome type 2 | KCNJ1 | #241200 | *600359 |
| Bartter syndrome type 4 | BSND | #602522 | *606412 |
| Blepharophimosis – ptosis – epicanthus inversus syndrome (BEPS) | FOXL2 | #110100 | *605597 |
| Brugada syndrome – long QT syndrome-3 | SCN5A | #601144 | *600163 |
| Bruton agammaglobulinaemia tyrosine kinase | BTK | +300300 | +300300 |
| Ceroid lipofuscinosis neuronal type 2 | CLN2 | #204500 | *607998 |
| Charcot–Marie–type 1A (CMT1A) | PMP22 | #118220 | *601097 |
| Charcot–Marie–Tooth type X (CMTX) | CMTX | #302800 | *304040 |
| Chronic granulomatous disease (CGD) | CYBB | #306400 | *300481 |
| Cystic fibrosis | CFTR | #219700 | *602421 |
| Citrullinaemia | ASS | #215700 | *603470 |
| Congenital adrenal hyperplasia (CAH) | CYP21A2 | 201910 | 201910 |
| Congenital disorder of glycosylation type Ia (CDG Ia) | PMM2 | #212065 | *601785 |
| Congenital fibrosis of extra-ocular muscles 1 (CFEOM1) | KIF21A | #135700 | *608283 |
| Crigler–Najjar syndrome | UGT1A1 | #218800 | *191740 |
| Deafness, autosomal recessive | CX26 | *121011 | *121011 |
| Diabetes mellitus insulin-resistant | INSR | #610549 | *147670 |
| Diamond–Blackfan anaemia (DBA) | RPS19 | #105650 | *603474 |
| Duchenne–Becker muscular dystrophy (DMD/DMB) | DMD | #310200 | *300377 |
| Duncan disease – X-linked lymphoproliferative syndrome (XLPD) | SH2D1A | #308240 | *300490 |
| Ectrodactyly ectodermal dysplasia and cleft lip/palate syndrome (EEC) | p63 | %129900 | *603273 |
| Epidermolysis bullosa dystrophica/pruriginosa | COL7A1 | #131750 | *120120 |
| Exostoses multiple type I (EXT1) | EXT1 | #133700 | *608177 |
| Exostoses multiple type II (EXT2) | EXT2 | #133701 | *608210 |
| Facioscapulohumeral muscular dystrophy | FRG1 | %158900 | *601278 |
| Factor VII deficiency | F7 | 227500 | 227500 |
| Familial Mediterranean fever (FMF) | MEFV | #249100 | *608107 |
| Fanconi anaemia A | FANCA | #227650 | *607139 |
| Fanconi anaemia G | FANCG | #227650 | +602956 |
| Fragile-X | FRAXA | 309550 | 309550 |
| Gangliosidosis (GM1) | GLB1 | 230500 | 230500 |
| Gaucher disease (GD) | GBA | #230800 | *606463 |
| Glanzmann thrombasthenia | ITGA2B | #273800 | *607759 |
| Glycogen storage disease type Ia | G6PC | +232200 | +232200 |
| Glycogen storage disease II | GAA | #232300 | *606800 |
| Glucose-6-phosphate dehydrogenase deficiency | G6PD | 305900 | 305900 |
| Glutaric acidaemia I | GCDH | #231670 | *608801 |
| Haemophagocytic lymphohistiocytosis familial, type 2 (FHL2) | PRF1 | #603553 | *170280 |
| Haemophilia A | F8 | 306700 | 306700 |
| Haemophilia B | F9 | 306900 | 306900 |
| Hand-foot-uterus syndrome | HOXD13 | #140000 | *142959 |
| Hypomagnesaemia primary | CLDN16 | #248250 | *603960 |
| Hypophosphatasia | ALPL | #241500 | *171760 |
| Holt–Oram syndrome (HOS) | TBX5 | #142900 | *601620 |
| Homocystinuria | MTHFR | #236250 | *607093 |
| Immune dysregulation, polyendocrinopathy, enteropathy, X-linked syndrome (IPEX) | FOXP3 | #304790 | *300292 |
| Incontinentia pigmenti | NEMO | #308300 | *300248 |
| Lesch–Nyhan syndrome | HPRT | #300322 | *308000 |
| Limb-girdle muscular dystrophy type 2C (LGMD2C) | SGCG | #253700 | *608896 |
| Long QT syndrome-1 | KCNQ1 | #192500 | *607542 |
| Mannosidosis alpha | MAN2B1 | #248500 | *609458 |
| Marfan syndrome | FBN1 | #154700 | *134797 |

**Table 1** *(continued)* Summary of the common monogenic disorders for which a PGD protocol has been established

| | | | |
|---|---|---|---|
| Methacrylic aciduria, deficiency of β-hydroxyisobutyryl-CoA deacylase | HIBCH | %250620 | %250620 |
| Mevalonic aciduria | MVK | 251170 | 251170 |
| Myotonic dystrophy (DM) | DMPK | #160900 | 605377 |
| Myotonic dystrophy type 2 (DM2) | ZNF9 | #602668 | *116955 |
| Mucopolysaccharidosis type I – Hurler syndrome | IDUA | #607014 | *252800 |
| Mucopolysaccharidosis type IIIA – Sanfilippo syndrome A (MPS3A) | SGSH | #252900 | *605270 |
| Mucopolysaccharidosis type IIIB – Sanfilippo syndrome B (MPS3B) | NAGLU | #252920 | 609701 |
| Mucopolysaccharidosis type VI (MPS VI) – Maroteaux–Lamy syndrome | ARSB | 253200 | 253200 |
| Nemaline myopathy type 7 | CFL2 | #610687 | *601443 |
| Neuro-axonal dystrophy, infantile | PLA2G6 | #256600 | *603604 |
| Neuronal ceroid lipofuscinosis 1 – Batten's disease (CLN1) | PPT1 | #256730 | *600722 |
| Niemann–Pick disease | SMPD1 | #257200 | 607608 |
| Noonan syndrome | PTPN11 | #163950 | *176876 |
| Oculocutaneous albinism type II | OCA2 | #203200 | *611409 |
| Omenn syndrome | RAG1 | #603554 | *179615 |
| Osteogenesis imperfecta | COL1A2 | #166200 | *120160 |
| Pancreatitis, hereditary (PCTT) | PRSS1 | #167800 | +276000 |
| Paramyotonia congenita (PMC) | SCN4A | #168300 | +603967 |
| Phenylketonuria | PAH | +261600 | +261600 |
| Pycnodysostosis | CTSK | #265800 | *601105 |
| Polycystic kidney disease type 1 (PKD1) | PKD1 | 601313 | 601313 |
| Polycystic kidney disease type 2 (PKD2) | PKD2 | +173910 | +173910 |
| Polycystic kidney and hepatic disease-1 (ARPKD) | PKHD1 | #263200 | *606702 |
| Propionic acidaemia | PCCB | #606054 | *232050 |
| Schwartz–Jampel/Stuve–Wiedemann syndrome | LIFR | #601559 | *151443 |
| Retinitis pigmentosa-3 | RPGR | #300389 | *312610 |
| Sickle cell anaemia | HBB | #603903 | 141900 |
| Synpolydactyly (SPD1) | HOXA13 | #186000 | *142989 |
| Smith–Lemli–Opitz syndrome | DHCR7 | #270400 | *602858 |
| Spastic paraplegia type 3 | SPG3A | #182600 | *606439 |
| Spinal muscular atrophy (SMA) | SMN | #253300 | *600354 |
| Spinocerebellar ataxia 3 (SCA3) | ATXN3 | #109150 | *607047 |
| Spinocerebellar ataxia 7 (SCA7) | ATXN7 | #164500 | *607640 |
| Stargardt disease | ABCA4 | #248200 | *601691 |
| Tay Sachs (TSD) | HEXA | #272800 | *606869 |
| α-Thalassemia mental retardation syndrome | ATRX | #301040 | *300032 |
| β-Thalassemia | HBB | 141900 | 141900 |
| Torsion dystonia, early onset (EOTD) | DYT1 | #128100 | *605204 |
| Treacher Collins syndrome | TCOF1 | #154500 | *606847 |
| Tyrosinaemia type 1 | FAH | +276700 | +276700 |
| Tuberosclerosis 1 | TSC1 | #191100 | *605284 |
| Tuberosclerosis 2 | TSC2 | #191100 | *191092 |
| van der Woude syndrome | IRF6 | #119300 | *607199 |
| Wiskott–Aldrich syndrome (WAS) | WAS | #301000 | *300392 |
| **PGD for inherited predisposition to cancer** | | | |
| Familial adenomatous polyposis | APC | +175100 | +175100 |
| Li–Fraumeni syndrome | p53 | #151623 | 191170 |
| Multiple endocrine neoplasia type I | MEN1 | 131100 | 131100 |
| Neurofibromatosis type 1 | NF1 | 162200 | 162200 |
| Retinoblastoma | RB1 | 180200 | 180200 |
| von Hippel-Lindau syndrome | VHL | #193300 | *608537 |
| **PGD for late on-set disorders** | | | |
| Alzheimer disease type 1 | APP | #104300 | *104760 |
| Huntington (HD) | HD | 143100 | 143100 |
| **Specific traits** | | | |
| Pre-implantation HLA Matching | HLA | | |
| SGD + pre-implantation HLA matching | Gene+HLA | | |

OMIN, Online Mendelian Inheritance in Man.
Table updated from Fiorentino and collaborators.[8]

spinal muscular atrophy. For autosomal dominant disorders, the most common indications are myotonic dystrophy and Charcot–Marie–Tooth disease type 1A. PGD for X-linked diseases has been performed mostly for fragile X syndrome, haemophilia A and Duchenne muscular dystrophy.[4,8]

Almost all genetically inherited conditions that are diagnosed prenatally can also be detected by PGD. It can theoretically be performed for any genetic disease with an identifiable gene. Diagnostic protocols now exist for more than 100 monogenic disorders (Table 1).

To establish a diagnostic PGD protocol, extensive preclinical experiments are carried out on single cells (lymphocytes, fibroblasts, cheek cells or spare blastomeres from research embryos) in order to evaluate the efficiency and reliability of the procedure.

Protocols for genotyping single cells for monogenic disorders are based on polymerase chain reaction (PCR). Amplified fragments can be then analysed according to the specific requirements of the test; procedures such as restriction enzyme digestion, single-strand conformation polymorphism (SSCP), denaturing gradient gel electrophoresis (DGGE), allele-specific amplification (ARMS), and recently minisequencing[21] have been used for mutation detection. The introduction of fluorescence multiplex PCR[22] allowed the incorporation of linked polymorphic markers, to improve the robustness of the PGD protocol or to be used as a tool for indirect mutation analysis in linkage-based protocols.

Originally, X-linked diseases were avoided by selection of female embryos, by using the fluorescence *in situ* hybridisation (FISH) procedure to identify embryos with two X chromosomes.[23] A disadvantage of this approach is that half of the discarded male embryos will be healthy, a fact that gives rise to ethical criticism and reduces the chances of pregnancy by depleting the number of embryos suitable for transfer. In addition, half of the female embryos transferred are carriers of the condition. In several X-linked dominant disorders (*e.g.* fragile X syndrome), there is also the possibility that, to a varying degree, carrier females may manifest the disease. For many X-linked diseases, the specific genetic defect has now been identified allowing a specific DNA diagnosis. Therefore, there is now a consensus that it is preferable to use PCR-based tests for sex-linked disorders for which the causative gene is known, instead of performing sex selection.[24]

Many genetic disorders can now be diagnosed using DNA from single cells. However, when using PCR in PGD, one is faced with a problem that only minute amounts of genomic DNA are available for routine genetic analysis. In fact, since PGD is performed on single cells, PCR has to be adapted and pushed to its physical limits. This implies a long process of fine-tuning of the PCR conditions in order to optimise and validate the PGD protocol before clinical application.

There are three main inherent difficulties associated with single-cell DNA amplification. The limited amount of template makes single-cell PCR very sensitive to contamination. The presence of extraneous DNA can easily lead to a misdiagnosis in clinical PGD. Cellular DNA from excess sperm or maternal cumulus cells that surround the oocyte are a potential source of contamination. These cells can be sampled accidentally during the biopsy procedure. For these reasons, oocytes used for PGD of single gene defects should always be stripped of their cumulus cells and fertilised by the use of intracytoplasmic

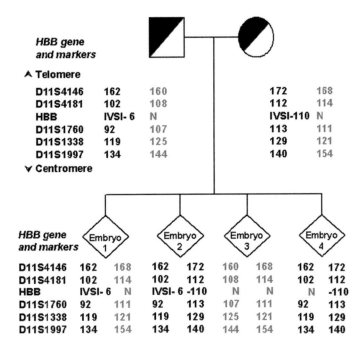

**Fig. 1** Pre-implantation genetic diagnosis for β-thalassemia. Pedigree of a couple carrying β-thalassemia mutations and examples of different results of the HBB gene mutation analysis. Informative STR markers are ordered from telomere (top) to centromere (bottom). The numbers in STR markers represent the size of PCR products in base pair. STR alleles linked to the paternal and maternal mutations are represented in bold. Embryo 1 is carrier for IVSI-6 T/C mutation, embryo 2 is compound heterozygote for the mutations IVSI-110 G-A and IVSI-6 T/C, embryo 3 is normal. Embryo 4 is also affected, although mutation analysis result shows a heterozygosity for mutation IVSI-110 G-A. In fact, linked STR markers highlight an allele drop-out (ADO) of the affected allele.

sperm injection (ICSI) in which only a single sperm is inserted into the oocyte. Furthermore, biopsied cells should be washed through a series of droplets of medium before transfer to the PCR tube, and the wash drop should be tested for contamination.

Other sources of contamination include skin cells from the operators performing the IVF/PGD procedure or 'carry over' contamination of previous PCR products.

Another problem specific to single-cell PCR is the allele drop out (ADO) phenomenon.[25] It consists of the random non-amplification of one of the alleles present in a heterozygous sample. ADO seriously compromises the reliability of PGD for single-gene disorders as a heterozygous embryo could potentially be diagnosed as either homozygous affected (in which case it would be lost from the cohort of available embryos) or homozygous normal (and, therefore, as suitable for replacement) depending on which allele would fail to amplify. This is particularly concerning in PGD for autosomal dominant disorders, where ADO of the affected allele could lead to the transfer of an affected embryo.

To obviate to the above-mentioned problems, PGD protocols now involve direct mutation(s) detection in combination with analysis of a panel of polymorphic short tandem repeat (STR) markers that are closely linked to the gene region containing the disease causing the mutation(s) (Fig. 1). This approach substantially increases the robustness of the diagnostic procedure and decreases the possibility of misdiagnosis, providing the added assurance of a partial 'fingerprint' of the embryo and confirming that the amplified fragment is of embryonic origin. In fact, determination of the specific STR haplotype associated with the mutation acts both as a diagnostic tool for indirect mutation analysis, providing an additional confirmation of the results obtained with the direct genotyping procedure, and as a control of misdiagnosis due to undetected ADO. Diagnosis is assigned only when haplotype profiles, obtained from linked STR markers, and mutation analysis profiles are concordant. The multiplex STR marker system also provides an additional control for contamination with exogenous DNA, as other alleles, differing in size from those of the parents, would be detected. The experience of a large series of PGD cycles[8] strongly suggests that PGD protocols for SGD are not appropriate for clinical practice without including a set of linked STR markers; consequently, this strategy is currently used by most PGD laboratories.

## CHROMOSOME TRANSLOCATION

Individuals who carry a balanced chromosomal translocation (reciprocal or Robertsonian), inversion, or other structural chromosomal re-arrangements, typically have no medical issues although some have reduced fertility. However, although the individual is healthy, there is increased risk that the egg or sperm of that individual can have an unbalanced chromosome make-up due to excess or missing genetic material. An embryo derived from the union of such an unbalanced gamete with a partner's normal gamete also will have an unbalanced genetic composition.[26] The presence of an unbalanced translocation can lead to an embryo not implanting, a pregnancy being lost or a child being born with mental and physical problems. Individuals with a translocation may, therefore, experience multiple pregnancy losses or have a child with a chromosomal abnormality.

The primary aim of PGD for translocation is to improve live-birth rates by either reducing the risk of recurrent spontaneous abortions or to improve pregnancy rate in infertile couples (*e.g.* after failed IVF attempts).[27]

Reciprocal translocations, characterised by the exchange of two terminal segments between different chromosomes, is the commonest form of chromosome abnormality, which occurs in about 1 in 500 live-births. Robertsonian translocations, in which a whole chromosome is translocated to another through centromeric fusion, are less common and occur in only about 1 in 1000 individuals.

FISH is the method of choice for diagnosing chromosome re-arrangements. This technique uses DNA probes labelled with distinctly coloured fluorochromes that bind to specific DNA sequences unique to each chromosome. Imaging systems enable the fluorescent probe signals to be identified and counted to detect missing or excess chromosomal material.

Analysis of reciprocal translocations for PGD is difficult since each translocation is effectively unique to the family or person within which it occurs, and the break-point may have arisen at any point on any chromosome; thus, different combinations of FISH probes are usually required for each couple. FISH strategies for assessment of reciprocal translocations use three differentially labelled probes, two probes that are specific for the subtelomeric regions of the translocated segments, combined with a centromeric probe.[5,26] Analysis of Robertsonian translocations is simpler, involving the use of specific probes chosen to bind at any point on the long arm of each chromosome that is involved in the translocation. The above combination of probes allows embryos that carry an unbalanced chromosome complement to be distinguished from healthy ones. However, both strategies do not discriminate between non-carrier embryos and those that carry the balanced form of the translocation.

A potential pitfall of PGD for chromosomal translocations is that, in some cases, FISH probes might cross-hybridise with other loci in the genome or polymorphisms might occur in some individuals, potentially leading to misdiagnosis. FISH probes should, therefore, always be tested on blood samples from both partners before being used for PGD.

By selecting and transferring embryos with unbalanced chromosome composition, it has been possible for translocation carriers to achieve normal pregnancies, and miscarriage rates in this patient group have been reduced.[28]

## GENETIC SCREENING FOR CHROMOSOME ANEUPLOIDY

Selection of the most competent embryo(s) for transfer is generally based on morphological criteria. However, many women fail to achieve a pregnancy after transfer of good-quality embryos. One of the presumed causes is that such morphologically normal embryos show an abnormal number of chromosomes (aneuploidies).[29] Aneuploid embryos have a lower survival rate than normal embryos and the majority fail to implant.

Aneuploidy screening of embryos derived from subfertile patients undergoing IVF is probably the most frequent indication for PGD.[4] Pre-implantation genetic diagnosis for aneuploidy screening, also named pre-implantation genetic screening (PGS), enables the assessment of the numerical chromosomal constitution of cleavage stage embryos. It aims to identify and select for transfer only chromosomally normal (euploid) embryos so to increase the implantation and pregnancy rate for IVF patients, lower the risk for miscarriage and reduce the risk of having a baby with an aneuploidy condition.[30]

PGS and PGD are often presented as similar treatments, although they have completely different indications: PGS aims to improve pregnancy rates in subfertile couples undergoing IVF/ICSI treatment; PGD aims to prevent the birth of affected children in fertile couples with a high risk of transmitting genetic disorders.

The detection of chromosomes in a single biopsied blastomere is usually achieved using FISH. Essentially, FISH probes to detect those aneuploidies most commonly observed after birth or in miscarriages (involving detection of chromosomes X, Y, 13, 16, 18, 21, and 22) are used. This panel of probes has the potential of detecting over 70% of the aneuploidies found in spontaneous abortions.[31] Aneuploidy conditions (involving chromosomes 8, 9, 15, and 17) that cause lack of implantation or can results in a miscarriage early in pregnancy are also tested.[32,33]

The main indications suggested for PGS are repeated implantation failure,[34] advanced maternal age,[34,35,37] repeated miscarriage in patients with normal karyotypes,[10,33,36,37] and severe male factor infertility.[38,39]

### Repeated implantation failure

Since the beginning of IVF, many efforts have been made to enhance success rates – the optimisation of embryo selection being one of the most evaluated strategies. Some couples, even after numerous IVF attempts, are unable to become pregnant. Recurrent implantation failure (RIF) has been defined as three or more unsuccessful embryo transfer procedures. Extensive evidence[34,40] has revealed a high incidence of numerical chromosomal abnormalities (60–70%) in embryos of patients with a poor outcome after IVF. This has been observed despite good embryo morphology, which offers a possible explanation for their low implantation potential. In women with repeated implantation failure, PGS has been proposed to minimise the likelihood of a chromosome abnormality in a future pregnancy and increase the chance of achieving an ongoing successful pregnancy.

### Advanced maternal age

It is well known that the chance of live birth after IVF treatment decreases dramatically with maternal age. It is widely accepted that reduced fertility with age is mostly egg related. Women of advanced maternal age (AMA; usually defined as maternal age $\geq 37$ years) are at a higher risk of producing aneuploid embryos, resulting in implantation failure, a higher risk of miscarriage or the birth of a child with a chromosome abnormality (e.g. Down syndrome). Aneuploidy is also believed to be a major reason for the decrease of fertility with age. Several studies have determined that approximately 70% of embryos from women of advanced maternal age may be aneuploid,[34,40,41] providing an explanation for their low implantation and high miscarriage rates after IVF treatment. The poor IVF success rate in this category of patients has been well documented and it was suggested that PGS could be used as a screening technique to detect the most common aneuploid syndromes (those involving chromosomes X, Y, 13, 18, 21 and also 16, 22, 15, 17, involved in spontaneous abortions) in an attempt to improve the on-going pregnancy rate, reduce miscarriage rates, and decrease the chance of a chromosomally abnormal pregnancies in these patients.

### Repeated miscarriage

Repeated miscarriage (RM), classically defined as three or more spontaneous pregnancy losses, affects about 1% of the population.[42] Approximately 5–8% of couples with a history of RM have an abnormal karyotype, usually a balanced translocation. Many couples have no identifiable cause or predisposing factor for their miscarriages and, therefore, no standard treatment options. Because women with a history of unexplained RM are more likely to have a high incidence (50–60%) of numerical chromosomal abnormalities in embryos,[10,36,37,43] PGS has been proposed as a means of reducing the risk of first-trimester miscarriage and of decreasing the risk of conceiving an aneuploid pregnancy.

## Severe male infertility

Meiotic disorders are reported to occur frequently in infertile males. Multiple studies have documented an increased aneuploidy rate in both testicular and epididymal spermatozoa from NOA and OA compared with normozoospermic men.[44,45] Increased aneuploidy and mosaicism rates have also been demonstrated for embryos derived from azoospermic men (NOA and OA) compared with embryos derived from fertile men.[38,39]

As the chromosomal defects in gametes can be transmitted to the resulting embryos, PGS has also been proposed for such categories of patients.

## Limitations of PGS

PGS currently has several disadvantages that limit its clinical value. The main concern is the elevated mosaicism rate observed at the human pre-implantation stage. Mosaicism is defined as the embryo having cells with different chromosome make-up and it has been found in up to 57% of day-3 biopsied embryos.[46,47] Mosaicism may represent a major source of misdiagnosis (60%) because of both false-positive and false-negative results.

Besides mosaicism, several technical limitations inherent to the FISH technique have been described. FISH is considered to have an error rate of 5–10%.[30,32] Overlapping signals may be a source of misdiagnosis resulting in false diagnosis of monosomies. Signal splitting has also been described, resulting in the detection of false trisomies. Finally, evidence suggests that up to half of all embryos identified as aneuploid at the cleavage stage and that survive to the blastocyst stage will 'self-correct';[48,49] therefore, an abnormal result may not necessarily indicate that the embryo is abnormal and ill-fated.

As a consequence of the above limitations, it has been questioned whether some normal embryos might be excluded from the cohort that is considered suitable for embryo transfer, which, especially in older women who might have small embryo cohorts, could result in the failure to reach embryo transfer.

## The debate on PGS usefulness

In the last few years, there has been a steady increase in the number of PGS cycles reported to the ESHRE PGD Consortium, from 116 cycles in the data collection from 1997–1998 to 1722 cycles in 2003.[4] The rapid increase in the use of this procedure has raised questions about its efficacy for routine use.

There have been a number of non-randomised, comparative studies of IVF/ICSI with or without PGS, for AMA or RIF. Most of these studies report that PGS increases the implantation rate,[9,10,34,35] decreases the abortion rate and reduces trisomic conceptions.[33,50,51]

Three randomised, controlled trials have been performed for AMA,[40,52,53] indicating that PGS does not improve on-going pregnancy or live-birth rates. In contrast, one of these studies showed that PGS decreased the chance of achieving an on-going pregnancy or live birth.[52] Furthermore, a randomised, controlled trial evaluating the effectiveness of PGS in women under the age of 35 years undergoing IVF treatment with single embryo transfer did not show a benefit for PGS.[54]

The two largest randomised trials for AMA have been criticised.[55–58] Staessen and collaborators[40] were criticised for biopsying two cells instead of one cell, which may have a negative impact on embryo survival.[59] The study by Mastenbroek and collaborators[52] was criticised for its high percentage of embryos without a diagnosis (20%), not including probes for chromosomes 15 and 22 and the low on-going pregnancy rate in the control group (39 pregnancies from 195 oocyte retrievals; 20%).

The debate on the usefulness of PGS continues. Further data are required to establish whether PGS results in enhanced live-birth rate and, if this is the case, to identify which patients may benefit. The only effective way to resolve this debate is to perform well-designed and well-executed randomised, controlled, clinical trials. The design of further studies should include an adequate randomisation protocol with a clear stratification concerning the indications to perform PGS, the replacement of the same number of embryos in both study and control groups and the healthy live-birth rate per treatment cycle as the main outcome measure. Additional points of interest for future research are which chromosomes should be evaluated (as well as the added value of using more probes) and the implementation of new technologies for chromosome analysis; for example, comparative genomic hybridisation (CGH) and array-CGH, that enable a complete assessment of the numerical chromosomal constitution of pre-implantational embryos.

## ETHICALLY DIFFICULT INDICATIONS

The proposed indications for use of PGD are being extended. New uses include PGD to detect mutations for susceptibility to cancer and for late-onset disorders. In addition, parents with children needing haematopoietic stem cell transplants have used PGD to ensure that their next child is free of disease and also to provide a good tissue match for an existing sick child.

### Late-onset disorders

One of the proposed uses of PGD is the identification of embryos at risk for late-onset or adult-onset diseases.[60,61] Many serious genetic disorders, such as Alzheimer's disease or Huntington disease, have their onset later in adult life, with the result that those affected remain healthy for years or even decades, until the onset of the disease, living a normal healthy life. However, some of these disorders are progressive and disabling, or even lethal, and account for serious ill health. On the other hand, the high probability or certainty of developing the disorders, and their incurable nature, can lead to a stressful life as the patient waits for the first symptoms to occur, and anticipates premature death.

Thus, late-onset disorders present a dilemma: at birth a child will be healthy and free of disease, but will carry the potential to develop ill health in later life. Ethically, the question is whether the burden of carrying susceptibility genes is so great for the child and parents that the burdens of IVF and PGD to screen embryos to avoid the affected children are justified. Many believe PGD is ethically acceptable for these indications because of the heavy burden imposed on patients who are carriers of one of these diseases.

The use of PGD for asymptomatic individuals with the Huntington mutation is one of the most common application of PGD for late-onset disorders.[4] 'Non-disclosure' PGD for Huntington disease is applied in those cases in which the prospective parent at risk does not wish to be informed about his or her own carrier status but wants to have offspring free of the disease.[62] Embryos can be tested for the presence of the mutation without revealing any of the details of the cycle or diagnosis to the prospective parents. Non-disclosure testing is controversial and not generally approved by professionals,[61,63] because it puts practitioners in an ethically difficult position, *i.e.* when no embryos are available for transfer and a mock transfer has to be carried out to avoid the patient suspecting that he/she is a carrier or having to undertake PGD cycles even when the results of previous cycles preclude the patient being a carrier.

The ESHRE Ethics Task Force[24] currently discourages non-disclosure testing, recommending the use of exclusion testing instead. Exclusion testing is based on a linkage analysis with polymorphic markers, in which the parental and grandparental origin of the chromosomes can be established. In this way, only embryos are replaced that do not contain the chromosome derived from the affected grandparent, avoiding the need to detect the mutation itself.[61]

However, exclusion testing PGD is also considered as ethically dubious by some because embryos with an allele from an affected grandparent will be excluded for transfer, although only in half of the cases will the allele be affected.

### Inherited cancer predisposition syndromes

Inherited cancer predisposition has become one of the emerging indications for PGD.[64] The use of PGD to screen out embryos carrying a mutation predisposing to cancer (*e.g.* breast/ovarian cancer – BRCA1, BRCA2 genes; Li–Fraumeni syndrome – p53 gene; neurofibromatosis – NF1 and NF2 genes; retinoblastoma – RB1 gene; familial adenomatous polyposis – APC gene; hereditary non-polyposys colon cancer – MSH2 and MLH1 genes; von Hippel–Lindau syndrome – VHL gene) prevents the birth of children who would face a greatly increased life-time risk of cancer, and hence require close monitoring, prophylactic surgery, or other preventive measures. Through PGD, couples with a familial history of cancer, where one partner has the high-risk gene, now have an opportunity to start a pregnancy knowing that their offspring will not carry the cancer-predisposing mutation.

Contrary to the monogenic late-onset diseases, which have full penetrance (*i.e.* a person found to have a mutation will inevitably get the symptoms in the future), having a predisposing mutation for a susceptibility gene only increases the risk of developing the disease (*e.g.* inheritance of a familial breast cancer mutation in the *BrCa1* gene is associated with an 80% life-time risk of breast cancer and other *BrCa1*-related cancers), since its effect is modified by other genes and other factors. For the hereditary forms of breast cancer (due to mutations in BRCA1 and BRCA2 genes) and for some hereditary forms of colorectal cancer (*e.g.* FAP and HNPCC), the absolute risk figures are relatively high but, unlike late-onset diseases, the above cancer predisposition syndromes can usually be treated or preventive measures can be adopted.

As couples present for PGD for heritable cancer genes, there is likely to be wide-spread debate in the community about the associated ethical issues, including disposal of embryos carrying the cancer-predisposition gene mutation and the practice of eugenics.[65] Although these indications do not involve diseases that manifest themselves in infancy or childhood, the conditions in question lead to substantial health problems for offspring in their thirties or forties. However, owing to the adult onset of hereditary cancer, prenatal diagnosis raises ethical issues surrounding the acceptability of terminating an affected pregnancy.

## Human leukocyte antigen matching

PGD of single gene disorders, combined with human leukocyte antigen (HLA) matching, represents one of the most recent applications of the technique in reproductive medicine.[11–14] This strategy has emerged as a tool for couples at risk of transmitting a genetic disease to allow them to select unaffected embryos of a HLA tissue type compatible with those of an existing affected child. In such cases, PGD is used not only to avoid the birth of affected children, but also to conceive healthy children who may also be potential HLA-identical donors of haematopoietic stem cells (HSC) for transplantation in siblings with a life-threatening disorder. At delivery, HSCs from the newborn umbilical cord blood are collected and used for the haematopoietic reconstruction of the affected sibling.

At present, allogenic HSC transplantation represents the only curative treatment for restoring normal haematopoiesis in severe cases of neoplastic (*e.g.* leukaemia) or congenital (*e.g.* β-thalassemia) disorders affecting the haematopoietic and/or the immune system. A critical factor associated with favourable outcome in stem cell transplantation is the use of HLA-genotype identical donors, and HLA-identical siblings provide the best chance to the recipient in the achievement of a successful transplantation. Unfortunately, because of the limited availability of HLA-matched sibling donors, most patients face the option of transplantation using a volunteer unrelated matched donor, identified from national or international registers. In these cases, the results are less favourable compared to the matched-sibling transplant. HLA mismatches are increased using unrelated donors, with a consequent higher incidence of both transplant-related mortality and graft-versus-host disease.

Therefore, if no HLA-identical donor is available in the family, an increasing number of couples with a child affected by an haematopoietic disorder are considering the use of IVF and PGD techniques for therapeutic intent. Before the existence of PGD, natural conception followed by prenatal diagnosis and possibly termination of pregnancy was the only option when trying to find a HLA matching future sibling.[66]

Verlinsky and collaborators[11] described the first pre-implantation HLA matching case in 2001. Since then, HLA typing has become an important PGD indication in four countries – the US,[11] Italy,[12,13] Turkey,[67,68] Belgium.[14]

The procedure is particularly indicated for patients with children affected by Fanconi anaemia, β-thalassemia, sickle cell anaemia, Wiscott–Aldrich syndrome (WAS), X-linked adrenoleukodystrophy (X-ALD), X-linked hyper-IgM syndrome (HIGM), X-linked hypohidrotic ectodermal dysplasia with immune deficiency (HED-ID) and other similar disorders, that require a HLA-compatible HSC or bone marrow donation to be treated effectively. The great difficulty in finding a HLA-matched donor, even among family members, led to the application of pre-implantation HLA matching also for diseases such as acute lymphoid leukaemia (ALL), acute myeloid leukaemia (AML), or

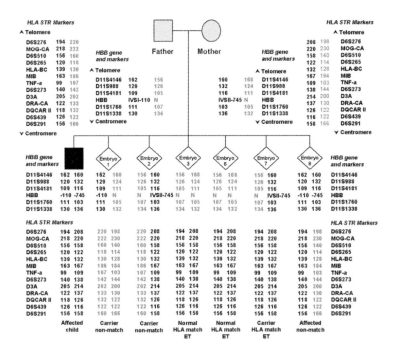

**Fig. 2** Pre-implantation HLA matching in combination with PGD for β-thalassemia, resulting in the birth of two twins, HLA matched with the affected sibling. Specific haplotypes were determined by genomic DNA analysis of HLA STR markers and β-globin (HBB) linked markers from father, mother (upper panel) and affected child (lower panel-left side, black square). Informative STR markers are ordered from telomere (top) to centromere (bottom). The numbers in STR markers represent the size of PCR products in base pair. Paternally and maternally derived HLA haplotypes matched to the affected child are shown in boldface. STR alleles linked to the paternal and maternal mutations are also represented in bold. Examples of different results of HBB mutation analysis and HLA haplotyping from biopsied blastomeres are shown in the lower panel. Paternally and maternally derived haplotypes from each embryo are shown on the left and the right, respectively. The HLA identity of the embryos with the affected sibling has been ascertained evaluating the inheritance of the matching haplotypes. Embryos 1, 2 (carriers) and 8 (affected) represent HLA non-identical embryos. Embryos 3 and 6 were diagnosed as normal, and embryo 7 as carrier, HLA matched with the affected sibling, and were transferred resulting in a HLA matched unaffected birth of two twins (babies have been originated from embryos 3 and 6). ET, embryo transfer.

sporadic Diamond–Blackfan anaemia (DBA).[13] For these conditions, not involving testing of a causative gene, PGD for HLA matching becomes the primary indication.

Technically, PGD for HLA typing is a difficult procedure due to the extreme polymorphism of the HLA region. Taking into account also the complexity of the region (presence of a large number of loci and alleles), the use of a direct HLA typing approach would require standardisation of a PCR protocol specific for each family, presenting different HLA allele combinations, making it time consuming and unfeasible. The use of a pre-implantation HLA matching protocol irrespective of the specific genotypes involved makes the procedure more straight-forward. Currently, PGD laboratories use a strategy based on a flexible indirect HLA typing protocol applicable to a wide spectrum

**Table 2** Different indications for pre-implantation HLA matching and clinical outcome

| Disease | No. of PGD cycles | No. of couples | No. of clinical pregnancies[a] (%)[b] | No. of pregnancies still going on | No. of pregnancies delivered | No. of babies born | No. of CBT |
|---|---|---|---|---|---|---|---|
| **HLA typing combined with PGD** | | | | | | | |
| β-Thalassemia | 164 | 84 | 39 (36.1) | 6 | 25 | 27 | 5 |
| Gaucher disease | 4 | 1 | 1 (33.3) | 0 | 0 | 0 | |
| Adrenoleukodystrophy | 3 | 2 | 1 (50.0) | 1 | 0 | 0 | |
| Duncan syndrome | 2 | 1 | 0 (0.0) | 0 | 0 | 0 | |
| Hurler syndrome | 2 | 2 | 0 (0.0) | 0 | 0 | 0 | |
| Sickle cell disease | 2 | 2 | 0 (0.0) | 0 | 0 | 0 | |
| Mannosidosis alpha | 2 | 1 | 0 (0.0) | 0 | 0 | 0 | |
| Chronic granulomatous disease | 1 | 1 | 1 (100.0) | 0 | 1 | 2 | |
| Wiskott–Aldrich syndrome | 1 | 1 | 1 (100.0) | 0 | 1 | 1 | 1 |
| Bruton agammaglobulinaemia | 1 | 1 | 1 (100.0) | 1 | 0 | 0 | |
| Glanzmann thrombasthenia | 1 | 1 | 0 (0.0) | 0 | 0 | 0 | |
| Fanconi anaemia – G | 1 | 1 | 0 (0.0) | 0 | 0 | 0 | |
| **HLA-only typing** | | | | | | | |
| Acute lymphoblastic leukaemia | 22 | 16 | 6 (37.5) | 3 | 2 | 2 | 1 |
| Diamond–Blackfan anaemia | 16 | 3 | 3 (27.3) | 1 | 0 | 0 | |
| Istiocitosis | 3 | 1 | 1 (33.3) | 0 | 1 | 1 | 7 |
| Total | 225 | 118 | 54 (35.5) | 12 | 30 | 33 | |

[a]Number of pregnancies evidenced by clinical or ultrasound parameters (ultrasound visualisation of a gestational sac).
[b]Pregnancy rate per embryo transfer.
Updated from Fiorentino and collaborators.[13]

of possible HLA genotypes.[11–14] The approach involves testing of single blastomeres by fluorescent multiplex PCR analysis of polymorphic STR markers, scattered throughout the HLA complex, obtaining a 'fingerprint' of the entire HLA region (Fig. 2).

Although several publications[11–14] on the argument have demonstrated the success and the usefulness of the PGD/HLA approach (Table 2), some limitations have to be considered. First, advanced maternal age as well as a poor ovarian response to hormonal hyperstimulation are known to have a major impact on the number of the retrievable oocytes and, consequently, on the number of embryos available for analysis, reducing the likelihood of finding transferable embryos. Thus, several IVF cycles may be necessary to obtain a pregnancy and a live birth. Second, the selection of a donor embryo for HSC transplantation before implantation is restricted by the intrinsic genetic constitution of the embryos: only a quarter or 25% (HLA typing), 3 of 16 or 19% (HLA typing and mutation analysis) of embryos will be transferable. Third, the clinical success rate of PGD/HLA typing is low. This is a common phenomenon in all centres offering HLA/PGD and couples should be counselled for this because they have put all their hope in this approach to cure their sick child.

Ethical discussions concerning PGD in combination with HLA are on-going, mainly because the procedure involves embryo selection.[66] In case of embryo selection based on HLA typing, the ethical discussion is even stronger since the selection here is based on a non-disease trait and opponents claim that the child to be born is instrumentalised, although some authors maintain that the Kantian imperative is not breached since the future donor child will not only be a donor but also become a loved individual within the family. However, if there would be an existing HLA-matched sibling, we would find it acceptable to use that child as a donor of haematopoietic stem cells. Unless the use as a donor would be the sole reason for creating the child, there would be no violation of its autonomy.

The question of the motivation of the couples also may raise concerns. They could be tempted to have an additional child solely for the purpose of furthering the interest of the existing sibling and not because they desire another baby. This difficult ethical issue can be partially addressed by careful genetic and psychological counselling of the couples to ascertain their real motivation. However, considering the efforts by the parents to save their sick child, it is very unlikely that they would not treat the saviour child as equal to the existing child.

Finally, considerable numbers of embryos are also needed to identify one closely matched with the sick sibling, although all resultant embryos not transferred to the patients are usually frozen for future possible use, in case the couples wish to have more unaffected children.

However, most consider the above criticisms a minor concern when compared with the possibility of saving a child's life from a devastating disease.

## FUTURE PERSPECTIVES

The most remarkable impact on PGD is likely to come from emerging new technologies. Using current FISH methods, less than half of the chromosome complement can be analysed in a single cell. New molecular cytogenetic techniques might allow a full analysis of all chromosomes, improving accuracy and reliability of chromosomal analysis.

The most promising new technique is array-CGH, in which CGH is performed using microarrays as the target DNA.[69] These microarrays are made up of DNA sequences specific to human chromosomes spotted onto a platform, usually a glass slide. Array-CGH enables the assessment of all the chromosomes by comparing the studied DNA with a normal sample and is appropriate for analysis of minute quantities of DNA and single cells, as for PGD.[70] This method has a high resolution and is amenable to automation. The array-CGH procedure detects imbalance across the genome allowing identification of whole-chromosome aneuploidies and even small structural aberrations. However, the technique is limited to detecting relative imbalance and, therefore, changes in whole ploidy cannot be identified.

The analysis of mutations in specific genes is also evolving. The principal advance has been the wider use of multiplex PCR. Other techniques aiming at maximising the data obtained from a single cell are also becoming increasingly important. One of the most exciting developments in single-cell analysis has been the introduction of protocols designed to amplify the entire genome from a single cell. A recent important evolution of these whole genome amplification (WGA) protocols is multiple displacement amplification (MDA), a technique that may offer greater accuracy and more rapid through-put in the future.[71] Aliquots of MDA products can be taken and used as a source of templates for subsequent locus-specific PCRs, allowing many individual DNA sequences or genes to be analysed in the same cell. The main limitations of using this method on single cells are the high ADO and preferential amplification rates compared with direct PCR on DNA from a single cell.[71,72] Moreover, WGA provides a sufficient supply of sample DNA available for other applications, such as aneuploidy screening by using array-CGH technique. It could be envisaged that, in the future, every embryo tested for a monogenic disorder is also routinely screened for aneuploidy, investigating all chromosomes.

## CONCLUSIONS

PGD is an effective clinical tool for assisted reproduction and genetic screening. From the patients' perspective, PGD is an important alternative to standard prenatal diagnosis. Low pregnancy and birth rates, and the high cost of the procedure, however, make it unlikely that PGD will supersede, completely, the more conventional methods of prenatal testing. PGD remains a complex combination of different technologies, which involve reproductive medicine as well as clinical and molecular genetics and require the close collaboration of a team of specialists. Rapid advances in molecular genetics are likely to stimulate further use of PGD and to encourage a substantial increase in the range of genetic conditions for which PGD is offered. The accuracy of procedures will be improved and its clinical application will be simplified. In the future, PGD will play an increasing role as a specialised clinical procedure, becoming a useful option for many more couples with a high risk of transmitting a genetic disease, to prevent the birth of affected children, and infertile couples to improve IVF success.

## Abbreviations

1PB, first polar body; 2PB, second polar body; ADO, allele drop out; ALL, acute lymphoid leukaemia; AMA, advanced maternal age; AML, acute myeloid leukaemia; ARMS, allele-specific amplification; CGH, comparative genomic hybridisation; CVS, chorionic villus sampling; DBA, sporadic Diamond–Blackfan anaemia; DGGE, denaturing gradient gel electrophoresis; FISH, fluorescence *in situ* hybridisation; HED-ID, X-linked hypohidrotic ectodermal dysplasia with immune deficiency; HIGM, X-linked hyper-IgM syndrome; HLA, human leukocyte antigen; HSCs, haematopoietic stem cells; ICSI, intracytoplasmic sperm injection; IVF, *in vitro* fertilisation; MDA, multiple displacement amplification; NOA, non-obstructive azoospermia; OA, obstructive azoospermia; PB, polar body; PCGD, pre-conception genetic diagnosis; PCR, polymerase chain reaction; PGD, pre-implantation genetic diagnosis; PGS, pre-implantation genetic screening; RIF, recurrent implantation failure; RM, repeated miscarriage; SGD, single gene disorder; SSCP, single-strand conformation polymorphism; STR, short tandem repeat; WAS, Wiscott–Aldrich syndrome; WGA, whole genome amplification; X-ALD, X-linked adrenoleukodystrophy

## References

1. Braude P, Pickering S, Flinter F, Ogilvie CM. Preimplantation genetic diagnosis. *Nat Rev Genet* 2002; **3**: 941–953.
2. Sermon K, Van Steirteghem A, Liebaers I. Preimplantation genetic diagnosis. *Lancet* 2004; **363**: 1633–1641.
3. Handyside AH, Kontogianni EH, Hardy K, Winston RM. Pregnancies from biopsied human preimplantation embryos sexed by Y-specific DNA amplification. *Nature* 1990; **344**: 769–770.
4. Sermon KD, Michiels A, Harton G *et al.* ESHRE PGD Consortium data collection VI: Cycles from January to December 2003 with pregnancy follow-up to October 2004. *Hum Reprod* 2007; **22**: 323–336.
5. Munne S, Sandalinas M, Escudero T *et al.* Outcome of preimplantation genetic diagnosis of translocations. *Fertil Steril* 2000; **73**: 1209–1218.
6. Vandervorts M, Staessen C, Sermon K *et al.* The Brussels' experience of more than 5 years of clinical preimplantation genetic diagnosis. *Hum Reprod Update* 2000; **6**: 364–373.
7. Pickering S, Polidoropoulos N, Caller J *et al.* Strategies and outcomes of the first 100 cycles of preimplantation genetic diagnosis at the Guy's and St Thomas' Center. *Fertil Steril* 2003; **79**: 81–90.
8. Fiorentino F, Biricik A, Nuccitelli A *et al.* Strategies and clinical outcome of 250 cycles of preimplantation genetic diagnosis for single gene disorders *Hum Reprod* 2006; **21**: 670–684.
9. Munne S, Cohen J, Sable D. Preimplantation genetic diagnosis for advanced maternal age and other indications. *Fertil Steril* 2002; **78**: 234–236.
10. Rubio C, Simon C, Vidal F *et al.* Chromosomal abnormalities and embryo development in recurrent miscarriage couples. *Hum Reprod* 2003; **18**: 182–188.
11. Verlinsky Y, Rechitsky S, Schoolcraft W, Strom C, Kuliev A. Preimplantation diagnosis for Fanconi anemia combined with HLA matching. *JAMA* 2001; **285**: 3130–3133.
12. Fiorentino F, Biricik A, Karadayi H *et al.* Development and clinical application of a strategy for preimplantation genetic diagnosis of single gene disorders combined with HLA matching. *Mol Hum Reprod* 2004; **10**: 445–460.
13. Fiorentino F, Kahraman S, Karadayi H *et al.* Short tandem repeats haplotyping of the HLA region in preimplantation HLA matching. *Eur J Hum Genet* 2005; **13**: 953–958.
14. Van de Velde H, Georgiou I, De Rycke M *et al.* Novel universal approach for preimplantation genetic diagnosis of b-thalassemia in combination with HLA matching of embryos. *Hum Reprod* 2004; **19**: 700–708.
15. Fiorentino F, Biricik A, Nuccitelli A *et al.* Rapid protocol for pre-conception genetic diagnosis of single gene mutations by first polar body analysis: a possible solution for the Italian patients. *Prenat Diagn* 2008; In press.
16. Verlinsky Y, Rechitsky S, Cieslak J *et al.* Preimplantation diagnosis of single gene disorders by two-step oocyte genetic analysis using first and second polar body. *Biochem Mol Med* 1997; **62**: 182–187.
17. Kuliev A, Rechitsky S, Laziuk K *et al.* Pre-embryonic diagnosis for Sandhoff disease.

*Reprod Biomed Online* 2006; **12**: 328–333.

18. Tomi D, Griesinger G, Schultze-Mosgau A *et al*. Polar body diagnosis for hemophilia a using multiplex PCR for linked polymorphic markers. *J Histochem Cytochem* 2005; **53**: 277–280.

19. Veiga A, Sandalinas M, Benkhalifa M *et al*. Laser blastocyst biopsy for preimplantation diagnosis in the human. *Zygote* 1997; **5**: 351–354.

20. Handyside AH, Lesko JG, Tarin JJ, Winston RM, Hughes MR. Birth of a normal girl after *in vitro* fertilization and preimplantation diagnostic testing for cystic fibrosis. *N Engl J Med* 1992; **327**: 905–909.

21. Fiorentino F, Magli MC, Podini D *et al*. The minisequencing method: an alternative strategy for preimplantation genetic diagnosis of single gene disorders. *Mol Hum Reprod* 2003; **9**: 399–410.

22. Findlay I, Quirke P, Hall J, Rutherford A. Fluorescent PCR: a new technique for PGD of sex and single-gene defects. *J Assist Reprod Genet* 1996; **13**: 96–103.

23. Harper JC, Coonen E, Ramaekers FC *et al*. Identification of the sex of human preimplantation embryos in two hours using an improved spreading method and fluorescent *in-situ* hybridization (FISH) using directly labelled probes. *Hum Reprod* 1994; **9**: 721–724.

24. Shenfield F, Pennings G, Devroey P, Sureau C, Tarlatzis B, Cohen J. Taskforce 5: preimplantation genetic diagnosis. *Hum Reprod* 2003; **18**: 649–651.

25. Findlay I, Ray P, Quirke P, Rutherford A, Lilford R. Allelic drop-out and preferential amplification in single cells and human blastomeres: implications for preimplantation diagnosis of sex and cystic fibrosis. *Hum Reprod* 1995; **10**: 1609–1618.

26. Scriven PN, Handyside AH, Ogilvie CM. Chromosome translocations: segregation modes and strategies for preimplantation genetic diagnosis. *Prenat Diagn* 1998; **18**: 1437–1449.

27. Scriven PN, Flinter F, Bickerstaff H, Braude P, Ogilvie MC. Robertsonian translocations – reproductive risks and indications for preimplantation genetic diagnosis. *Hum Reprod* 2001; **16**: 2267–2273.

28. Munne S, Morrison L, Fung J *et al*. Spontaneous abortions are reduced after preconception diagnosis of translocations. *J Assist Reprod Genet* 1998; **15**: 290–296.

29. Marquez C, Sandalinas M, Bahçe M, Alikani M, Munné S. Chromosome abnormalities in 1255 cleavage-stage human embryos. *Reprod BioMed Online* 2000; **1**: 17–26.

30. Wilton L. Preimplantation genetic diagnosis for aneuploidy screening in early human embryos: a review. *Prenat Diagn* 2002; **22**: 512–518.

31. Simpson JL, Bombard AT. Chromosomal abnormalities in spontaneous abortion: frequency, pathology and genetic counselling. In: Edmonds K, Bennett MJ. (eds) *Spontaneous Abortion*. London: Blackwell, 1987; 51.

32. Munné S, Magli C, Bahçe M *et al*. Preimplantation diagnosis of the aneuploidies most commonly found in spontaneous abortions and live births: XY, 13, 14, 15, 16, 18, 21, 22. *Prenat Diagn* 1998; **18**: 1459–1466.

33. Munné S, Chen S, Fischer J *et al*. Preimplantation genetic diagnosis reduces pregnancy loss in women aged 35 years and older with a history of recurrent miscarriages. *Fertil Steril* 2005; **84**: 331–335.

34. Gianaroli L, Magli MC, Ferraretti AP, Munne S. Preimplantation diagnosis for aneuploidies in patients undergoing *in vitro* fertilization with a poor prognosis: identification of the categories for which it should be proposed. *Fertil Steril* 1999; **72**: 837–838.

35. Munné S, Magli MC, Cohen J *et al*. Positive outcome after preimplantation diagnosis of aneuploidy in human embryos. *Hum Reprod* 1999; **14**: 2191–2199.

36. Pellicer A, Rubio C, Vidal F *et al*. *In vitro* fertilization plus preimplantation genetic diagnosis in patients with recurrent miscarriage: an analysis of chromosome abnormalities in human preimplantation embryos. *Fertil Steril* 1999; **71**: 1033–1039.

37. Munné S, Chen S, Fischer J *et al*. Preimplantation genetic diagnosis reduces pregnancy loss in women aged 35 years and older with a history of recurrent miscarriages. *Fertil Steril* 2005; **84**: 331–335.

38. Platteau P, Staessen C, Michiels A *et al*. Comparison of the aneuploidy frequency in embryos derived from testicular sperm extraction in obstructive azoospermic men. *Hum*

*Reprod* 2004; **19**: 1570–1574..

39. Silber S, Escudero T, Lenahan K. Chromosomal abnormalities in embryos derived from testicular sperm extraction. *Fertil Steril* 2003; **79**: 30–38.

40. Staessen C, Platteau P, Van Assche E *et al*. Comparison of blastocyst transfer with or without preimplantation genetic diagnosis for aneuploidy screening in couples with advanced maternal age: a prospective randomized controlled trial. *Hum Reprod* 2004; **19**: 2849–2858.

41. Platteau P, Staessen C, Michiels A *et al*. Preimplantation genetic diagnosis for aneuploidy screening in women older than 37 years. *Fertil Steril* 2005; **84**: 319–324.

42. Li TC, Makris M, Tomsu M, Tuckerman E, Laird S. Recurrent miscarriage: aetiology management and prognosis. *Hum Reprod Update* 2002; **8**: 463–481.

43. Platteau P, Staessen C, Michiels A *et al*. Preimplantation genetic diagnosis for aneuploidy screening in patients with unexplained recurrent miscarriages. *Fertil Steril* 2005; **83**: 393–397.

44. Egozcue S, Blanco J, Vendrell JM *et al*. Human male infertility: chromosome anomalies, meiotic disorders, abnormal spermatozoa and recurrent abortion. *Hum Reprod Update* 2000; **6**: 93–105.

45. Calogero A, Burello N, De Palma A *et al*. Sperm aneuploidy in infertile men. *Reprod Biomed Online* 2003; **6**: 310–317.

46. Baart E, Van Opstal D, Los F, Fauser B, Martini E. Fluorescence *in situ* hybridization analysis of two blastomeres from day 3 frozen-thawed embryos followed by analysis of the remaining embryo on day 5. *Hum Reprod* 2004; **19**: 685–693.

47. Coonen E, Derhaag JG, Dumoulin JC *et al*. Anaphase lagging mainly explains chromosomal mosaicism in human preimplantation embryo. *Hum Reprod* 2004; **19**: 316–324.

48. Li M, DeUgarte C, Surrey M *et al*. Fluorescence *in situ* hybridization reanalysis of day-6 human blastocysts diagnosed with aneuploidy on day 3. *Fertil Steril* 2005; **84**: 1395–1400.

49. Munne S, Velilla E, Colls P *et al*. Self-correction of chromosomally abnormal embryos in culture and implications for stem cell production. *Fertil Steril* 2005; **84**: 1328–1334.

50. Munné S, Fischer J, Warner A *et al*. Preimplantation genetic diagnosis significantly reduces pregnancy loss in infertile couples: a multi-center study. *Fertil Steril* 2006; **85**: 326–332.

51. Colls P, Escudero T, Cekleniak N *et al*. Increased efficiency of preimplantation genetic diagnosis for infertility using 'no result rescue'. *Fertil Steril* 2007; **88**: 53–61.

52. Mastenbroek S, Twisk M, Van Echten-Arends J *et al*. *In vitro* fertilization with preimplantation genetic screening. *N Engl J Med* 2007; **357**: 9–17.

53. Stevens J, Wale P, Surrey ES, Schoolcraft WB. Is aneuploidy screening for patients aged 35 or over beneficial? A prospective randomized trial. *Fertil Steril* 2004; **82 (Suppl 2)**: 249.

54. Staessen C, Michiels A, Verpoest W *et al*. Does PGS improve pregnancy rates in young patients with single embryo transfer? *Hum Reprod* 2007; **22 (Suppl)**: i32.

55. Handyside AH, Thornhill AR. *In vitro* fertilization with preimplantation genetic screening. *N Engl J Med* 2007; **357**: 1770.

56. Wilton LJ. *In vitro* fertilization with preimplantation genetic screening. *N Engl J Med* 2007; **357**: 1770.

57. Munné S, Cohen J, Simpson JL. *In vitro* fertilization with preimplantation genetic screening. *N Engl J Med* 2007; **357**: 1769–1770.

58. Munné S, Gianaroli L, Tur-Kaspa I *et al*. Substandard application of preimplantation genetic screening may interfere with its clinical success. *Fertil Steril* 2007; **88**: 781–784.

59. Cohen J, Wells D, Munné S. Removal of 2 cells from cleavage stage embryos is likely to reduce the efficacy of chromosomal tests that are used to enhance implantation rates. *Fertil Steril* 2007; **87**: 496–503.

60. Verlinsky Y, Rechitsky S, Verlinsky O *et al*. Preimplantation diagnosis for early-onset Alzheimer disease caused by V717L mutation. *JAMA* 2002; **287**: 1018–1021.

61. Sermon K, De Rijcke M, Lissens W *et al*. Preimplantation genetic diagnosis for Huntington's disease with exclusion testing. *Eur J Hum Genet* 2002; **10**: 591–598.

62. Stern H, Harton G, Sisson M *et al*. Non-disclosing preimplantation genetic diagnosis for Huntington disease. *Prenat Diagn* 2002; **22**: 303–307.

63. Braude PR, de Wert GMWR, Evers-Kiebooms G, Pettigrew RA, Geraedts JP. Non-

disclosure preimplantation genetic diagnosis for Huntington's disease: practical and ethical dilemma. *Prenat Diagn* 1998; **18**: 1422–1426.

64. Rechitsky S, Verlinsky O, Chistokhina A *et al.* Preimplantation genetic diagnosis for cancer predisposition. *Reprod BioMed Online* 2002; **4**: 148–155.

65. Robertson J. Extending preimplantation genetic diagnosis: the ethical debate – ethical issues in new uses of preimplantation genetic diagnosis. *Hum Reprod* 2003; **18**: 465–471.

66. Pennings G, Schots R, Liebaers I. Ethical considerations on preimplantation genetic diagnosis for HLA typing to match a future child as a donor of haematopoietic stem cells to a sibling. *Hum Reprod* 2002; **17**: 534–538.

67. Kahraman S, Findikli N, Karliklaya G *et al.* Medical and social perspectives of PGD for single gene disorders and human leukocyte antigen typing. *Reprod BioMed Online* 2007; **14 (Suppl 1)**: 104–108.

68. Kahraman S, Karlikaya G, Serteyl S *et al.* Clinical aspects of preimplantation genetic diagnosis for single gene disorders combined with HLA matching. *Reprod BioMed Online* 2004; **9**: 529–532.

69. Pinkel D, Segraves R, Sudar D *et al.* High resolution analysis of DNA copy number variation using comparative genomic hybridization to microarrays. *Nat Genet* 1998; **20**: 207–211.

70. Le Caignec C, Spits C, Sermon K *et al.* Single-cell chromosomal imbalances detection by array CGH. *Nucleic Acids Res* 2006; **34**: e68.

71. Handyside AH, Robinson MD, Simpson RJ *et al.* Isothermal whole genome amplification from single and small numbers of cells: a new era for preimplantation genetic diagnosis of inherited disease. *Mol Hum Reprod* 2004; **10**: 767–772.

72. Spits C, Le Caignec C, De Rycke M *et al.* Optimization and evaluation of single-cell whole-genome multiple displacement amplification. *Hum Mutat* 2006; **27**: 496–503.

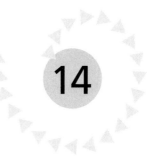

*Alka Prakash  William L. Ledger*

# 14

# Recurrent miscarriage

Recurrent miscarriage is defined as three or more consecutive spontaneous miscarriages. It occurs in about 0.5–3% of women trying to conceive.[1] Patients with recurrent miscarriage are frequently treated conservatively leading to patient dissatisfaction with a perceived lack of useful intervention. Identifiable causes can be found in only about 30–50% of these women.[2] Possible causes of recurrent miscarriage include chromosomal anomaly, prothrombotic states, uterine malformations, primary endometrial defects and endocrinological abnormalities. Treatment depends on the underlying cause of the miscarriage.

## CHROMOSOMAL ANOMALY

Chromosomal anomaly may be parental or fetal. Parental chromosomal anomalies appear to be directly associated with recurrent miscarriage[3] and occur in around 4% of couples with recurrent miscarriage as compared to 0.2% in the general population.[4] Chromosomal translocation is the commonest anomaly seen in these patients including Robertsonian translocations which lead to unbalanced translocations in the fetus, leading to miscarriage. Recent studies have also identified lethal X chromosome mutations, which occur as a result of non-random X chromosome inactivation, which may lead to recurrent pregnancy loss.[5] Studies have also shown that sperm defects may be associated with recurrent pregnancy loss, with significantly increased sperm chromosome aneuploidy, apoptosis, and abnormal sperm morphology in partners of women with recurrent pregnancy loss.[6]

**Alka Prakash** MD MRCOG  (for correspondence)
Sub-speciality Registrar in Reproductive Medicine, Cambridge University Hospitals at Addenbrooke's Hospital, Hills Road, Cambridge CB2 0QQ, UK
E-mail: alkaprakash@hotmail.com

**Willam L. Ledger** MA DPhil FRCOG
Professor and Head of Department, Academic Unit of Reproductive and Developmental Medicine, University of Sheffield, Jessop Wing, Tree Root Walk, Sheffield S10 2SF, UK

Fetal chromosomal abnormality accounts for a significant proportion of recurrent miscarriage and was detected in 60% of samples of chorionic villous trophoblast tested after miscarriage.[7] Recurrent fetal chromosomal anomalies due to aneuploidies, associated with increased maternal age is also responsible for a significant number of cases of recurrent miscarriage. Cytogenetic study of the products of conception may be misleading due to contamination from maternal tissue and there is a need for refinement in assessment of pregnancy loss tissue.

It is possible to apply pre-implantation genetic diagnosis (PGD) in conjunction with IVF to reduce the likelihood of a further miscarriage. *In vitro* fertilisation allows pre-implantation embryos to be screened for aneuploidy, using fluorescent *in situ* hybridisation. Although the embryo aneuploidy rate is higher in women with recurrent miscarriage than in age-matched controls, aneuploidy screening and the replacement of chromosomally normal embryos does not improve the rate of live-births.[8] Moreover, women with recurrent miscarriage aged less than 37 years only had a 26% live-birth rate after *in vitro* fertilisation and aneuploidy screening. By contrast, after spontaneous conception, the live-birth rate is 75%. At the present time, PGD can only be offered for commonly abnormal chromosomes. Patients with chromosomal anomalies are offered genetic counselling; in selected cases, consideration should be given to the use of donor gametes.

## PROTHROMBOTIC STATES

Prothrombotic states may be acquired or hereditary. An example of an acquired form of prothrombotic state is antiphospholipid syndrome whereas there are various types of hereditary thrombophilias such as deficiencies of antithrombin III, protein C or protein S as well as factor V Leiden and prothrombin 2010A variant.[4] Antiphospholipid syndrome has now been recognised as a cause of recurrent miscarriage and is reported to occur in 7–42% of women with recurrent pregnancy loss. The wide variation in results of different studies is due to diverse criteria for patient selection, the temporary fluctuation of antiphospholipid antibody titres in individual patients, transient positivity secondary to infections, suboptimal sample collection and preparation and lack of standardisation of laboratory tests for their detection.[9]

The cause for pregnancy failure in women with antiphospholipid antibodies has been suggested to be defective endovascular trophoblast invasion.[10] It can, in turn, impair placentation by increasing apoptosis and attenuating mitosis and leading to abnormal trophoblast differentiation.[11]

Antiphospholipid antibodies consist of about 20 antibodies directed against negatively charged phospholipid binding proteins. Of these, only lupus anticoagulant and anticardiolipin antibodies are believed to be of clinical significance. Antiphospholipid antibody syndrome is now accepted as an established and treatable cause of recurrent miscarriage. There has been inconsistency in the diagnosis of antiphospholipid syndrome, both clinically and by laboratory parameters. The diagnosis of antiphospholipid syndrome requires fulfilment of at least one of the following clinical criteria:[12]

1. Three or more unexplained consecutive spontaneous abortions before the 10th week of gestation, with maternal anatomical or hormonal abnormalities and paternal and maternal chromosomal abnormalities excluded.

2. One or more unexplained deaths of a morphologically normal fetus at or beyond the 10th week of gestation, with normal fetal morphology documented by ultrasound or by direct examination of the fetus.

3. One or more premature births of a morphologically normal neonate at or before the 34th week of gestation because of severe pre-eclampsia or eclampsia or severe placental insufficiency.

In addition, persistent abnormality of one of the following tests when measured at least twice, > 6 weeks apart:

1. *Lupus anticoagulant* – this can be detected in a number of ways using coagulation-based assays.

2. *Antiphospholipid antibodies* – these are IgG or IgM antibodies against cardiolipin and are usually detected using the enzyme-linked immunosorbent assay technique.

The hereditary thrombophilias include deficiencies of antithrombin III, protein C, protein S, factor V Leiden and prothrombin 20210 variant. Research suggests that prothrombotic state not only results in an exaggerated haemostatic response during pregnancy, leading to thrombosis of uteroplacental vasculature and subsequent fetal loss,[13] but also confers a risk of ischaemic heart disease in later life.[14] In the European prospective cohort study on thrombophilias (EPCOT), a significant association between thrombophilias and miscarriage was reported.[15] Another study reported significantly reduced live-birth rates in women with a history of recurrent miscarriage who carried the factor V Leiden allele.[16] Since then, various smaller studies have shown conflicting results. In a recent study, the prevalence of thrombophilic genetic mutations was similarly distributed in women with recurrent miscarriage and parous controls. However, in women with recurrent miscarriage, presence of multiple mutations increases the risk of future miscarriage.[17] It is uncertain if heritable thrombophilias cause recurrent miscarriage and routine testing in women with recurrent miscarriage is desirable but not currently advocated.[18]

Most centres treat women with antiphospholipid antibodies by thromboprophylaxis using low-dose aspirin and/or heparin. The debate continues as to which is better. While one study reported that a combination of heparin and aspirin significantly improves live-birth rates,[19] another study reported no improvement in pregnancy outcome with addition of low molecular heparin over and above the use of aspirin in this group of women.[20] At present, most centres would treat these women with a combination of aspirin and heparin based on the Royal College of Obstetricians and Gynaecologists guidelines.

Most previous studies have used unfractionated heparin in their protocol but more use is now made of low molecular weight heparins, which can be given as once-daily instead of twice-daily injections. Aspirin is usually started as soon as a pregnancy test is positive, with addition of heparin at the detection of fetal heart pulsations on ultrasound scan.[21] The ideal treatment length is difficult to define but it is reasonable to stop treatment at 34–40 weeks' gestation depending on previous history and the type of pregnancy loss. Post partum thromboprophylaxis is required for women with history of thrombosis and is continued up to 6 weeks' postpartum.[4]

## ENDOMETRIAL DEFECT

'Luteal phase defect' has been reported to be associated with recurrent miscarriage for some time. Luteal phase defect may be found in 17–28% of women with recurrent miscarriage.[22] The large variation in incidence can be explained by differences in endometrial dating criteria or patient selection.

Endometrial defects were initially thought to reflect suboptimal progesterone production but sometimes appear when serum concentration of progesterone is normal.[22] The latter may represent a suboptimal response of an inadequately primed endometrium.

Immunohistochemical studies of expression of steroid receptors in the endometrium have shown abnormalities in the 'unexplained' group of women with recurrent miscarriage. However, further studies are needed to establish the possible contribution of steroid receptor defects to recurrent miscarriage. Initial investigations have revealed conflicting results between oestrogen and progesterone receptor status and luteal phase defects. Li et al.[23] found variation in staining patterns in different parts of the same endometrial biopsy specimen. The wide regional variation in the intensity and pattern of staining make identification of abnormal patterns of oestrogen receptors by immunohistochemistry difficult. Furthermore, their data suggested altered progesterone receptor expression may be present in about a third of women with recurrent miscarriage. Endometrial androgen receptor expression was not found to be different in women with recurrent miscarriage compared to a fertile control group.[23] In summary, preliminary results using immunohistochemistry suggest that differences in steroid receptors unrelated to luteal phase defect may be present in a small subpopulation of women with unexplained recurrent miscarriage. However, these studies need strengthening by further investigations using techniques such as in situ hybridisation, RT–PCR and RNase protection assays which will detect the differences in mRNA expression.

The biochemistry of the endometrium has been investigated in recurrent miscarriage. Some studies have shown reduced levels of glycoprotein MUC-1 in the endometrium[24] and lower levels of PP14 (glycodelin A) in plasma and endometrial flushings of women with recurrent miscarriage.[25] MUC-1 is a major epithelial apical surface glycoprotein in human endometrium. It may be involved in the very early stage of human implantation and play a role in the attachment of the embryo to the luminal epithelium. Glycodelin appears to have immunosuppressive function thereby aiding implantation.

Inhibin, activin and follistatin are glycoprotein hormones which play an integral role in decidualisation process during the reproductive cycle. In a recent study, we found a significantly reduced expression of beta-A-subunit and follistatin in the endometrial stroma at the time of implantation in women with recurrent miscarriage.[26] The stroma is the prime site for decidualisation, and the decreased expression of beta-A-subunit (which is a constituent of activin A) and follistatin in the stroma in the women with recurrent miscarriage supports the view that decidualisation may be impaired in these women which may reflect as early pregnancy failure.

Gonadotropin treatment may be used to treat luteal phase defect associated with recurrent miscarriage. In a preliminary study by Li and Cooke,[27] gonadotropins were employed for ovarian stimulation to increase oestrogen production. This was based on the observation that the majority of cases with luteal phase defect are associated with suboptimal response of the endometrium to normal levels of circulating progesterone.[27] Gonadotropins were employed to increase oestrogen production in the follicular phase to prime the endometrium adequately, and the miscarriage rate in the treatment group (2 of 13) was significantly lower than the untreated group (7 of 13). Adequately powered studies are still lacking to confirm the benefit of gonadotropin treatment in women with recurrent pregnancy loss.

Progesterone induces secretory changes in the endometrium which are essential for implantation of the embryo. It has been suggested that some cases of miscarriage might be due to inadequate secretion of progesterone, either in the postovulatory phase of the menstrual cycle or in early pregnancy. Hence, progestational agents have been used, beginning in the early first trimester of pregnancy, in an attempt to prevent miscarriage. A meta-analysis of the use of progesterone showed that it did not reduce the miscarriage rate for women with sporadic miscarriage. However, a subgroup analysis of women with recurrent miscarriage suggested that progesterone use in the first trimester might be of benefit with a trend towards improved birth rates.[28]

## UTERINE PATHOLOGY

This may be congenital (such as uterine septum) or acquired, for example uterine fibroid and intra-uterine adhesions (Asherman's syndrome). Women with sub-septate uterus have been reported to have a higher proportion of first trimester loss.[29] In the septate uterus, defective implantation on the septate portion of the uterus may lead to recurrent miscarriage.[30] A recent study using 3-dimensional scanning reported congenital anomalies to be more severe in women with a history of recurrent miscarriage as compared with a control group.[31] Asherman's syndrome is the development of post-traumatic intra-uterine fibrosis which may obliterate all or part of the cavity leading to miscarriage. This may be mechanical or due to reduced responsiveness of the fibrosed endometrium to circulating steroids.

Uterine fibroids, especially submucous in location, may reduce pregnancy rates and increase miscarriage rates. However, their effect on reproductive potential is controversial.[32] Removal of submucous and intramural fibroids decreases the risk of subsequent miscarriage.[33] The mechanism by which fibroids cause early pregnancy loss is unclear. The expression of HOX10, a gene that controls differentiation and is involved in implantation, has now been shown to be lower in uteri with fibroids than those without.[34]

Cervical weakness is a common cause of second trimester miscarriage, presenting typically with painless dilatation of the cervix leading to miscarriage. It may be associated with congenital uterine anomalies such as bicornuate uterus, or in isolation. The objective diagnostic test for this in the non-pregnant state is not yet clearly established and diagnosis is usually based on the clinical history.

Congenital uterine malformations such as septate uterus are best treated with hysteroscopic resection while bicornuate uterus is treated with laparotomy and Strassman's metroplasty. Acquired abnormalities such as fibroids or synechia should be removed hysteroscopically to reduce miscarriage rates.[33] Cervical weakness is treated by cervical cerclage, which reduces the incidence of preterm birth but has no significant effect on perinatal survival.[35] A Cochrane Review identified no conclusive evidence that prophylactic cervical cerclage reduces the risk of recurrent mid-trimester miscarriage.[36] Therefore, the value of serial ultrasound assessments of cervical shortening and the insertion of a rescue cerclage for prevention of late miscarriage and preterm delivery are questionable.[37]

## ENDOCRINOLOGICAL ABNORMALITIES

It is estimated that approximately 8–12% of all pregnancy losses are the result of endocrine factors.[38] Endocrine factors may, in turn, affect endometrial development, the normality of which is a pre-requisite for successful implantation and establishment of the fetomaternal unit. Putative endocrine abnormalities that may lead to recurrent miscarriage include hypersecretion of luteinising hormone (LH) as may occur in polycystic ovary syndrome (PCOS). Hypersecretion of LH may be present in about 50% of women with PCOS. The prevalence of raised LH in the follicular phase in patients with recurrent miscarriage has been found to vary between 0–50% in various studies.[2,39] This may reflect the use of different assay methods or differences in the populations studied. However, high LH and testosterone concentrations did not appear to have a significant relation to pregnancy outcome.[39] Rai et al.[40] found the prevalence of ultrasound appearance of polycystic ovary in women with recurrent miscarriage at 41%, but the live-birth rate was similar in these women compared with those without ultrasonographical features of polycystic ovary.

Hence, prepregnancy suppression of raised LH is not recommended based on current understanding and there does not appear to be any value in measuring LH in the follicular phase of women presenting with recurrent miscarriage.

Laparoscopic ovarian drilling is a recognised treatment option for polycystic ovarian disease. This procedure improves reproductive outcome in women with polycystic ovaries with anovulation. However, randomised studies are required for assessing the effect of ovarian drilling on patients with history of recurrent miscarriage with polycystic ovaries.

Metformin is an oral biguanide insulin sensitising agent that reduces insulin resistance and improves implantation rate after IVF.[41] Its effect on women with recurrent miscarriage and PCOS is unclear. A prospective pilot study reported that metformin, reduced miscarriage rates in women with polycystic ovary syndrome. Ten women with PCOS with 22 previous pregnancies and 16 first-trimester spontaneous miscarriages in the past had 10 pregnancies with one spontaneous miscarriage after being treated with metformin. In a retrospective study, metformin administration during pregnancy reduced first-trimester pregnancy loss significantly.[42] The early pregnancy loss in the metformin group was 8.8% compared with 41.9% in the control group.

Although large, randomised, controlled trials are required to confirm these findings, the preliminary data suggest that therapeutic measures that correct the endocrinological imbalance in PCOS by the use of metformin may help to reduce miscarriage rates. However, larger studies are required to confirm this and metformin should be used in pregnancy with caution.

## THYROID DYSFUNCTION AND DIABETES

Maternal endocrine abnormalities such as diabetes or thyroid dysfunction have been linked to miscarriages. However, well-controlled diabetes or thyroid dysfunction does not appear to increase the risk of recurrent miscarriage. A recent study reported an increased incidence of insulin resistance in women with recurrent miscarriage compared with age-matched controls.[43] Thyroid antibodies have also been studied in women with recurrent miscarriage but the presence or absence of thyroid antibodies do not appear to have any prognostic value on the outcome of future pregnancy in this subgroup of women.[44] Routine screening for occult diabetes and thyroid disease is, therefore, not justified at present.[45]

## ANDROGENS

Elevated circulating concentrations of androgens have also been measured in women with recurrent miscarriage, independent of association with PCOS. Raised androgens appear to affect endometrial glandular function adversely[46] and, therefore, may affect the implantation process. In a recent study, Nardo et al.[39] examined 344 women with a history of recurrent miscarriage and reported no difference in pregnancy outcome of women with raised follicular phase testosterone concentrations compared with those that had normal concentrations.

## PROLACTIN

Elevation of prolactin in the circulation may be associated with recurrent miscarriage, as there is in vitro evidence that prolactin reduces the secretion of HCG from early human placenta. However, this has not yet been confirmed by rigorous in vivo studies. The role of hyperprolactinaemia as a risk factor for recurrent miscarriage is unclear, with conflicting evidence regarding its role in recurrent pregnancy loss.[22] In a randomised control trial including 64 women with hyperprolactinaemia and recurrent miscarriage, a higher rate of successful pregnancy outcome was seen in women who received treatment for hyperprolactinaemia.[47] In another study, in which plasma prolactin levels were measured daily from the mid-luteal to early follicular phase, there was no association of hyperprolactinaemia with recurrent miscarriage.[22] At present, there is insufficient evidence for routine testing of prolactin levels in women being investigated for recurrent miscarriage.[45]

## IMMUNOLOGICAL ABNORMALITIES

Adaptation of the maternal immunological response is required for successful implantation of the embryo. This depends on a link between the fetal antigen presentation and maternal recognition and response to this antigen. The role of endometrial immunity is currently under study. Although it has been implicated that endometrial immune factors such as cytokines and leukocytes which act at the fetomaternal interface may affect implantation, this is still in its research phase and more investigations are required to establish the precise role of these immune factors in recurrent pregnancy loss.[45]

Alloimmune response has been implicated in recurrent miscarriage by the increased sharing of human leukocyte antigens (HLA) with the male partner, which may inhibit the production of anti-paternal cytotoxic antibodies, anti-idiotype antibodies and mixed lymphocyte reaction blocking antibodies.[48]

Some studies have reported high levels of various autoantibodies in women with recurrent miscarriage but prospective data on pregnancy outcome for women with or without autoantibodies are also conflicting with most studies suggesting no association.[44] Autoantibodies are found in 18–43% of patients with recurrent miscarriage.[4] Apart from antiphospholipid antibodies, the significance of other autoantibodies is unknown. Thyroid autoantibodies, for example, have been studied in depth but research so far has generated conflicting results. The antibodies may affect pregnancy in two ways, either by a direct effect on fetal tissue or as a reflection of a more wide-spread underlying autoimmune response. The prognostic value of thyroid antibodies has been studied; while some investigators found it a good prognostic marker,[49] other studies did not.[44]

The role of cellular immunity has recently been a subject to significant research in recurrent miscarriage. Natural killer cells were found to be higher in the circulation[50] and CD56+ leukocytes were found to be higher in the endometrium of women with recurrent miscarriage.[51] Due to the intrinsic differences in peripheral and uterine natural killer cells, measurement of peripheral natural killer cells is unlikely to reflect on uterine function accurately.[52] These studies are still in the early stage of research and further work is required before routine testing can be recommended.

The immunological relationship shared by the mother and developing embryo is unique and bidirectional. It depends on the fetal antigen presentation on one hand and the recognition of these antigens by the maternal immune system on the other. Immunotherapy is designed to reduce an inappropriate immune response mounted by the mother to the fetus. Immunotherapy may be active, in which paternal leukocytes are injected in the mother, or passive, injecting immunoglobulins that help neutralise circulating autoantibodies. Recent studies have shown that steroid therapy helped in reducing the number of endometrial natural killer cells in women with recurrent miscarriage.[53] Studies to evaluate the maternal response to paternal leukocyte injection and intravenous immunoglobulin infusion are also conflicting with some studies reporting benefit whilst and others do not. A Cochrane systematic review of randomised controlled trials has shown that the use of various forms of immunotherapy, including paternal cell immunisation, third-party donor leukocytes, trophoblast membranes and immunoglobulins given parenterally, in women with unexplained recurrent miscarriage provides no significant beneficial effect over placebo in preventing further miscarriage.[54] Such treatments are not evidence-based and should not be used outside a research setting.[55]

## MISCELLANEOUS

In women with unexplained miscarriages, advice is often given regarding a healthy diet and avoidance of coffee, alcohol and smoking. A significant proportion of women with recurrent miscarriage have been shown to have levels of anxiety similar to women attending psychiatric out-patient departments.[56] Maternal stress has been linked to increased risk of miscarriage. This has been shown in studies suggesting increased urinary cortisol levels in the initial post-conception period in women who had miscarriages.[57] It has been suggested that stress may lead to increased miscarriages by altering the endocrine system, which triggers an immune bias towards an abortogenic cytokine profile; this has been established in murine models and recently been implicated in humans.[58] Women with recurrent miscarriage are in need of re-assurance and psychological support termed 'tender loving care' (TLC). The mechanism by which constant re-assurance may help in improving pregnancy outcome may be related to the reduction of stress in these women.

Infection has long been believed to be a cause of recurrent miscarriage; however, recent studies do not support this hypothesis, and women with recurrent miscarriage do not benefit from extensive infection screening.[45]

Nutrition-related studies have, in the past, implicated consumption of coffee in sporadic miscarriage and smoking in recurrent miscarriage.[59] Recently, hyperhomocysteinaemia has been implicated with defective chorionic villous vascularisation leading to recurrent pregnancy loss.[60]

Obesity has a wide impact on reproductive health. It is another factor that has been implicated in increasing the risk of recurrent miscarriage. The suggested reason for the increased risk of miscarriage in obese women is unclear; it could be due to poor egg quality or abnormal endometrial development. Obesity may also affect metabolism of steroids and proteins such as leptin, adeponectin and affect secretion of androgen and sex hormone binding globulin thereby affecting pregnancy outcome.[61]

The effects of environmental exposure on pregnancy have concentrated on the rate of sporadic miscarriage rather than recurrent miscarriage. The results are conflicting – biased by difficulties in controlling for confounding factors and the lack of accurate data on exposure or toxin dose. Cigarette smoking has an adverse effect on trophoblast function and is associated with a dose-dependent increased risk of miscarriage.[62] Alcohol has adverse effects on fertility and fetal development: even moderate consumption of 3–5 units per week has been shown to heighten the risk of miscarriage.

## CONCLUSIONS

Recurrent miscarriage is a complex situation in which the pathophysiology is not clearly understood in a significant proportion of cases. This makes it extremely difficult to devise ways of treating the problem effectively. There is a rapid increase of interest within this field, which may help to resolve some of the controversies surrounding the causes and management of this condition.

## Key points for clinical practice

- Recurrent miscarriage occurs in 0.5% of pregnancy and identifiable causes can be seen in about 50% of these. Treatment depends on the cause of recurrent miscarriage.

- Antiphospholipid antibodies are a known cause which is treated with aspirin and low molecular weight heparin.

- Fetal chromosomal anomalies are the commonest cause and cytogenetic studies of products of conception may help in diagnosing the type of anomaly. Pre-implantation genetic diagnosis is a possible option, currently used only in research settings.

- Uterine pathology such as septum and synechia can be successfully treated by hysteroscopic surgery with good outcome.

- Current research shows that endometrial biochemistry plays an important role in successful implantation and may in future lead to prognostication and treatment of women with recurrent miscarriage. At the moment, this is in the research phase and should not be used in routine practice.

- Natural killer cells appear to be reduced in the endometrium of women with recurrent miscarriage; however, their value in prognostication and treatment of these women is still under study.

- The modern-day epidemic of obesity is likely to affect reproductive outcome by affecting metabolism of various steroids and proteins; hence, advice regarding life-style change can benefit these women in more than one way.

### References

1. Daya S. Evaluation and management of recurrent spontaneous abortion. *Curr Opin Obstet Gynecol* 1993; **8**: 188–192.
2. Clifford K, Rai R, Watson H, Regan L. An informative protocol for the investigation of recurrent miscarriage: preliminary experience of 500 consecutive cases. *Hum Reprod* 1994; **9**: 1328–1332.
3. Franssen MT, Korevaar JC, Leschot NJ *et al*. Selective chromosome analysis in couples with two or more miscarriages: case-control study. *BMJ* 2005; **331**: 137–141.
4. Li TC, Makris M, Tomsu M, Tuckerman E, Laird S. Recurrent miscarriage: aetiology, management and prognosis. *Hum Reprod Update* 2002; **8**: 463–481.
5. Robinson WP, Beever C, Brown CJ, Stephenson MD. Skewed X inactivation and recurrent spontaneous abortion. *Semin Reprod Med* 2001; **19**: 175–181.
6. Carrell DT, Wilcox AL, Lowy L *et al*. Elevated sperm chromosome aneuploidy and apoptosis in patients with unexplained recurrent pregnancy loss. *Obstet Gynecol* 2003; **101**: 1229–1235.
7. Stern JJ, Dorfmann AD, Gutierrez-Najar AJ, Cerrillo M, Coulam CB. Frequency of abnormal karyotypes among abortuses from women with and without a history of recurrent spontaneous abortion. *Fertil Steril* 1996; **65**: 250–253.
8. Platteau P, Staessen C, Michiels A *et al*. Preimplantation genetic diagnosis for aneuploidy screening in patients with unexplained recurrent miscarriages. *Fertil Steril* 2005; **83**: 393–397, quiz 525–526.
9. Robert JM, Macara LM, Chalmers EA, Smith GC. Inter-assay variation in antiphospholipid antibody testing. *Br J Obstet Gynaecol* 2002; **109**: 348–349.
10. Sebire NJ, Fox H, Backos M *et al*. Defective endovascular trophoblast invasion in primary antiphospholipid antibody syndrome-associated early pregnancy failure. *Hum Reprod* 2002; **17**: 1067–1071.

11. Bose P, Kadyrov M, Goldin R et al. Aberrations of early trophoblast differentiation predispose to pregnancy failure: lessons from the anti-phospholipid syndrome. *Placenta* 2006; **27**: 869–875.

12. Wilson WA, Gharavi AE, Koike T et al. International consensus statement on preliminary classification criteria for definite antiphospholipid syndrome: report of an international workshop. *Arthritis Rheum* 1999; **42**: 1309–1311.

13. Rai R, Shlebak A, Cohen H et al. Factor V Leiden and acquired activated protein C resistance among 1000 women with recurrent miscarriage. *Hum Reprod* 2001; **16**: 961–965.

14. Smith GC, Pell JP, Walsh D. Spontaneous loss of early pregnancy and risk of ischaemic heart disease in later life: retrospective cohort study. *BMJ* 2003; **326**: 423–424.

15. Preston FE, Rosendaal FR, Walker ID et al. Increased fetal loss in women with heritable thrombophilia. *Lancet* 1996; **348**: 913–916.

16. Rai R, Backos M, Elgaddal S, Shlebak A, Regan L. Factor V Leiden and recurrent miscarriage – prospective outcome of untreated pregnancies. *Hum Reprod* 2002; **17**: 442–445.

17. Jivraj S, Rai R, Underwood J, Regan L. Genetic thrombophilic mutations among couples with recurrent miscarriage. *Hum Reprod* 2006; **21**: 1161–1165.

18. Walker ID, Greaves M, Preston FE. Investigation and management of heritable thrombophilia. *Br J Haematol* 2001; **114**: 512–528.

19. Rai R, Cohen H, Dave M, Regan L. Randomised controlled trial of aspirin and aspirin plus heparin in pregnant women with recurrent miscarriage associated with phospholipid antibodies (or antiphospholipid antibodies). *BMJ* 1997; **314**: 253–257.

20. Farquharson RG, Quenby S, Greaves M. Antiphospholipid syndrome in pregnancy: a randomized, controlled trial of treatment. *Obstet Gynecol* 2002; **100**: 408–413.

21. Greaves M, Cohen H, MacHin SJ, Mackie I. Guidelines on the investigation and management of the antiphospholipid syndrome. *Br J Haematol* 2000; **109**: 704–715.

22. Li TC, Spuijbroek MD, Tuckerman E et al. Endocrinological and endometrial factors in recurrent miscarriage. *Br J Obstet Gynaecol* 2000; **107**: 1471–1479.

23. Li TC, Tuckerman EM, Laird SM. Endometrial factors in recurrent miscarriage. *Hum Reprod Update* 2002; **8**: 43–52.

24. Hey NA, Li TC, Devine PL et al. MUC1 in secretory phase endometrium: expression in precisely dated biopsies and flushings from normal and recurrent miscarriage patients. *Hum Reprod* 1995; **10**: 2655–2662.

25. Dalton CF, Laird SM, Serle E et al. The measurement of CA 125 and placental protein 14 in uterine flushings in women with recurrent miscarriage; relation to endometrial morphology. *Hum Reprod* 1995; **10**: 2680–2684.

26. Prakash A, Li TC, Tuckerman E et al. A study of luteal phase expression of inhibin, activin, and follistatin subunits in the endometrium of women with recurrent miscarriage. *Fertil Steril* 2006; **86**: 1723–1730.

27. Li TC, Cooke ID. Evaluation of the luteal phase. *Hum Reprod* 1991; **6**: 484–499.

28. Oates-Whitehead RM, Haas DM, Carrier JA. Progestogen for preventing miscarriage. Cochrane Database Syst Rev 2003; (4): CD003511.

29. Woelfer B, Salim R, Banerjee S et al. Reproductive outcomes in women with congenital uterine anomalies detected by three-dimensional ultrasound screening. *Obstet Gynecol* 2001; **98**: 1099–1103.

30. Homer HA, Li TC, Cooke ID. The septate uterus: a review of management and reproductive outcome. *Fertil Steril* 2000; **73**: 1–14.

31. Salim R, Regan L, Woelfer B, Backos M, Jurkovic D. A comparative study of the morphology of congenital uterine anomalies in women with and without a history of recurrent first trimester miscarriage. *Hum Reprod* 2003; **18**: 162–166.

32. Hart R, Khalaf Y, Yeong CT et al. A prospective controlled study of the effect of intramural uterine fibroids on the outcome of assisted conception. *Hum Reprod* 2001; **16**: 2411–2417.

33. Bajekal N, Li TC. Fibroids, infertility and pregnancy wastage. *Hum Reprod Update* 2000; **6**: 614–620.

34. Rackow B, Taylor H. Uterine leiomyomas affect endometrial HOXA10 expression. *J Soc Gynecol Invest* 2006; **13 (Suppl 2)**: 654.

35. Royal College of Obstetricians and Gynaecologists. Final report of the Medical Research Council/Royal College of Obstetricians and Gynaecologists multicentre randomised trial of cervical cerclage. MRC/RCOG Working Party on Cervical Cerclage. *Br J Obstet Gynaecol* 1993; **100**: 516–523.

36. Drakeley AJ, Roberts D, Alfirevic Z. Cervical stitch (cerclage) for preventing pregnancy loss in women. Cochrane Database Syst Rev 2003; (1): CD003253.

37. Rust OA, Atlas RO, Jones KJ, Benham BN, Balducci J. A randomized trial of cerclage versus no cerclage among patients with ultrasonographically detected second-trimester preterm dilatation of the internal os. *Am J Obstet Gynecol* 2000; **183**: 830–835.

38. Arredondo F, Noble LS. Endocrinology of recurrent pregnancy loss. *Semin Reprod Med* 2006; **24**: 33–39.

39. Nardo LG, Rai R, Backos M, El-Gaddal S, Regan L. High serum luteinizing hormone and testosterone concentrations do not predict pregnancy outcome in women with recurrent miscarriage. *Fertil Steril* 2002; **77**: 348–352.

40. Rai R, Backos M, Rushworth F, Regan L. Polycystic ovaries and recurrent miscarriage – a reappraisal. *Hum Reprod* 2000; **15**: 612–615.

41. Costello MF, Eden JA. A systematic review of the reproductive system effects of metformin in patients with polycystic ovary syndrome. *Fertil Steril* 2003; **79**: 1–13.

42. Jakubowicz DJ, Iuorno MJ, Jakubowicz S, Roberts KA, Nestler JE. Effects of metformin on early pregnancy loss in the polycystic ovary syndrome. *J Clin Endocrinol Metab* 2002; **87**: 524–529.

43. Craig LB, Ke RW, Kutteh WH. Increased prevalence of insulin resistance in women with a history of recurrent pregnancy loss. *Fertil Steril* 2002; **78**: 487–490.

44. Rushworth FH, Backos M, Rai R *et al.* Prospective pregnancy outcome in untreated recurrent miscarriers with thyroid autoantibodies. *Hum Reprod* 2000; **15**: 1637–1639.

45. Royal College of Obstetricians and Gynaecologists. *The investigation and treatment of couples with recurrent miscarriage* (Guideline No. 17). London: RCOG, 2003.

46. Tuckerman EM, Okon MA, Li T, Laird SM. Do androgens have a direct effect on endometrial function? An *in vitro* study. *Fertil Steril* 2000; **74**: 771–779.

47. Hirahara F, Andoh N, Sawai K *et al.* Hyperprolactinemic recurrent miscarriage and results of randomized bromocriptine treatment trials. *Fertil Steril* 1998; **70**: 246–252.

48. Pandey MK, Thakur S, Agrawal S. Lymphocyte immunotherapy and its probable mechanism in the maintenance of pregnancy in women with recurrent spontaneous abortion. *Arch Gynecol Obstet* 2004; **269**: 161–172.

49. Wilson R, Ling H, MacLean MA *et al.* Thyroid antibody titer and avidity in patients with recurrent miscarriage. *Fertil Steril* 1999; **71**: 558–561.

50. Ntrivalas EI, Kwak-Kim JY, Gilman-Sachs A *et al.* Status of peripheral blood natural killer cells in women with recurrent spontaneous abortions and infertility of unknown aetiology. *Hum Reprod* 2001; **16**: 855–861.

51. Clifford K, Flanagan AM, Regan L. Endometrial CD56+ natural killer cells in women with recurrent miscarriage: a histomorphometric study. *Hum Reprod* 1999; **14**: 2727–2730.

52. Moffett A, Regan L, Braude P. Natural killer cells, miscarriage, and infertility. *BMJ* 2004; **329**: 1283–1285.

53. Quenby S, Kalumbi C, Bates M, Farquharson R, Vince G. Prednisolone reduces preconceptual endometrial natural killer cells in women with recurrent miscarriage. *Fertil Steril* 2005; **84**: 980–984.

54. Scott JR. Immunotherapy for recurrent miscarriage. Cochrane Database Syst Rev 2000; (2): CD000112.

55. ASRM. Intravenous immunoglobulin (IVIG) and recurrent spontaneous pregnancy loss. *Fertil Steril* 2006; **86 (Suppl)**: S226–S227.

56. Craig M, Tata P, Regan L. Psychiatric morbidity among patients with recurrent miscarriage. *J Psychosom Obstet Gynaecol* 2002; **23**: 157–164.

57. Nepomnaschy PA, Welch KB, McConnell DS *et al.* Cortisol levels and very early pregnancy loss in humans. *Proc Natl Acad Sci USA* 2006; **103**: 3938–3942.

58. Arck P. [Stress and embryo implantation]. *J Gynecol Obstet Biol Reprod (Paris)* 2004; **33**: S40–S42.

59. Dominguez-Rojas V, de Juanes-Pardo JR, Astasio-Arbiza P, Ortega-Molina P, Gordillo-Florencio E. Spontaneous abortion in a hospital population: are tobacco and coffee intake risk factors? *Eur J Epidemiol* 1994; **10**: 665–668.

60. Nelen WL, Blom HJ, Steegers EA, den Heijer M, Eskes TK. Hyperhomocysteinemia and recurrent early pregnancy loss: a meta-analysis. *Fertil Steril* 2000; **74**: 1196–1199.

61. Eshre WG. Nutrition and reproduction in women. *Hum Reprod Update* 2006; **12**: 193–207.

62. Lindbohm ML, Sallmen M, Taskinen H. Effects of exposure to environmental tobacco smoke on reproductive health. *Scand J Work Environ Health* 2002; **28 (Suppl 2)**: 84–96.

*Gaity Ahmad Andrew J.S. Watson*

# 15

# Evidence-based management of endometriosis

Endometriosis is a chronic condition characterised by growth of endometrial tissue in sites other than the uterine cavity. The condition is found in women of reproductive age from all ethnic and social groups. The most commonly affected sites are the pelvic organs and peritoneum, including the ovaries, uterosacral ligaments, and pouch of Douglas, although occasionally other parts of the body such as bowel, bladder and lung may be affected. There can be extensive fibrosis and adhesion formation causing a marked distortion of pelvic anatomy. The disease severity can be assessed by describing the findings at surgery or by using a classification of severity of endometriosis at laparoscopy published by The American Society for Reproductive Medicine.[1]

Minimal (stage I) and mild (stage II) disease are both characterized by scattered, superficial implants on structures other than uterus, tubes or ovaries, with no associated scarring or significant adhesions and, at worst, superficial implants on the ovaries. Moderate (stage III) disease is characterized by multiple implants or small endometriomas ($\leq 2$ cm) involving one or both ovaries, minimal peritubular or peri-ovarian adhesions, and scattered, scarred implants on other structures. Severe (stage IV) disease is characterized by large ovarian endometriomas, significant tubal or ovarian adhesions, tubal obstruction, obliteration of the cul-de-sac, major uterosacral involvement, and significant bowel or urinary tract disease (revised American Fertility Society [AFS] Score).

Common symptoms of endometriosis include dysmenorrhoea, dyspareunia, non-cyclical pelvic pain, and sub fertility. Other symptoms may include cyclical bowel or bladder symptoms such as pain with or without abnormal

**Gaity Ahmad** MRCOG
Specialist Registrar, Department of Obstetrics and Gynaecology, Stepping Hill Hospital, Stockport SK2 7JE, UK. E-mail: gaityahmad@hotmail.com

**Andrew J.S. Watson** MRCOG (for correspondence)
Consultant Obstetrician and Gynaecologist, Tameside General Hospital, Ashton under Lyne OL6 9RW, UK. E-mail: andy.watson@tgh.nhs.uk

bleeding. The clinical presentation is variable, with some women experiencing several severe symptoms and others having no symptoms at all.

The incidence of endometriosis is 40–60% in women with dysmenorrhoea and 20–30% in women with subfertility. Symptoms and laparoscopic appearance do not always correlate. Vaginal endometriosis is frequently associated with deep dyspareunia[2] and the presence of rectal or vaginal lesions are significantly related to the severity of dysmenorrhoea.[3] The type of pelvic pain is related to the anatomical location.[4] This group demonstrates that the frequency of dyspareunia increases with the presence of uterosacral invasion, painful defecation with bowel and vaginal lesions and severe dysmenorrhoea with increased obliteration of the pouch of Douglas. In summary, the severity and nature of the symptoms of endometriosis are associated with the location and depth of the lesions but probably not with the revised AFS score.

It is widely accepted that endometriosis of sufficient severity to cause pelvic adhesions (AFS Stages III and IV) impairs fertility by interfering with oocyte pick-up and transport. The association is less clear in Stage I (minimal) and Stage II (mild) endometriosis. Although it has been recognized that endometriosis is more prevalent in nulliparous women, it is unclear if mild endometriosis causes infertility or if it is simply a marker for an underlying pathology which itself reduces fertility.

## AETIOLOGY

Several factors are thought to be involved in the development of endometriosis. Retrograde menstruation remains the dominant theory for the development of pelvic disease. Although this is almost universally accepted, it is unlikely to be the only explanation.[5] The quantity and quality of endometrial cells, failure of immunological mechanisms, angiogenesis and the production of antibodies against endometrial cells may also have a role.[6] Embryonic cells may give rise to deposits in distant sites such as the umbilicus, the pleural cavity, and even the brain.[7,8]

## DIAGNOSIS

### HISTORY AND EXAMINATION

In women of reproductive age who present with recurrent dysmenorrhoea or pelvic pain, a full history should be taken and pelvic examination should be carried out. Cyclical pain and a relation to menstruation point to a diagnosis of endometriosis. Painful micturition and defecation and dyspareunia are also associated. The predictive value of any one symptom or group of symptoms remains uncertain as there is considerable overlap with other conditions such as irritable bowel syndrome and pelvic inflammatory disease and a significant proportion of women may be asymptomatic. In young women, consideration should be given to other diagnoses such as pelvic infection, problems in early pregnancy, ectopic pregnancy, ovarian cyst accidents and appendicitis. During pelvic examination, tenderness in the posterior fornix or adnexae, nodules in the posterior fornix or adnexal masses may indicate the presence of endometriotic disease.

## INVESTIGATIONS

Laparoscopy is the only diagnostic test that can reliably diagnose pelvic endometriosis. Transvaginal ultrasonography can detect endometrioma, but failure to reveal cystic structures does not exclude a diagnosis of endometriosis.[9] Magnetic resonance imaging (MRI) is increasingly being used to identify deep pelvic endometriosis. One study using MRI showed high accuracy in the detection of deep pelvic endometriosis. The sensitivity, specificity and accuracy of MR imaging are 80%, 97% and 96% respectively, for the diagnosis of rectovaginal disease, 88%, 97% and 94% in rectosigmoid disease and 88%, 98% and 97% in bladder disease.[10]

Although concentrations of the cancer antigen CA125 are slightly raised in some women with endometriosis, the test is neither sensitive nor specific for the condition. The threshold for surgery is unlikely to be influenced by the CA125 concentration.

## TREATMENT

The treatment of endometriosis is closely linked to, and highly dependent on, the wishes of the patient. This particularly relates to their decisions concerning the conservation of fertility or requirements for contraception. Other factors include age, degree of symptoms and personal preferences. Clinically, endometriosis has been classified into two distinct subtypes by the presence or absence of palpable nodules in the deep pelvis. Patients with such nodules with or without associated ovarian endometrioma usually have severe symptoms with significant risks of bowel and urinary tract involvement. The rectosigmoid colon is affected by deep pelvic endometriosis in 3–37% of cases. Patients without such palpable lesions usually have the classic superficial sub-peritoneal lesions. This group often have less severe symptoms and little risk of developing serious associated problems.[11] Broadly, treatment can be classified according to presenting symptom (pain or sub-fertility), severity of the disease (superficial or nodular disease with or without endometrioma), and the patient's wishes.

## MANAGEMENT OF EARLY STAGE DISEASE

### PAIN AS THE PRESENTING SYMPTOM

There are no randomised controlled trials comparing medical versus surgical treatments for the management of endometriosis. Management options at the time of diagnosis will depend on several factors including patient choice, the availability of laparoscopic surgery, the desire for fertility, and concerns about long-term medical therapy.

#### Conservative management
Predicting the natural course of disease is difficult because studies would require second-look laparoscopy. Two studies in which laparoscopy was repeated after treatment in women given placebo reported spontaneous resolution of endometrial deposits in a third of cases, deterioration in nearly

half and no change in the remainder over a 6–12 month period.[12,13] Clearly, it is justified not to treat endometriosis found accidentally at laparoscopy in asymptomatic women.

### Medical treatment

Endometriosis is a recurring disease and medical therapy should be viewed as symptomatic control rather than curative. All treatments suppress ovarian activity and menstruation, leading to atrophy of endometriotic implants. These drugs are equally effective but side effects and costs differ. Recurrence of symptoms after 6 months of medical treatment may be as high as 50% in the 12–24 months after treatment is stopped.[14] Recurrence may, in part, be due to the poor response of large lesions to medical treatment.

Treatment options for medical therapy include oral contraceptives, progestogens, androgenic agents, and gonadotropin releasing hormone (GnRH) analogues. There have been few randomised controlled trials of medical treatment versus placebo, although many trials have compared different types of medical treatment.

For some time there has also been epidemiological evidence that the current use of the oral contraceptive is associated with a reduced incidence of endometriosis. The clinical observation of apparent symptom resolution during pregnancy gave rise to the concept of treating patients with a pseudo pregnancy regimen.[15] High doses of oestrogen and progestogen are now only very rarely prescribed and modern, low-dose, combined, oral contraceptive pills are used in clinical practice in the management of endometriosis without much high-level evidence of their effectiveness. The oral contraceptive has been observed to reduce menstrual flow and decidualisation of endometriotic implants with decreased cell proliferation and increased apoptosis.[16] For women at risk, oral contraceptives may prevent endometriosis by limiting the relentless heavy monthly bleeding that predisposes to endometriosis by retrograde menstruation. It is logical to believe that they have increased effectiveness when used continuously rather than cyclically. Moreover, the oral contraceptive has the great advantage over other hormonal treatments in that it can be taken indefinitely in non-smokers and is generally more acceptable to women than alternative hormonal treatments, thus improving compliance.

The only randomised control trial of the use of oral contraceptive in the management of endometriosis included in a recent Cochrane review found that although goserelin was more effective at relieving dysmenorrhoea and possibly dyspareunia during treatment, symptom relief with the oral contraceptive is at least as good 6 months after treatment has ended. Since significantly more side effects occur with goserelin (for example, osteoporosis and menopausal-like symptoms), the oral contraceptive might be preferable overall.[17]

The side-effect profiles are important in deciding treatment choice. The hormonal dependence of endometrial implants has provided the basis for medical management of endometriosis. Progestins such as medroxyprogestrone acetate have been used to create 'pseudo pregnancy'.[18] Several studies have shown objective and subjective improvement in endometriosis-associated pain with progestestogen use.[18,19] Progestogens are associated with irregular menstrual bleeding, acne, weight gain, mood swings, and decreased libido.

The observation that menopause typically 'cures' endometriosis has led many to recommend the induction of a sustained hypo-oestrogenic state to promote the regression of existing endometriosis. Danazol (an isoxazol derivative of 17-α-ethinyl testosterone) was the first medication approved by the US Food and Drug Administration for the treatment of endometriosis. Danazol has numerous actions that in combination explain its efficacy in the management of this disease. Danazol suppresses the pituitary gonadotropins to a modest degree, binds to both androgen and progesterone receptors, and inhibits various steroidogenic enzymes. The drug has high affinity for androgen receptors and exerts androgenic effects via these receptors as well as by displacing testosterone from sex hormone-binding globulin and decreasing production of sex hormone-binding globulin.[20]

In addition to its hormonally mediated effects, evidence indicates that Danazol has immunosuppressive properties, including inhibition of lymphocyte proliferation *in vitro* and suppression of auto-antibody production. Several studies have demonstrated beneficial effects of Danazol on the extent of endometriosis and symptoms of pelvic pain.[21–23] Unfortunately, the androgenic effects of Danazol produce many undesirable side effects, including hot flushes, acne, reduced libido, oily hair and skin, weight gain, nausea, and lowering of the voice.

The mechanism of action of GnRH agonists derives from pituitary down-regulation of GnRH receptors which desensitizes the pituitary and decrease the gonadotrophin secretion. This results in ovarian quiescence, an induced hypogonadotrophic hypogonadism that mimics menopause (with regard to serum oestrogen levels) and decreases the size and activity of endometriotic implants *in vivo*.[24]

Gonadotrophin releasing hormone agonists have proved effective in the treatment of pain associated with endometriosis,[25–28] although symptoms may flare with the first injection. Pre-operative treatment with GnRH agonists has been shown to reduce the incidence of disease after laparoscopic resection of endometriomas.[29] The side effects of GnRH agonists result from the induced hypogonadal state and are largely limited to vasomotor instability and other symptoms of hypo-oestrogenism. This has raised concerns regarding the effect of hypo-oestrogenism on bone mineral density. Approaches to counteract the problems of prolonged treatment have included the use of 'add-back' therapy. This approach entails the addition of small concentrations of oestradiol or progestins, which prevent bone mineral resorption without re-activation of endometriosis.

At present in the UK, licensed use of GnRH agonist is limited to 6 months because of the associated bone loss. A previous review has shown no difference in efficacy between medical treatments for pain associated with endometriosis.[30] However, reduction in bone mineral density is an important side effect since a reduction of one standard deviation (SD) in bone mass is associated with an increase of 50–100% in the incidence of fractures.[31] In the randomised controlled trials comparing subcutaneous depot medroxyprogesterone acetate (SC-DMPA) with GnRH agonists, bone loss was less during treatment with progesterone.[32,33] A Cochrane review on GnRH agonists and add-back therapy in the treatment of endometriosis has shown that Danazol/gestrinone and progesterone + oestrogen add-back are protective against the reduction of bone mineral density caused by GnRH agonists in the short term. However, 2 years after treatment is stopped, no difference was seen between the group receiving GnRH agonist only and the group receiving GnRH agonist + HRT add-back.[34]

The duration of other medical treatments is also limited to 6 months in the first instance because of unwanted metabolic effects. The oral contraceptive has the great advantage that it can be taken indefinitely. Although serious side effects, such as thrombo-embolic episodes, may occur with treatment the risk is low and not cumulative.

The levonorgestrel intra-uterine system (LNG-IUS) provides an alternative means of administering progestogens. This system is an established treatment for heavy menstrual bleeding but can also be used for dysmenorrhoea and endometriosis.[35]

Its effects are predominantly localized to the endometrium where the high concentrations of levonorgestrel induce atrophy and pseudo-decidualization.[36–38] One trial[13] of 82 women with endometriosis compared the LNG-IUS with a gonadotropin-releasing hormone agonist and found both treatments to be equally effective in the treatment of endometriosis-related pain. However, the authors concluded that the advantage of the LNG-IUS over the GnRH agonist was the avoidance of low oestrogen levels and the need for only one medical intervention every 5 years. It has also been used in women with rectovaginal disease.[39]

In the future, aromatase inhibitors may have a therapeutic role in endometriosis as they selectively inhibit oestrogen production in endometriotic lesions, without affecting ovarian function.[40] Aromatase enzyme demonstrated locally in endometriotic implants is indicative of oestrogen synthesis. Local oestrogen production by these implants could contribute to the progression of endometriosis even during treatment with GnRH agonists which only inhibit ovarian production of oestrogen.[41] On the other hand, normal oestrogen-producing peripheral tissues (*e.g.* skin and adipose tissue) also contain aromatase and continue to generate significant circulating levels of $E_2$ during GnRH agonist treatment.[42] Thus, extra-ovarian aromatase is likely to cause a resistance to GnRH agonist treatment via persistence of local and peripheral oestrogen production during such treatment.

## Surgical treatment

The surgical treatment of early-stage disease includes excision of all visible endometriosis, or ablation using laser energy or electrodiathermy. The relationship between the degree of endometriosis and the amount of pain experienced by the patient is not always easy to correlate. Sutton *et al.*,[43] in a randomised control trial, compared diagnostic laparoscopy to laser treatment, adhesiolysis and uterine nerve transaction in women with pain and minimal-to-moderate endometriosis. Seventy-four women were randomised at the time of laparoscopy to laser ablation of endometriotic deposits and laparoscopic uterine nerve ablation or to expectant management. Pain symptoms were recorded by asking subjectively how pain had changed and results presented as visual analogue scores. The authors concluded a beneficial effect of combined surgical modalities of laser treatment, adhesiolysis, and uterine nerve transaction. This study did not include women with Stage IV disease as it was considered unethical to withhold treatment from this group. There were

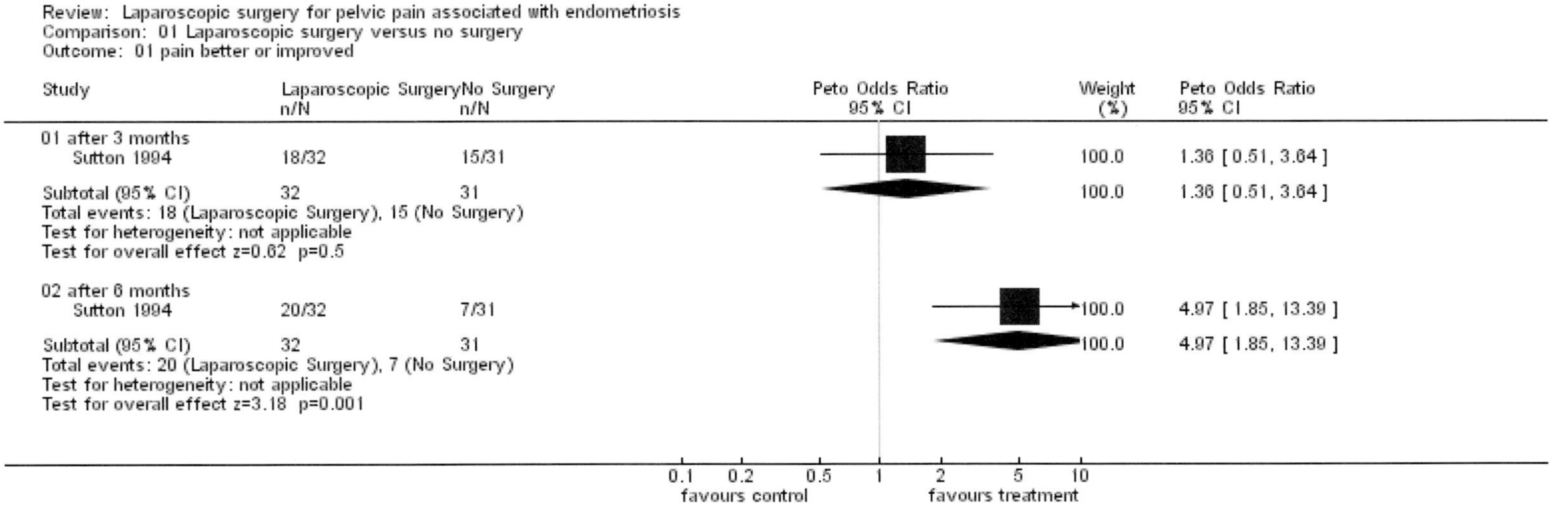

**Fig. 1** Laparoscopic surgery for pelvic pain associated with endometriosis.

very few women in the moderate (Stage III) group (three cases in each arm of the trial); therefore, any conclusions from this trial regarding treatment of moderate or severe endometriosis should be made with caution (Fig. 1). The study used the revised AFS score to ascertain the severity of endometriosis. As discussed earlier, it is important to realise that this may not assess the types of endometriosis that are associated with strong pain such as deep lesions. The revised AFS score is more directed to the severity of adhesions which may be a consequence of old, rather than active, endometriosis

Hysterectomy with bilateral salpingophorectomy (BSO) is well-established treatment for pelvic endometriosis. Hysterectomy alone would not provide symptomatic relief. Effort should be made to excise all evident endometriosis at the time of pelvic clearance.

Studies concerning HRT after BSO or after total hysterectomy and BSO for endometriosis are scant. Most are retrospective, and the follow-up evaluations and diagnosis lack standardization. Most employ therapeutic regimens that are no longer used. In 1971, Ranney et al.[44] reported a 3.1% recurrence rate among 96 women with total hysterectomy and BSO, employing only ethinyl-oestradiol as HRT. In another series of 85 women receiving implants of oestradiol and testosterone, a recurrence rate of 1.2% per woman (0.2% per year) was reported.[45] A randomized prospective study concerning HRT in endometriosis, involving 21 women studied over 12 months, suggested that tibolone may be a safe HRT in women with residual endometriosis.[46] Matorras et al.,[42] in another randomized control trial, reported a 3.5% recurrence rate with oestrogen plus progesterone HRT following hysterectomy and BSO in women with endometriosis.

## ROLE OF HORMONAL TREATMENT BEFORE SURGERY FOR ENDOMETRIOSIS

There is insufficient evidence to support the hypothesis that medical therapy for hormonal suppression of endometriosis prior to surgery is more effective than surgery alone. In the only study[47] comparing presurgical medical therapy with surgery alone, AFS scores were the only outcomes reported. The significant improvement in AFS scores in the medical therapy group may or may not be associated with better outcomes for the patients.

## ROLE OF HORMONAL TREATMENT AFTER CONSERVATIVE SURGERY

There was no evidence of improved pain relief with postoperative hormonal treatment (including Danazol, GnRH agonists, oral contraceptives, and medroxyprogesterone acetate) up to 12 months after surgery. The studies included were small, with insufficient follow-up to rule out a benefit.[35]

## WHEN SUB-FERTILITY IS THE PRESENTING SYMPTOM

### Medical treatment

A systematic review of medical treatment for women with infertility and endometriosis did not find evidence of benefit, and it is not recommended for women trying to conceive.[48]

The Flush trial was conducted to assess the effectiveness of flushing with oil-soluble contrast medium lipoidol in women with unexplained infertility.[49] Lipoidal flushing resulted in a significant increase in pregnancy and live birthrate versus no intervention for women with endometriosis. Two-year follow-up of this trial suggested a transient benefit in pregnancy rate in women with endometriosis but sustained benefit in women with unexplained sub-fertility and no endometriosis.[50] The authors speculated this might result from an immunobiological fertility-enhancing effect either on the intraperitoneal environment or on the endometrial environment to enhance implantation.

### Surgical treatment

A systematic review of laparoscopic treatment of endometriosis in women with sub-fertility suggested an improvement in pregnancy rate in the 9–12 months after surgery.[51] Of the two included studies, one reported live birth. Prazzini et al.[52] found a non-significantly reduced chance of live birth and pregnancy. The other study[53] claimed a statistically significant benefit following laparoscopic surgery with an increased chance of pregnancy and on-going pregnancy after 20 weeks following laparoscopic surgery.

Combining live birth and on-going pregnancy from the two studies would suggest a benefit of surgery and an overall increase in clinical pregnancy rate (Fig. 2). No randomised controlled trials have compared laser versus electrosurgical removal of endometriosis.

## MANAGEMENT OF ENDOMETRIOMA

### WHEN PAIN IS THE PRESENTING SYMPTOM

#### Medical management

The evidence suggests that medical treatment may reduce the size of endometrioma; however, surgical treatment is still considered to be more effective.[5] Furthermore, if they are left, as with any ovarian cyst they have a risk of rupture and torsion.

#### Surgical management

Surgical treatment may involve drainage of the endometrioma with or without diathermy to the base, stripping of the cyst wall or ophorectomy. Incision and drainage of the cyst entails an increased risk of recurrence. There is no other evidence to suggest that any one technique is superior to another.

### MANAGEMENT OF ENDOMETRIOMA IN WOMEN WITH SUB-FERTILITY

#### Medical treatment

There is no evidence to suggest that medical treatment of endometrioma improves fertility.

#### Surgical management

Cohort studies of women with moderate and severe endometriosis undergoing operative treatment with laparoscopy or laparotomy suggest that

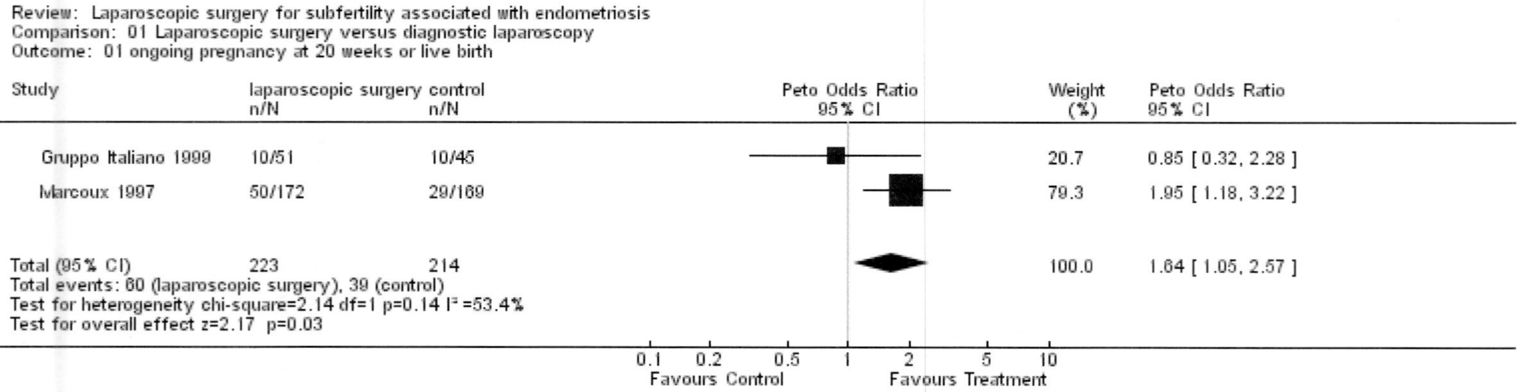

Review: Laparoscopic surgery for subfertility associated with endometriosis
Comparison: 01 Laparoscopic surgery versus diagnostic laparoscopy
Outcome: 01 ongoing pregnancy at 20 weeks or live birth

| Study | laparoscopic surgery n/N | control n/N | Peto Odds Ratio 95% CI | Weight (%) | Peto Odds Ratio 95% CI |
|---|---|---|---|---|---|
| Gruppo Italiano 1999 | 10/51 | 10/45 | | 20.7 | 0.85 [ 0.32, 2.28 ] |
| Marcoux 1997 | 50/172 | 29/169 | | 79.3 | 1.95 [ 1.18, 3.22 ] |
| Total (95% CI) | 223 | 214 | | 100.0 | 1.64 [ 1.05, 2.57 ] |

Total events: 60 (laparoscopic surgery), 39 (control)
Test for heterogeneity chi-square=2.14 df=1 p=0.14 I²=53.4%
Test for overall effect z=2.17 p=0.03

0.1  0.2  0.5  1  2  5  10
Favours Control        Favours Treatment

**Fig. 2** Laparoscopic surgery for subfertility associated with endometriosis.

pregnancy rates may be the same or increased in those treated by laparoscopy (54–66% with operative laparoscopy versus 36–45% with laparotomy).[54–57]

One RCT found that laparoscopic cystectomy increased cumulative pregnancy rates at 24 months when compared with drainage and coagulation treatment of large ovarian endometrioma (66.7% versus 23.5%; OR, 2.83; 95% CI, 1.01–7.50).[58]

Several techniques have been described for the treatment of ovarian endometrioma: cyst wall laser vaporization (destruction by burning) drainage and coagulation, and stripping. Excision of the cyst involves the opening of the endometrioma either with or without the use of electrosurgical or laser energy. Ablation of the endometrioma also involves opening and draining the endometrioma or fenestration (making a window in the wall of the cyst), followed by the destruction of the cyst wall using either cutting or coagulating current, or a form of laser energy. Whatever the surgical modality employed to treat the cyst, a sample of the endometrioma must be sent for histological assessment as there is a need to confirm the clinical diagnosis. The risk of malignant transformation of the cyst is ~0.7%.

There is on-going debate about the best way to manage endometrioma in women presenting with sub-fertility. Meta-analysis of two randomized control trials comparing excision versus ablation of endometrioma revealed a favourable outcome for the excision group in terms of reduced chance of recurrence of endometrioma, recurrence of pain, and improved spontaneous pregnancy rate in previously infertile women.[59] The National Institute for Health and Clinical Excellence (NICE) recommends surgery if endometrioma are 4 cm or more in diameter.

Data on the impact of endometriosis on the results of IVF treatment are controversial. Olivennes et al.[60] found that pregnancy rates were no different from those of women with tubal infertility, whereas Bergendal et al.[61] found that patients with endometriosis had a reduced response to ovarian stimulation, a lower number of oocytes and a reduced fertilization rate, but not a reduced pregnancy rate. In a meta-analysis of 22 published studies,[62] the conclusion was that women with endometriosis have a reduced pregnancy rate (< 35%) compared with women with tubal infertility.

Several studies reported a lower ovarian response to gonadotrophins in women with endometriosis.[63–65] Excision of endometrioma may result in reduced ovarian reserve and thus an increase in the dose of gonadotrophins required for ovarian hyperstimulation. Al-Azemi et al.[64] found that women with endometriosis needed more human menopausal gonadotrophin (HMG) ampoules per cycle, while the control group of tubal factor subjects maintained a constant ovarian response over the five analyzed cycles. In contrast, Donnez et al.[66] reported no difference in the ovarian response to stimulation in women in whom endometrioma had been treated with vaporization of the internal cyst wall as compared to women with tubal factor infertility. Aboulghar et al.[64] investigated women with severe endometriosis who had had previous surgical treatment and reported 29.7% discontinuation of treatment as compared to 1.1% for women with tubal factor infertility.

Furthermore, the severity of endometriosis is likely to affect the outcome of assisted reproduction, women with Stages III and IV disease having lower fertilization rates compared with those with Stages I and II disease. Overall, the data from the study carried out by Barnhart *et al.*[62] suggest that endometriosis affects infertility not only by distorting normal pelvic anatomy but also by having effects on developing follicles, oocytes and embryos.

## MANAGEMENT OF RECTOVAGINAL DISEASE

### WHEN PAIN IS THE PRESENTING SYMPTOM

#### Medical management
One small study of the levonorgestrel intra-uterine system in women with rectovaginal endometriosis found improved dysmenorrhoea, pelvic pain, and dyspareunia after 1 year. A trial comparing oestrogen and progesterone combination with low dose progestogen in 90 women with rectovaginal disease reported substantial reductions at 12 months in all types of pain without major differences between groups.[12] Overall, two-thirds of patients were satisfied with this approach.

#### Surgical management
Rectovaginal endometriosis presents surgical challenges because of difficult access and the risk of injury to the bowel. Although up to 70% improvement has been reported in pelvic symptoms with advanced laparoscopic surgery, there are few prospective studies and no randomised controlled trials.[67,68] Another study reported improvement in quality of life with persistence of results in patients who have failed to respond to medical treatment with complete surgical resection of deep infiltrative endometriosis.[57]

### MANAGEMENT OF RECTOVAGINAL DISEASE IN WOMEN WITH SUB FERTILITY

Conservative surgery for rectovaginal endometriosis in infertile women may not modify the reproductive prognosis; however, significant differences in pain-free intervals in favour of the surgery group have been reported in terms of relief of dysmenorrhoea, dyspareunia, and dyschezia.[68]

Recurrence of endometriosis after laparoscopic surgery is common.[68] Even with experienced laparoscopic surgeons, the cumulative rate of recurrence after 5 years is nearly 20%.[67]

## CONCLUSIONS

In women presenting with sub-fertility, dysmenorrhoea, dyspareunia or chronic pelvic pain, a diagnosis of endometriosis should be considered. Laparoscopy can reliably identify pelvic endometriosis. Surgery should be the first choice of treatment in women who wish to conceive. In women with endometrioma, the cyst wall should be excised, instead of drainage and ablation, as the recurrences are fewer and pregnancy rates improved. Surgical and medical options of treatment can be offered to women who present with pelvic pain. Surgical treatment may be offered to women with rectovaginal disease. At present, there is no evidence of benefit of postoperative medical treatment but the levonorgestrel intra-uterine system has the potential for long-term use.

## Key points for clinical practice

- Retrograde menstruation remains the dominant theory for the development of pelvic disease.

- In women of reproductive age who present with recurrent dysmenorrhoea or cyclical pelvic pain, a diagnosis of endometriosis should be considered.

- Laparoscopy is the only diagnostic test that can reliably diagnose pelvic endometriosis. Transvaginal ultrasonography can reliably detect endometrioma.

- The treatment of endometriosis is closely linked to, and highly dependent on, the wishes of the patient.

- All forms of medical treatment are equally effective in relieving pelvic symptoms.

- Medical or surgical treatment can be offered to women who present with pelvic pain.

- Laparoscopic surgery is the treatment of choice for women with early-stage disease who wish to conceive.

- There is insufficient evidence to support the use of medical treatment pre- and post-surgery for endometriosis.

- Surgical treatment is considered effective in the management of endometrioma.

- Advanced laparoscopic surgery may be offered to women with rectovaginal disease.

## References

1. American Society for Reproductive Medicine. Revised American Society for Reproductive Medicine classification of endometriosis: 1996. *Fertil Steril* 1997; **67**: 817–821.
2. Vercellini P, Trespidi L, De Giorgi O, Cortesi I, Parazzini F, Crosignani PG. Endometriosis and pelvic pain: relation to disease stage and localization. *Fertil Steril* 1996; **65**: 299–304.
3. Chapron C, Fauconnier A, Dubuisson JB, Barakat H, Vieira M, Breart G. Deep infiltrating endometriosis: relation between severity of dysmenorrhoea and extent of disease. *Hum Reprod* 2003; **18**: 760–766.
4. Fauconnier A, Chapron C, Dubuisson JB, Vieira M, Dousset B, Breart G. Relation between pain symptoms and the anatomic location of deep infiltrating endometriosis. *Fertil Steril* 2002; **78**: 719–726.
5. Farquhar C, Sutton C. The evidence for the management of endometriosis. *Curr Opin Obstet Gynecol* 1998; **10**: 321–332.
6. Crosignani PG, Vercellini P, Biffignandi F, Costantini W, Cortesi I, Imparato E. Laparoscopy versus laparotomy in conservative surgical treatment for severe endometriosis. *Fertil Steril* 1996; **66**: 706–711.
7. Prentice A, Deary AJ, Bland E. Progestogens and anti-progestogens for pain associated with endometriosis. Cochrane Database Syst Rev. 2000; (2): CD002122.
8. Selak V, Farquhar C, Prentice A, Singla A. Danazol for pelvic pain associated with endometriosis. Cochrane Database Syst Rev. 2001; (4): CD000068.

9. Alcazar JL, Laparte C, Jurado M, Lopez-Garcia G. The role of transvaginal ultrasonography combined with color velocity imaging and pulsed Doppler in the diagnosis of endometrioma. *Fertil Steril* 1997; **67**: 487–491.

10. Bazot M, Darai E, Hourani R *et al.* Deep pelvic endometriosis: MR imaging for diagnosis and prediction of extension of disease. *Radiology* 2004; **232**: 379–389.

11. Garry R. The endometriosis syndromes: a clinical classification in the presence of aetiological confusion and therapeutic anarchy. *Hum Reprod* 2004; **19**: 760–768.

12. Vercellini P, Pietropaolo G, De Giorgi O, Pasin R, Chiodini A, Crosignani PG. Treatment of symptomatic rectovaginal endometriosis with an estrogen-progestogen combination versus low-dose norethindrone acetate. *Fertil Steril* 2005; **84**: 1375–1387.

13. Petta CA, Ferriani RA, Abrao MS *et al.* Randomized clinical trial of a levonorgestrel-releasing intrauterine system and a depot GnRH analogue for the treatment of chronic pelvic pain in women with endometriosis. *Hum Reprod* 2005; **20**: 1993–1998.

14. Matorras R, Elorriaga MA, Pijoan JI, Ramon O, Rodriguez-Escudaro FJ. Recurrence of endometriosis in women with bilateral adnexectomy (with or without total hysterectomy) who received hormone replacement therapy. *Fertil Steril* 2002; **77**: 303–308.

15. Kistner RW. Conservative management of endometriosis. *Lancet* 1959; **79**: 179–183.

16. Meresman GF, Auge L, Baranao RI, Lombardi E, Tesone M, Sueldo C. Oral contraceptives suppress cell proliferation and enhance apoptosis of eutopic endometrial tissue from patients with endometriosis. *Fertil Steril* 2002; **77**: 1141–1147.

17. Davis L, Kennedy SS, Moore J, Prentice A. Modern combined oral contraceptives for pain associated with endometriosis. Cochrane Database Syst Rev. 2007; (3): CD001019.

18. Moghissi KS, Boyce CR. Management of endometriosis with oral medroxyprogesterone acetate. *Obstet Gynecol* 1976; **47**: 265–267.

19. Luciano AA, Turksoy RN, Carleo J. Evaluation of oral medroxyprogesterone acetate in the treatment of endometriosis. *Obstet Gynecol* 1988; **72**: 323–327.

20. Barbieri RL. Danazol: molecular, endocrine, and clinical pharmacology. *Prog Clin Biol Res* 1990; **323**: 241–252.

21. Buttram VC, Reiter RC, Ward S. Treatment of endometriosis with Danazol: report of a 6 year prospective study. *Fertil Steril* 1985; **43**: 353–358.

22. Dmowski WP, Cohen MR. Treatment of endometriosis with an antigonadotropin, Danazol. A laproscopic and hysteroscopic evaluation. *Obstet Gynecol* 1975; **46**: 147–154.

23. Bayer SR, Seibel MM, Saffan DS, Berger MJ, Taymor ML. Efficacy of Danazol treatment for minimal endometriosis in infertile women. A prospective, randomized study. *J Reprod Med* 1988; **33**: 179–183.

24. Hurst BS, Schlaff WD. Treatment options for endometriosis in clinics of North America. *Infertil Reprod Med* 1992; **3**: 645–655.

25. Dlugi AM, Miller JD, Knittle J. Lupron depot (leuprolide acetate for depot suspension) in the treatment of endometriosis: a randomized, placebo-controlled, double-blind study. Lupron Study Group. *Fertil Steril* 1990; **54**: 419–427.

26. Zorn JR, Mathieson J, Risquez, Comaru Schally AM, Schally AV. Treatment of endometriosis with a delayed release preparation of the agonist D-Trp6-luteinizing hormone-releasing hormone: long-term follow-up in a series of 50 patients. *Fertil Steril* 1990; **53**: 401–406.

27. Lemay A, Maheux R, Faure N, Jean C, Fazekas ATA. Reversible hypogonadism induced by a luteinizing hormone-releasing hormone (LHRH) agonist (buserelin) as a new therapeutic approach for endometriosis. *Fertil Steril* 1984; **41**: 863–871.

28. Henzl MR, Corson SL, Moghissi K, Buttram C, Berqvist C, Jacobson J. Administration of nasal nafarelin as compared with oral Danazol for endometriosis. A multicenter double-blind comparative clinical trial. *N Engl J Med* 1988; **318**: 485–489.

29. Muzii L, Marana R, Caruana P, Mancuso S. The impact of preoperative gonadotropin-releasing hormone agonist treatment on laparoscopic excision of ovarian endometriotic cysts. *Fertil Steril* 1996; **65**: 1235–1237.

30. Prentice A, Deary AJ, Goldbeck-Wood S, Farquhar C, Smith SK. Gonadotrophin-releasing hormone analogues for pain associated with endometriosis. The Cochrane Library 2003; Issue 1: CD000346.

31. Dawood MY, Ramos J, Khan-Dawood FS. Depot leuprolide acetate versus Danazol for the treatment of pelvic endometriosis: changes in vertebral bone mass and serum estrodiol and calcitonin. *Fertil Steril* 1995; **63**: 1177–1183.

32. Wong BC, Gillman NC, Oehninger S, Gibbons WE, Stadtmauer LA. Results of *in vitro* fertilization in patients with endometriomas: is surgical removal beneficial? *Am J Obstet Gynecol* 2004; **191**: 597–607.

33. Vercellini P, Frontino G, De Giorgi O, Aimi G, Zaina B, Crosignani PG. Comparison of a levonorgestrel-releasing intrauterine device versus expectant management after conservative surgery for symptomatic endometriosis: a pilot study. *Fertil Steril* 2003; **80**: 305–309.

34. Sagsveen M, Farmer JE, Prentice A, Breeze A. Gonadotrophin-releasing hormone analogues for endometriosis: bone mineral density. Cochrane Database Syst Rev 2003; (4): CD001297.

35. Yap C, Furness S, Farquhar C. Pre and post operative medical therapy for endometriosis surgery. Cochrane Database Syst Rev 2004; (3): CD003678.

36. Maruo T, Laoag-Fernandez JB, Pakarinen P, Murakoshi H, Spitz IM, Johansson E. Use of a levonorgestrel intrauterine system on proliferation and apoptosis in the endometrium. *Hum Reprod* 2001; **16**: 2103–2108.

37. Nilsson CG, Luukkainen T, Arko H. Endometrial morphology of women using a D-norgestrel releasing intrauterine device. *Fertil Steril* 1978; **29**: 297–401.

38. Silverberg SG, Haukkamaa M, Arko H, Nilsson CG, Luukkainen T. Endometrial morphometry of women during long term use of levonorgestrel intrauterine system. *Int J Gynecol Pathol* 1986; **5**: 235–241.

39. Abbott J, Hawe J, Hunter D, Holmes M, Finn P, Garry R. Laparoscopic excision of endometriosis: a randomized, placebo-controlled trial. *Fertil Steril* 2004; **82**: 878–884.

40. Ailawadi RK, Jobanputra S, Kataria M, Gurates B, Bulun SE. Treatment of endometriosis and chronic pelvic pain with letrozole and norethindrone acetate: a pilot study. *Fertil Steril* 2004; 81: 290–296.

41. Bulun SE, Zeitoun K, Takayama K *et al.* Estrogen production in endometriosis and use of aromatase inhibitors to treat endometriosis. *Endo Rel Cancer* 1999; **6**: 293–301.

42. Matorras R, Elorriaga MA, Pijoan JI *et al.* The essential role of the aromatase/p450arom. *Semin Reprod Med* 2002; **20**: 277–284.

43. Sutton CJ, Ewen SP, Whitelaw N, Haines P. Prospective, randomized, double-blind, controlled trial of laser laparoscopy in the treatment of pelvic pain associated with minimal, mild, and moderate endometriosis. *Fertil Steril* 1994; **62**: 696–700.

44. Ranney B. Endometriosis III: complete operations, reason, sequelae and treatment. *Am J Obstet Gynecol* 1971; **109**: 1137–1114.

45. Henderson AF, Studd JWW, Watson N. A retrospective study of oestrogen replacement therapy following hysterectomy for the treatment of endometriosis. In: Shaw RW. (ed) *Advances in Reproductive Endocrinology*. Lancaster: Parthenon, 1990; 131–138.

46. Fedele L, Bianchi, S, Raffaelli R, Zanconato G. Comparison of transdermal estradiol and tibolone for the treatment of oophorectomized women with deep residual endometriosis. *Maturitas* 1999; **92**: 189–193.

47. Donnez J, Nisolle M, Gillerot S, Anaf V, Clerckx-Braun F, Casanas-Roux F. Ovarian endometrial cysts: the role of gonadotropin-releasing hormone agonist and/or drainage. *Fertil Steril* 1994; **62**: 63–66.

48. National Institute for Health and Clinical Excellence. NICE guidelines for Management of Infertile Couple. 2004 <www.nice.org.uk>.

49. Johnson NP, Farquhar CM, Hadden WE, Suckling J, Yu Y, Sadler. The FLUSH trial – flushing with lipiodol for unexplained (and endometriosis-related) subfertility by hysterosalpingography: a randomized trial. *Hum Reprod* 2004; **19**: 2043–2051.

50. Johnson NP, Kwok R, Stewart AW, Saththianathan M, Hadden WE, Chamley LW. Lipiodol fertility enhancement: two-year follow-up of a randomized trial suggests a transient benefit in endometriosis, but a sustained benefit in unexplained fertility. *Hum Reprod* 2007; **22**: 2857–2862.

51. Jacobson TZ, Barlow DH, Koninckx PR, Olive D, Farquhar C. Laparoscopic surgery for subfertility associated with endometriosis. Cochrane Database Syst Rev. 2002; (4): CD001398.

52. Parazzini F. Ablation of lesions or no treatment in minimal-mild endometriosis in infertile women: a randomized trial. Gruppo Italiano per lo Studio dell'Endometriosi. *Hum Reprod* 1999; **14**: 1332–1334.

53. Marcoux S, Maheux R, Berube S. Laparoscopic surgery in infertile women with minimal or mild endometriosis. Canadian Collaborative Group on Endometriosis. *N Engl J Med* 1997; **337**: 217–222.

54. Adamson GD, Hurd SJ, Pasta DJ, Rodriguez BD. Laparoscopic endometriosis treatment: is it better? *Fertil Steril* 1993; **59**: 35–44.

55. Busacca M, Fedele L, Bianchi S *et al*. Surgical treatment of recurrent endometriosis: laparotomy versus laparoscopy. *Hum Reprod* 1998; **13**: 2271–2274.

56. Fayez JA, Collazo LM. Comparison between laparotomy and operative laparoscopy in the treatment of moderate and severe stages of endometriosis. *Int J Fertil* 1990; **35**: 272–279.

57. Crosignani P, Olive D, Bergqvist A, Luciano A. Advances in the management of endometriosis: an update for clinicians. *Hum Reprod Update* 2006; **12**: 179–189.

58. Beretta P, Franchi M, Ghezzi F, Busacca M, Zupi E, Bolis P. Randomized clinical trial of two laparoscopic treatments of endometriomas: cystectomy versus drainage and coagulation. *Fertil Steril* 1998; **70**: 1176–1180.

59. Hart R, Hickey M, Maouris P, Buckett W, Garry R. Excisional surgery versus ablative surgery for ovarian endometriomata: a Cochrane Review. *Hum Reprod* 2005; **20**: 3000–3007.

60. Olivennes F, Feldberg D, Liu HC, Cohen J, Moy F, Rosenwaks Z. Endometriosis: a stage by stage analysis – the role of in vitro fertilization. *Fertil Steril* 1995; **64**: 392–398.

61. Bergendal A, Naffah S, Nagy C, Bergqvist A, Sjoblom P, Hillensjo T. Outcome of IVF in patients with endometriosis in comparison with tubal-factor infertility. *J Assist Reprod Genet* 1998; **15**: 530–534.

62. Barnhart K, Dunsmoor-Su R, Coutifaris C. Effect of endometriosis on *in vitro* fertilization. *Fertil Steril* 2002; **77**: 1148–1155.

63. Azem F, Lessing JB, Geva E *et al*. Patients with stages III and IV endometriosis have a poorer outcome of *in vitro* fertilization-embryo transfer than patients with tubal infertility. *Fertil Steril* 1999; **72**: 1107–1109.

64. Al-Azemi M, Bernal AL, Steele J, Gramsbergen I, Barlow D, Kennedy S. Ovarian response to repeated controlled stimulation in *in-vitro* fertilization cycles in patients with ovarian endometriosis. *Hum Reprod* 2000; **15**: 72–75.

65. Aboulghar MA, Mansour RT, Serour GI, Al-Inany HG, Aboulghar MM. The outcome of *in vitro* fertilization in advanced endometriosis with previous surgery: a case-controlled study. *Am J Obstet Gynecol* 2003; **188**: 371–375.

66. Donnez J, Wyns C, Nisolle M. Does ovarian surgery for endometriomas impair the ovarian response to gonadotropin? *Fertil Steril* 2001; **76**: 662–665.

67. Redwine DB, Wright JT. Laparoscopic treatment of complete obliteration of the cul-de-sac associated with endometriosis: long-term follow-up of *en bloc* resection. *Fertil Steril* 2001; **76**: 358–365.

68. Fedele L, Bianchi S, Zanconato G, Bettoni G, Gotsch F. Long-term follow-up after conservative surgery for rectovaginal endometriosis. *Am J Obstet Gynecol* 2004; **190**: 1020–1024.

69. Vercellini P, Pietropaolo G, De Giorgi O, Daguati R, Pasin R, Crosignani PG. Reproductive performance in infertile women with rectovaginal endometriosis: is surgery worthwhile? *Am J Obstet Gynecol* 2006; **195**: 1303–1310.

*Saad A.K. Amer*

**16**

# Laparoscopic ovarian surgery for polycystic ovarian syndrome

Polycystic ovarian syndrome (PCOS) is a common endocrine disorder affecting 6–8% of women of reproductive age,[1] and the most common cause (~75%) of anovulatory infertility.[2] According to the 2003 ESHRE/ASRM (Rotterdam) criteria, PCOS is defined as a syndrome of ovarian dysfunction along with the cardinal features of hyperandrogenism and polycystic ovary morphology.[3] It is characterised by a varied combination of clinical (oligo/amenorrhoea, hirsutism and obesity), biochemical (increased serum levels of luteinizing hormone and androgens), and sonographic (enlarged polycystic ovaries) features. PCOS is also associated with insulin resistance and compensatory hyperinsulinaemia.[3]

In women with PCOS presenting with anovulatory infertility, clomifene citrate is the standard first-line treatment for induction of ovulation. Patients, who either remain anovulatory (clomifene citrate resistant) or fail to conceive despite ovulation on clomifene citrate, can be offered laparoscopic ovarian surgery (LOS), gonadotrophin ovarian stimulation or metformin. Since its introduction in the late 1970s, laparoscopic ovarian surgery has been widely accepted in many reproductive centres as the treatment of choice in clomifene citrate-resistant PCOS patients. More recently, the efficacy of LOS in inducing ovulation and generating pregnancies has been confirmed in large randomised clinical trials.[4,5] LOS has also been shown to offer several advantages over gonadotrophin therapy such as reducing the costs and avoidance of the complexity and complications of medical ovulation induction.

This chapter will present an overview of the current role of LOS in the management of PCOS. The chapter will also discuss the techniques, clinical outcomes, possible mechanisms of action, complications and predictors of success of LOS.

**Saad A.K. Amer** MBChB MSc MD MRCOG
Associate Professor in Obstetrics and Gynaecology and Consultant Gynaecologist, University of Nottingham, Derby City General Hospital, Uttoxeter Road, Derby DE22 3DT, UK
E-mail: saad.amer@nottingham.ac.uk

**Table 1** History of important developments in the treatment of anovulation associated with PCOS

| Date | Treatment |
|------|-----------|
| 1930 | Bilateral ovarian wedge resection[6] |
| 1961 | Clomiphene citrate[8] |
| 1967 | Laparoscopic ovarian biopsies[9] |
| 1978 | Laparoscopic ovarian drilling (diathermy)[10] |
| 1988 | Laparoscopic ovarian drilling (laser)[11] |

## HISTORICAL BACKGROUND

Although the main features of PCOS were defined early in the 20th century by Stein and Leventhal,[6] there was no mention in the literature of any treatment for infertility associated with this syndrome until 1930. Stein and Leventhal[6] first reported the success of ovarian wedge resection in inducing ovulation in women with PCOS in 1935. Ovarian wedge resection then became widely accepted as the only treatment for infertility associated with PCOS and remained so for many years. In the 1960s, with the introduction of medical ovulation induction, ovarian wedge resection was largely abandoned due to its associated morbidity.[7] Instead; clomifene citrate became the standard treatment in anovulatory PCOS.[8] The development of operative laparoscopy in the late 1960s led to a revival of the surgical treatment of PCOS carried out laparoscopically. The laparoscopic approach was claimed to reduce the morbidity associated with laparotomy. The initial laparoscopic procedures included wedge resections similar to the earlier open techniques. With the evolution of the laparoscopic techniques, the amount of injury to the ovary gradually decreased from excision of large biopsies to making a number of punctures on the surface of the ovary. Several techniques have been described including ovarian biopsy, ovarian electrocautery and ovarian laser treatment. Electrocautery and laser treatment result in thermal injury to the ovary via a number of punctures hence the term 'ovarian drilling' was used. In Table 1, the evolution of the different laparoscopic techniques is summarised.

## INDICATIONS OF LAPAROSCOPIC OVARIAN SURGERY

### OVULATION INDUCTION

Currently, the only established indication for LOS is ovulation induction after failure of clomifene citrate to achieve a successful pregnancy in women with PCOS. Three types of failure with clomifene treatment can be identified:

Type 1    *Clomifene resistance*, defined as failure to ovulate on incremental doses (50–150 mg) of clomifene citrate. In this case, LOS results in ovulation in about 80% and conception in 50–60% of patients.[4,5,12] Furthermore, it renders the ovaries more sensitive to clomifene citrate and gonadotrophins.[10]

Type 2    *Clomifene failure*, defined when pregnancy does not occur despite regular ovulation on clomifene citrate for 6–9 cycles. In this case, LOS allows the patient to ovulate spontaneously and avoids the untoward peripheral anti-oestrogenic effect of clomifene citrate on: (i) endometrial development, which may adversely affect implantation;[13] and (ii) cervical mucus, which may impede passage of sperm through the cervix.[14] Also, LOS avoids the possible abnormal hormonal response to clomifene citrate (abnormally high levels of mid-follicular luteinising hormone [LH] with premature luteinisation), which may be responsible for clomifene citrate failure.[15]

Type 3  *Clomifene pregnancy failure*, defined as failure to maintain a pregnancy conceived with clomifene citrate. Although still debatable, several studies reported an increase in miscarriage rates (30–40%) in PCOS women possibly due to the high serum levels of LH and/or androgens.[16,17] In a long-term follow-up study after LOS, we have shown a reduction of the miscarriage rate from 54% to 17% after LOS.[12] This lower risk of miscarriage after LOS is possibly due to normalisation of the serum levels of LH and/or androgens.

## OTHER POTENTIAL INDICATIONS FOR LOS

### Recurrent miscarriages

The relationship between PCOS and recurrent miscarriage remains uncertain: whereas earlier reports suggested that PCOS is a significant cause of recurrent miscarriage,[16–18] more recent reports have questioned the importance of PCOS as a cause of recurrent miscarriage.[19,20] In our long-term follow-up study involving 116 women with PCOS who underwent LOS, we reported a reduction of recurrent miscarriage from 6% to < 1% after LOS.[12]

### Acne and hirsutism associated with PCOS resistant to medical treatment

LOS results in a significant and persistent fall of the serum levels of androgens.[21–23] However, the impact of this reduction in androgens on acne and hirsutism has not been investigated.

### Menstrual irregularities associated with PCOS

The beneficial effect of LOS on menstrual pattern is well documented by many authors.[12,21,22] LOS may, therefore, be considered as a treatment option if the hormonal methods (combined oral contraceptives or progestogens) are contraindicated or not suitable in women with PCOS presenting with menstrual irregularities.

### Prevention of long-term morbidity

Available literature data do not support the use of LOS for this indication. Lemieux and co-workers[24] reported that LOS does not improve insulin resistance or lipoprotein abnormalities associated with PCOS. This indicates that LOS does not eliminate the associated risk for diabetes and cardiovascular disease. Furthermore, in a long-term follow-up study after ovarian wedge resection, Dahlgren and co-workers[25] reported a significant increase in the prevalence of hypertension and diabetes mellitus in a cohort of PCOS patients ($n = 33$) aged 40–59 years who underwent ovarian wedge resection 22–31 years previously as compared to a group of age-matched, non-PCOS women ($n = 132$).

The authors also found that this group of PCOS patients had increased metabolic and cardiovascular risks. Assuming that LOS and wedge resection produce similar clinical, biochemical and metabolic effects in PCOS women, the results observed by Dahlgren and co-workers may be extrapolated to LOS.[25]

## CURRENT ROLE OF LOS IN ANOVULATORY INFERTILITY ASSOCIATED WITH PCOS

All overweight and obese PCOS women should first be encouraged to loose weight through life-style measures before any medical treatment. Whilst there is a consensus on the use clomifene citrate as the standard first-line treatment in anovulatory PCOS women, the second-line treatment has been the subject of much debate, with competition between LOS, gonadotrophin and metformin as the preferred choice (Fig. 1). Perhaps, with the increasing awareness of the predictors of success/failure of each of these treatments, it may now be possible to apply an individually tailored treatment according to each patient's pretreatment characteristics. The initial reports on the efficacy of metformin in ovulation induction in PCOS were encouraging.[26,27] However, more recent data from large randomised trials showed metformin not to be as effective as initially thought.[28,29] LOS and gonadotrophins have been shown to be equally effective in inducing ovulation and producing high pregnancy and live-birth rates in women with PCOS (Table 2).[4,5] Whilst some reproductive medicine specialists (including the author) advocate LOS for clomifene citrate resistant PCOS women, others are in favour of gonadotrophin ovulation induction. LOS may be seen as a preferred second line for ovulation induction as it offers several advantages over gonadotrophin therapy (Table 3). Importantly, in contrast to gonadotrophin therapy, LOS results in mono-ovulation, with no risk of ovarian hyperstimulation syndrome (OHSS) and with an incidence of multiple pregnancies no higher than background rates.[4,5] Moreover, LOS is less costly and does not require complex monitoring. The cost per term pregnancy

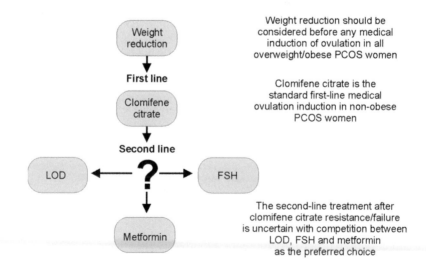

**Fig. 1** Management options for anovulatory infertility associated with PCOS.

has been estimated to be 14,489 euros for gonadotrophin and 11,301 euros for LOS (22% lower).[30] In addition, with LOS, a single treatment leads to repeated physiological ovulatory cycles and potentially repeated pregnancies without the need for repeated courses of medical treatment. The main drawback of LOS is the need for general anaesthetic and surgery. Other complications, such as iatrogenic adhesion formation and a theoretical risk of premature ovarian failure appear to be of little clinical significance.

More recently, we have investigated the possible role of LOS as a first-line method of ovulation induction in anovulatory women with PCOS. We conducted a randomised controlled trial including 72 PCOS women comparing LOS with clomifene citrate. LOS was effective as a first-line method of ovulation induction but offered no advantages over clomifene citrate (unpublished data). Therefore, we recommended that clomifene citrate should remain the standard first line for ovulation induction in PCOS. However, LOS could be offered as a first line if laparoscopy is carried out for other indications in women with PCOS.

Table 2 LOD versus rFSH in clomiphene citrate resistant women with PCOS (RCT by Bayram and co-workers[5])

| | LOD strategy[a] (n = 83) n (%) | rFSH[b] (n = 85) n (%) |
|---|---|---|
| Ovulation (per cycle) | 70% | 69% |
| Conception at 12/12 | 63 (76%) | 64 (75%) |
| Multiple pregnancies | 1[c] (< 2%) | 9 (14%) |
| Miscarriage rate | 7 (11%) | 7 (11%) |
| Live-birth rate | 53 (64%) | 51 (60%) |

[a]LOD strategy
    LOD alone (n = 36) — 31/83 pregnancies (37%)
    LOD followed by clomifene citrate and/or rFSH (n = 47) as follows
        LOD followed by clomifene citrate only (n = 24) — 14/83 pregnancies (17%)
        LOD followed by clomifene citrate then rFSH (n = 21)
        LOD followed by rFSH directly (n = 2) — 18/83 pregnancies (22%)

[b]rFSH: chronic low-dose step-up protocol.
[c]One patient had quintuplets after rFSH. A successful embryo reduction led to the live birth of twins.

Table 3 Advantages and disadvantages of LOD compared to FSH

| Advantages | |
|---|---|
| | At least as effective as gonadotrophin treatment |
| | Less costly |
| | Avoids intensive, inconvenient and complex monitoring |
| | Single treatment produces repeated ovulatory cycles and potentially repeated pregnancies |
| | Avoids OHSS |
| | No increase in multiple pregnancies |
| Disadvantages | |
| | The need for surgery under general anaesthetic |
| | Iatrogenic adhesion formation |
| | Theoretical risk of premature ovarian failure |

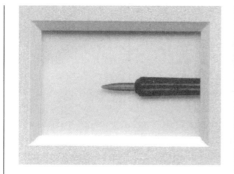

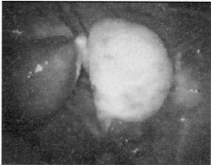

**Fig. 2** The Rockett of London ovarian diathermy needle probe. The distal stainless steel needle measures 8 mm in length and 2 mm in diameter and projects from an insulated solid cone of 6 mm maximum diameter.

**Fig. 3** Stabilising the ovary for LOD. The utero-ovarian ligament is grasped with atraumatic grasping forceps and the ovary is lifted up away from the bowel.

## TECHNIQUES OF LAPAROSCOPIC OVARIAN SURGERY

Several techniques of laparoscopic ovarian surgery to induce ovulation in PCOS have been described in the literature. Most of the techniques involve either taking ovarian biopsies or making multiple punctures on the surface of the ovary using electrocautery or laser. More recently, there have been several attempts to use a transvaginal route to perform the ovarian surgery utilising either a fertiloscopy or an ultrasound-guided approach. Currently, the most widely used technique for ovarian surgery is laparoscopic ovarian diathermy (LOD) using electrocautery due to its simplicity, effectiveness, relative safety and low cost.

### LOD USING ELECTROCAUTERY

Three-puncture laparoscopy is established, the pelvis is thoroughly inspected for any pathology and the ovaries examined for the features of PCO. A specially designed monopolar electrocautery probe (ovarian diathermy needle, Rockett of London; Fig. 2) is used to penetrate the ovarian capsule at a number of points. The probe has a distal stainless steel needle measuring 8 mm in length and 2 mm in diameter and projecting from an insulated solid cone of 6 mm maximum diameter. The insulated cone prevents deep penetration and minimises thermal damage to the ovarian surface. The utero-ovarian ligament is grasped with a pair of atraumatic grasping forceps and the ovary is lifted up and stabilised in position away from the bowel (Fig. 3). This is essential to avoid direct or indirect thermal injury to the bowel. The needle is applied to the antimesenteric surface of the ovary at right angles to avoid slippage and to minimise surface damage (Fig. 4). The site of application should be away from the ovarian hilum and the fallopian tube. This is necessary to avoid damage of the hilum (which can lead to ovarian atrophy) and the fallopian tube (which can cause mechanical infertility). After insertion of the needle through the ovarian capsule (Fig. 5), monopolar coagulation electricity current is activated for 5 s with a power setting of 30 W. Electricity should not be activated before

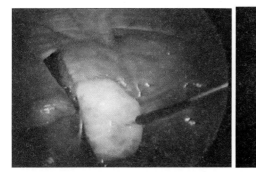

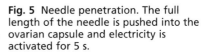

**Fig. 4** Needle application. With the ovary stabilised in position, the needle is applied to the antimesenteric surface at right angles.

**Fig. 5** Needle penetration. The full length of the needle is pushed into the ovarian capsule and electricity is activated for 5 s.

penetrating the surface of the ovary to avoid arcing and to minimise the damage to the ovarian surface due to the charring effect, which may later cause adhesion formation. However, it may be necessary to facilitate the needle insertion by a short burst of diathermy. The ovary is then irrigated using Hartmann's solution before releasing it to its normal position. The techniques are summarised in Table 4.

### How much energy should be used for LOD?

The amount of thermal energy used and number of punctures made in each ovary varied considerably in different studies (3–25 punctures with power settings of 30–400 W).[10,22,31,32] In a retrospective review of 161 women who underwent LOD, we found that two punctures resulted in poor outcome and three punctures seemed to represent plateau dose, above which no further improvement of the outcome was observed. Seven or more punctures seemed to be associated with reduction of the ovarian reserve suggesting excessive ovarian destruction (Fig. 6).[33] More recently, in a prospective dose finding study utilising an 'up-and-down design' and involving 30 women with

**Table 4** Techniques of LOD using electrocautery

- Three-puncture laparoscopy
- Utero-ovarian ligament is grasped with a pair of atraumatic forceps
- The ovary is lifted up away from the bowel and stabilised
- A specially designed monopolar electrocautery needle probe is used
- The probe is applied at right angles to the antimesenteric surface of the ovary
- The probe should be away from ovarian hilum and the fallopian tube
- Power is set at 30 W (coagulating)
- The full length of the needle is pushed into the capsule to a depth of 6–8 mm
- Electricity is activated for 5 s
- Four punctures are made in each ovary
- The ovary is irrigated with saline before releasing the ovarian ligament
- A crystalloid solution is instilled at the end of the procedure

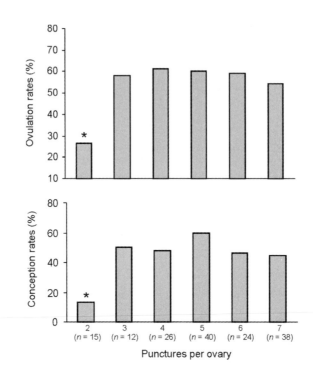

**Fig. 6** The rates of spontaneous ovulation and conception in women with PCOS after laparoscopic ovarian diathermy using different numbers of punctures (*$P < 0.05$).[33]

anovulatory PCOS undergoing LOD, we have found four punctures per ovary at 30 W for 5 s (150 J) per puncture to be the optimum number required to achieve the best result (Fig. 7).[34]

### Other techniques of ovarian electrocautery

Some authors made craters on the ovarian surface with biopsy or sterilisation forceps or scissors connected to monopolar current (200–300 W) and pressed against ovarian surface for 2–4 s.[10,21,24,31] Other techniques involved making linear incisions into the ovarian tissue to a depth of 5–7 mm or coagulating all the visible cysts. The overall results of these techniques are encouraging and the success rates are comparable. However, techniques producing significant damage to the ovarian surface may increase the chances of adhesion formation and should be discouraged. LOD (described above) may be superior to other procedures as it produces deep stromal injury with minimal surface damage.

### LASER OVARIAN SURGERY

Four different modalities of laser, including Nd:YAG, $CO_2$, argon and KTP have been used to perform ovarian drilling in women with PCOS. Nd:YAG laser is delivered via a fine quartz fibre and can be used in the contact and non-contact mode. In the non-contact mode, the laser fibre is applied at a distance of 5–10 mm of the antimesenteric surface of the ovary with a power setting of 30–100 W. It has been used to make incisions[11] or punctures[35] or to coagulate a wedge-like area.[36] In the contact mode, with a sapphire tip screwed on the

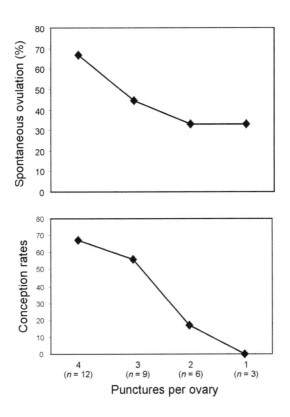

**Fig. 7** The rates of spontaneous ovulation, conception and conversion of oligo/amenorrhoea to regular cycles in women with PCOS after laparoscopic ovarian diathermy (LOD) using different doses of thermal energy (numbers of punctures).[34]

flexible laser fibre, the probe can be introduced into the ovarian capsule to create punctures[37] or to cut out a wedge-shaped portion (5 mm) of the ovary.[38] $CO_2$ laser has been used to drill 10–40 craters in the ovarian tissue and to vaporise the visible subcapsular follicles. With a power setting of 10–30 W in a continuous mode, the laser beam is focused to a spot size of 0.2 mm for 5–10 s

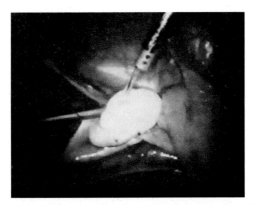

**Fig. 8** Laparoscopic ovarian drilling with argon laser. The argon laser fibre is introduced through a suction irrigation probe and is pushed into the ovarian capsule. Laser is activated for 1 s at 6–16 W. Twenty to forty punctures are usually made.

per puncture. Argon and potassium-titanyl-phosphate (KTP) lasers are delivered by flexible fibres, which are used in the contact mode without special tips. With a power setting of 6–16 W, all the visible subcapsular cysts can be vaporised and 20–40 punctures can be made in each ovary (Fig. 8).

## LASER VERSUS ELECTROCAUTERY

It appears that electrocautery is superior to laser for LOS for a number of reasons. First, electrocautery is more effective than laser in achieving ovulation and pregnancy.[35,39,40] Second, laser, especially $CO_2$ laser, may be associated with a higher risk of adhesion formation because it produces more surface injury than electrocautery. Third, electrocautery is less costly, easier to set up and carries fewer hazards. In addition, the effect of diathermy may last longer than the laser effect.[39]

## TRANSVAGINAL OVARIAN SURGERY

In a search for less invasive ovarian surgery for PCOS, some authors have a described transvaginal approach to apply diathermy, laser or hydrocoagulation to the ovarian stroma. Other authors used transvaginal mini-laparoscopy (fertiloscopy) to perform ovarian drilling. Mio and co-workers[41] were the first to report on the efficacy of transvaginal ultrasound (TVS)-guided follicular aspiration in women with PCOS. Syritsa[42] performed TVS-guided ovarian drilling using a specially designed monopolar needle, which has a polyester coating except the 2-mm tip.[42] More recently, Zhu and co-workers[43] described TVS-guided ovarian interstitial YAG-laser-coagulation. They introduced the YAG fibre through an egg-pickup needle (used for *in vitro* fertilisation [IVF]) into the ovarian substance under sedation to coagulate 3–5 points. Fernandez and co-workers[44] described the use of fertiloscopy to perform ovarian drilling. Ramzy and co-workers[45] injected warm saline (75°C) into the ovarian stroma using IVF pickup needle under TVS-guidance. These early reports have shown encouraging results, although the efficacy and safety of these new techniques need to be adequately assessed before they can be recommended for clinical use. The main concern of any transvaginal approach applying any form of energy (*e.g.* electrocautery or laser) is the risk of thermal injury to adjacent organs such as the bowel. Chiesa-Montadou and co-workers[46] reported two severe adverse events with fertiloscopic ovarian drilling.

## CLINICAL OUTCOME OF LOS

### SHORT-TERM OUTCOME

A very rapid response has been reported following LOS in several studies, with ovulation occurring within 2–4 weeks and menstruation within 4–6 weeks in the responders.[47] Restoration of regular ovulatory cycles occurs in about two-thirds of cases.[10] Recently, in a large randomised controlled trial involving 168 clomifene citrate-resistant PCOS women, Bayram and co-workers[4] reported an ovulation rate of 70% per cycle and cumulative conception and live-birth rates of 76% and 64%, respectively, following LOS (Table 2).

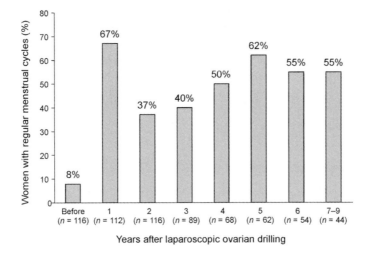

**Fig. 9** The proportion of women with regular menstrual cycles before and at yearly intervals following laparoscopic ovarian drilling.[12]

## LONG-TERM OUTCOME

In our long-term follow-up study involving 116 women with anovulatory PCOS who underwent LOS, we found that about two-thirds of women responded to the treatment shortly after surgery (Fig. 9). In about half of the responders (*i.e.* a third of the total number of women), the effects were sustained for many years. Of these women, 49% conceived within the first year after LOS with a miscarriage rate similar to the general population. The improvement in the reproductive performance seems to last for many years in about a third of cases.[12]

## ENDOCRINE EFFECTS OF LOS

### IMMEDIATE EFFECTS

The main hormonal changes consistently observed after LOS include a rapid and persistent fall of circulating androgens (testosterone and androstenedione) with a transient increase of gonadotrophins (LH and FSH) during the first 24–48 h followed later by a gradual fall.[21,22] Preliminary data suggest that insulin sensitivity and lipoprotein abnormalities associated with PCOS are not improved by LOS.[23] This indicates that the risk factors for diabetes and cardiovascular disease persist after LOS. Circulating inhibin B concentrations do not change in response to LOS.[48]

### LONG-TERM EFFECTS

Naether and co-workers[39] reported that the effects of LOS lasted for up to 6 years. In another study, Gjonnaess[22] showed that LOS effects were stable for up to 20 years in 50 women with PCOS. However, Elting and co-workers[49] reported that women with PCOS gain regular menstrual cycles as they become older. It is, therefore, possible that the favourable late effects demonstrated by the above two studies could have been the effect of advancing age rather than LOS. In order to investigate this further, we have recently compared the results of long-term follow-up of 116 women with PCOS who underwent LOS with that of a comparison group of age-matched PCOS women ($n = 38$), who did not undergo LOS. We have confirmed the long-term beneficial effects of LOS. In addition, we have shown that LOS contributed significantly to these long-term improvements.[12]

## MECHANISM OF ACTION OF LOS

The mechanism of action of LOS remains largely unexplained. It is likely that LOS exerts its effects via the destruction of androgen-producing tissue in the ovary. The resulting decrease in circulating androgen concentrations may result in a fall in oestrone (E1) due to decreased peripheral aromatisation of androgens. This fall in E1 then results in decreased positive feedback on LH and decreased negative feedback on FSH at the level of the pituitary. The resulting rise in serum FSH concentrations occurring in the postoperative period results in increased aromatase activity within the follicles. This effect, coupled with a decrease in local androgen concentrations, would convert the intrafollicular environment from being androgen dominant to one that is oestrogenic. This may remove an intra-ovarian block to follicular maturation, allowing follicular development to proceed to subsequent ovulation.

It has previously been hypothesised that LOS results in reduction of circulating inhibin B level and resumption of its pulsatility. This, in turn, leads to an increase in circulating FSH triggering an ovulatory cycle.[50] However, in a recent study involving 50 women with anovulatory PCOS, we reported that serum inhibin B concentrations did not change in response to LOS.[48] This finding makes it unlikely that inhibin B has any role to play in the mechanism of action of LOS.

It has also been suggested that ovarian injury leads to the production of non-steroidal factors which affect the ovarian-pituitary feedback. Another theory explaining the action of LOS is the ovarian production of a number of growth factors (such as IGF-I) in response to tissue injury, which sensitise the ovary to circulating FSH resulting in stimulation of follicular growth.

## PREDICTORS OF THE OUTCOME OF LOS

In a recent study, we investigated various clinical and biochemical factors that may predict the clinical outcome of LOS in 200 women with PCOS.[51] We found that ovulation and pregnancy rates significantly decreased with increasing duration of infertility, body mass index, serum testosterone concentration and free androgen index (Fig. 10). Women with marked obesity (BMI $\geq 35$ kg/m$^2$), marked hyperandrogenism (testosterone $\geq 4.5$ nmo/l or FAI $\geq 15$) and/or long duration of infertility (> 3 years) seemed to be resistant to LOS. Multiple logistic regression analysis showed the duration of infertility to be the most important independent predictor of ovulation after LOD followed by FAI then BMI. We also reported that high pre-operative LH concentration ($\geq 10$ IU/l) in

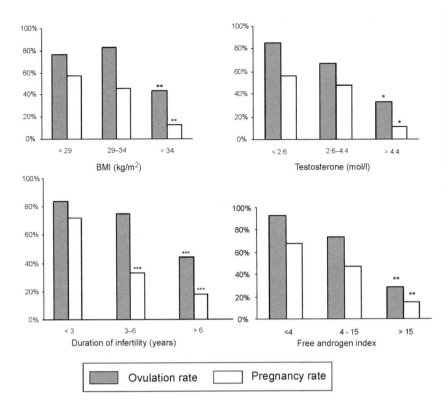

**Fig. 10** Ovulation and pregnancy rates after LOD related to different categories of body mass index (BMI), testosterone, free androgen index and duration of infertility Contingency table analysis was used to compare between the groups (*P < 0.05; **P < 0.01).[51]

women who ovulated after LOS appeared to predict higher probability of pregnancy. Age, the presence or absence of acne, the menstrual pattern, LH:FSH ratio and ovarian volume did not seem to predict the outcome of LOS.[51]

More recently, we have investigated the impact of insulin resistance as determined by homeostasis model assessment resistance index ($HOMA_{RI}$) on the outcome of LOS (unpublished data). We found insulin resistance ($HOMA_{RI}$ ≥ 2.1) to be associated with significantly lower ovulation and pregnancy rates (67% and 33%) compared with that of women with normal $HOMA_{RI}$ (96% and 65%) after LOS. Multiple logistic regression analysis showed $HOMA_{RI}$ to be more important than FAI and BMI in determining the outcome of LOS. Using ROC curves, we found $HOMA_{RI}$ to be useful in predicting ovulation (but not pregnancy) after LOS, with AUC of 0.826. An $HOMA_{RI}$ cut-off value of 2.43 was found to have a sensitivity of 86% and specificity of 81%.

## COMPLICATIONS OF LAPAROSCOPIC OVARIAN SURGERY

Intra-operative complications of LOS are rare and include damage to the utero-ovarian ligament, bleeding from the ovary at the cautery points and thermal injury to the bowel. Postoperatively, the main drawback of LOS is iatrogenic adhesion formation. An incidence of 30–40% has been reported.[52,53] Most studies reported only mild and moderate adhesions which do not seem to affect the pregnancy rate after LOS. Nevertheless, all precautions should be taken to minimise adhesion formation. This can be achieved by minimising thermal injury to the ovarian surface (as described above), ample irrigation and instillation of crystalloid solution at the end of the procedure.[53] Another theoretical risk associated with LOS is premature ovarian failure possibly due to excessive destruction of the normal ovarian follicles or the inadvertent damage of the ovarian blood supply. In our cohort of 116 patients with PCOS who were followed up for up to 9 years after LOS, no case of premature ovarian failure was observed.[12] This risk can be largely avoided by minimising the number of punctures made and by delivering the energy away from the ovarian hilum.

## FAILURE OF LAPAROSCOPIC OVARIAN SURGERY

Women are considered to have failed after LOS if they do not ovulate within 6–8 weeks, if they experience recurrence of the anovulatory status after an initial response or if they fail to conceive despite regular ovulation for 12 months. For anovulatory patients, clomifene citrate may be restarted. Many studies have demonstrated that LOS renders the ovaries more sensitive to clomifene citrate.[10] If the patient is still anovulatory on clomifene citrate, the treatment options are: (i) gonadotrophin ovarian stimulation; (ii) metformin; (iii) IVF; or (iv) repeat LOS. We have recently reported encouraging success rates after repeat LOS in women who previously responded to their first LOS. On the other hand, repeat LOS does not seem to be effective in previous non-responders.[54]

## CONCLUSIONS

Laparoscopic ovarian surgery is widely accepted as the preferred second line for induction of ovulation after clomifene citrate resistance/failure, although some reproductive specialists advocate gonadotrophin ovarian stimulation as the treatment of choice. LOS is as effective as gonadotrophins for ovulation induction and has the advantage of avoiding complications such as multiple pregnancies and OHSS. The most widely used technique for laparoscopic ovarian surgery is ovarian drilling using monopolar diathermy needle. Four punctures per ovary at 30 W applied for 5 s per puncture seem to be the optimum amount of energy required for LOS. About two-thirds of women ovulate in response to LOS. Of the responders, 50% (*i.e.* about one-third of the total number of patients undergoing LOS) will continue to benefit for several years. About 50% of women are expected to conceive during the first year after LOS. The main drawback of LOS is the need for general anaesthetic, adhesion formation and a theoretical risk of premature ovarian failure.

## Key points for clinical practice??

- LOS is used for ovulation induction in women with PCOS after CC resistence/failure.

- Evidence from RCTs and meta-analysis indicate that LOS is as effective as gonadotrophins for ovulation induction and has the advantage of avoiding complications such as multiple pregnancies and OHSS.

- Four punctures per ovary at 30w for 5 seconds per puncture using a monopolar diathermy needle seems to be the optimum amount of energy reqired for LOS.

- About two-thirds of women ovulate after LOD and 50% conceive within 12 months.

- About one-third of the patients continue to benefit from LOD for many years.

- Postoperative adhesion formation can be minimized by avoiding thermal injury to the ovarian surface and by ample irrigation.

- Women with BMI≥35 kg/m$^2$, testesterone ≥4.5 nmol/l, FAI ≥15 and/or infertility for >3 years are resistant to LOS.

## References

1. Asuncion M, Calvo RM, San Millan JL *et al.* A prospective study of the prevalence of the polycystic ovary syndrome in unselected Caucasian women from Spain. *J Clin Endocrinol Metab* 2000; **85**: 2434–2438.
2. Hull MG. Epidemiology of infertility and polycystic ovarian disease: endocrinological and demographic studies. *Gynecol Endocrinol* 1987; **1**: 235–245.
3. Rotterdam ESHRE/ASRM-Sponsored PCOS Consensus Workshop Group. Revised 2003 consensus on diagnostic criteria and long-term health risks related to polycystic ovary syndrome. *Fertil Steril* 2004; **81**: 19–25.
4. Bayram N, van Wely M, Kaaijk EM *et al.* Using an electrocautery strategy or recombinant follicle stimulating hormone to induce ovulation in polycystic ovary syndrome: randomised controlled trial. *BMJ* 2004; **328**: 192–195.
5. Farquhar C, Lilford RJ, Marjoribanks J *et al.* Laparoscopic "drilling" by diathermy or laser for ovulation induction in anovulatory polycystic ovary syndrome. Cochrane Database Syst Rev 2005; 20: CD001122.
6. Stein IF, Leventhal ML. Amenorrhea associated with bilateral polycystic ovaries. *Am J Obstet Gynecol* 1935; **29**: 181–191.
7. Buttram VC, Vaquero C. Post-ovarian wedge resection adhesive disease. *Fertil Steril* 1975; **26**: 874–876.
8. Greenblatt RB. Chemical induction of ovulation. *Fertil Steril* 1961; **12**: 402–404.
9. Palmer R, de Brux J. Résulats histologiques, biochemiques et therapeutiques obtenus ches les femmes dont les ovaries avaient été diagnostiqués Stein-Leventhal à la coelioscpie. *Bulletin Federation Societes de Gynecologie et Obstetrique de Langue Française* 1967; **19**: 405–412.
10. Gjonnaess H. Polycystic ovarian syndrome treated by ovarian electrocautery through the laparoscope. *Fertil Steril* 1984; **41**: 20–25.
11. Huber J, Hosmann J, Spona J. Polycystic ovarian syndrome treated by laser through the laparoscope [letter]. *Lancet* 1988; **2**: 215.
12. Amer S, Li TC, Gopalan V, Ledger WL, Cooke ID. Long term follow up of patients with

polycystic ovarian syndrome after laparoscopic ovarian drilling: clinical outcome. *Hum Reprod* 2002; **17**: 2035–2042.

13. Gonen Y, Casper RF. Sonographic determination of an adverse effect of clomiphene citrate on endometrial growth. *Hum Reprod* 1990; **5**: 670–674.

14. Randall JM, Templeton A. Cervical mucus score and *in vitro* sperm mucus interaction in spontaneous and clomiphene citrate cycles. *Fertil Steril* 1991; **56**: 465–468.

15. Shoham Z, Borenstein R, Lunenfeld B, Pariente C. Hormonal profiles following clomiphene citrate therapy in conception and nonconception cycles. *Clin Endocrinol* 1990; **33**: 271–278.

16. Sagle M, Bishop K, Ridley N *et al*. Recurrent early miscarriage and polycystic ovaries. *BMJ* 1988; **297**: 1027–1028.

17. Regan L, Owen EJ, Jacobs HS. Hypersecretion of luteinising hormone, infertility and miscarriage. *Lancet* 1990; **336**: 1141–1144.

18. Tulppala M, Stenman UH, Cacciatore B, Ylikorkala O. Polycystic ovaries and levels of gonadotrophins and androgens in recurrent miscarriage: prospective study in 50 women. *Br J Obstet Gynaecol* 1993; **100**: 348–352.

19. Li TC, Spuijbroek MDEH, Tuckerman E *et al*. Endocrinological and endometrial factors in recurrent miscarriage. *Br J Obstet Gynaecol* 2000; **107**: 1471–1479.

20. Rai R, Backos M, Rushworth F, Regan L. Polycystic ovaries and recurrent miscarriage – a reappraisal. *Hum Reprod* 2000; **15**: 612–615.

21. Greenblatt E, Casper RF. Endocrine changes after laparoscopic ovarian cautery in polycystic ovarian syndrome. *Am J Obstet Gynecol* 1987; **156**: 279–285.

22. Armar NA, McGarrigle HHG, Honour J *et al*. Laparoscopic ovarian diathermy in the management of anovulatory infertility in women with polycystic ovaries: endocrine changes and clinical outcome. *Fertil Steril* 1990; **53**: 45–49.

23. Gjonnaess H. Late endocrine effects of Ovarian electrocautery in of women with polycystic ovary syndrome. *Fertil Steril* 1998; **69**: 697–701.

24. Lemieux S, Lewis GF, Ben-Chetrit A, Steiner G, Greenblatt EM. Correction of hyperandrogenemia by laparoscopic ovarian cautery in women with polycystic ovarian syndrome is not accompanied by improved insulin sensitivity or lipid-lipoprotein levels. *J Clin Endocrinol Metab* 1999; **84**: 4278–4282.

25. Dahlgren E, Johansson S, Lindstedt G *et al*. Women with polycystic ovary syndrome wedge resected in 1956 to 1965: a long-term follow-up focusing on natural history and circulating hormones. *Fertil Steril* 1992; **57**: 505–513.

26. Lord JM, Flight IH, Norman RJ. Metformin in polycystic ovary syndrome: systematic review and meta-analysis. *BMJ* 2003; **327**: 951–953.

27. Palomba S, Orio Jr F, Nardo LG *et al*. Metformin administration versus laparoscopic ovarian diathermy in clomiphene citrate-resistant women with polycystic ovary syndrome: a prospective parallel randomized double-blind placebo-controlled trial. *J Clin Endocrinol Metab* 2004; **89**: 4801–4809.

28. Moll E, Bossuyt PM, Korevaar JC *et al*. Effect of clomifene citrate plus metformin and clomifene citrate plus placebo on induction of ovulation in women with newly diagnosed polycystic ovary syndrome: randomised double blind clinical trial. *BMJ* 2006; **24**: 1485–1488.

29. Legro RS, Barnhart HX, Schlaff WD *et al*. Clomiphene, metformin, or both for infertility in the polycystic ovary syndrome. *N Engl J Med* 2007; **356**: 551–566.

30. Farquhar CM. An economic evaluation of laparoscopic ovarian diathermy versus gonadotrophin therapy for women with clomiphene citrate-resistant polycystic ovarian syndrome. *Curr Opin Obstet Gynecol* 2005; **17**: 347–353.

31. Naether OGJ, Fischer R, Weise HC *et al*. Laparoscopic electrocoagulation of the ovarian surface in infertile patients with polycystic ovarian disease. *Fertil Steril* 1993; **60**: 88–94.

32. Felemban A, Tan SL, Tulandi T. Laparoscopic treatment of polycystic ovaries with insulated needle cautery: a reappraisal. *Fertil Steril* 2000; **73**: 266–269.

33. Amer SA, Li TC, Cooke ID. Laparoscopic ovarian diathermy in women with polycystic ovarian syndrome: a retrospective study on the influence of the amount of energy used on the outcome. *Hum Reprod* 2002; **17**: 1046–1051.

34. Amer S, Li TC, Cooke ID. A prospective dose finding study of the amount of energy required for laparoscopic ovarian diathermy in women with polycystic ovarian

syndrome. *Hum Reprod* 2003; **18**: 1693–1698.

35. Gurgan T, Kisnisci H, Yarali H *et al.* Evaluation of adhesion formation after laparoscopic treatment of polycystic ovarian disease. *Fertil Steril* 1991; **56**: 1176–1178.

36. Keckstein G, Rossmanith W, Spatzier K *et al.* The effect of laparoscopic treatment of polycystic ovarian disease by $CO_2$-laser or Nd:YAG laser. *Surg Endosc* 1990; **4**: 103–107.

37. Keckstein J. Laparoscopic treatment of polycystic ovarian syndrome. *Baillières Clin Obstet Gynaecol* 1989; **3**: 563–581.

38. Kojima E, Yanagibori A, Otaka K *et al.* Ovarian wedge resection with contact Nd:YAG laser irradiation used laparoscopically. *J Reprod Med* 1989; **34**: 444–446.

39. Naether OGJ, Baukloh V, Fischer R *et al.* Long-term follow-up in 206 infertility patients with polycystic ovarian syndrome after laparoscopic electrocautery of the ovarian surface. *Hum Reprod* 1994; **9**: 2342–2349.

40. Li TC, Saravelos H, Chow MS *et al.* Factors affecting the outcome of laparoscopic ovarian drilling for polycystic ovarian syndrome in women with anovulatory infertility. *Br J Obstet Gynaecol* 1998; **105**: 338–344.

41. Mio Y, Toda T, Tanikawa M *et al.* Transvaginal ultrasound-guided follicular aspiration in the management of anovulatory infertility associated with polycystic ovaries. *Fertil Steril* 1991; **56**: 1060–1065.

42. Syritsa A. Transvaginal ultrasound-guided electrocautery of the ovaries in infertile patients with polycystic ovarian disease. *Int J Gynaecol Obstet* 1998; **63**: 293–294.

43. Zhu W, Li X, Chen X, Lin Z, Zhang L. Ovarian interstitial YAG-laser: an effective new method to manage anovulation in women with polycystic ovary syndrome. *Am J Obstet Gynecol* 2006; **195**: 458–463.

44. Fernandez H, Watrelot A, Alby JD *et al.* Fertility after ovarian drilling by transvaginal fertiloscopy for treatment of polycystic ovary syndrome. *J Am Assoc Gynecol Laparosc* 2004; **11**: 374–378.

45. Ramzy AM, Al-Inany H, Aboulfoutouh I *et al.* Ultrasonographic guided ovarian stroma hydrocoagulation for ovarian stimulation in polycystic ovary syndrome. *Acta Obstet Gynecol Scand* 2001; **80**: 1046–1050.

46. Chiesa-Montadou S, Rongieres C, Garbin O, Nisand I. [About two complications of ovarian drilling by fertiloscopy]. *Gynecol Obstet Fertil* 2003; **31**: 844–846.

47. Liguori G, Tolino A, Moccia G, Scognamiglio G, Nappi C. Laparoscopic ovarian treatment in infertile patients with polycystic ovarian syndrome (PCOS): endocrine changes and clinical outcome. *Gynecol Endocrinol* 1996; **10**: 257–264.

48. Amer S, Laird S, Ledger WL, Li TC. Effect of laparoscopic ovarian diathermy on circulating inhibin B in women with anovulatory polycystic ovarian syndrome. *Hum Reprod* 2007; **22**: 389–394.

49. Elting MW, Korsen TJM, Rekers-Mombarg LTM, Schoemaker J. Women with polycystic ovary syndrome gain regular menstrual cycles when ageing. *Hum Reprod* 2000; **15**: 24–28.

50. Lockwood GM, Muttukrishna S, Groome NP, Matthews DR, Ledger WL. Mid-follicular phase pulses of inhibin B are absent in polycystic ovarian syndrome and are initiated by successful laparoscopic ovarian diathermy: a possible mechanism regulating emergence of the dominant follicle. *J Clin Endocrinol Metab* 1998; **83**: 1730–1735.

51. Amer S, Li TC, Ledger WL. Ovulation induction using laparoscopic ovarian drilling in women with polycystic ovarian syndrome: predictors of success. *Hum Reprod* 2004; **19**: 1719–1724.

52. Greenblatt EM, Casper RF. Adhesion formation after laparoscopic ovarian cautery for polycystic ovarian syndrome: lack of correlation with pregnancy rate. *Fertil Steril* 1993; **60**: 766–770.

53. Naether OGJ. Significant reduction of adnexal adhesions following laparoscopic electrocautery of the ovarian surface (LEOS) by lavage and artificial ascites. *Gynaecol Endosc* 1995; **4**: 17–19.

54. Amer S, Li TC, Cooke ID. Repeated laparoscopic ovarian diathermy is effective in women with anovulatory infertility due to polycystic ovarian syndrome. *Fertil Steril* 2003; **79**: 1211–1215.

*Tom O'Gorman  Tony Hollingworth*

# 17

# Postmenopausal bleeding

The menopause is defined by the World Health Organization (WHO) as the permanent cessation of menstruation resulting from the loss of ovarian follicular activity.[1] This definition of the menopause is unhelpful in determining when an episode of bleeding can be described as postmenopausal. From a symptomatic perspective, postmenopausal bleeding describes the occurrence of vaginal bleeding following a woman's last menstrual cycle. Vaginal bleeding that occurs after 6 months of amenorrhoea from presumed menopause should be considered as suspicious and warrants investigation.

Postmenopausal bleeding accounts for a significant proportion of gynaecological referrals and occurs in approximately 3% of postmenopausal women. The use of hormones increases the likelihood of bleeding by a factor of more than 5.[2] The amount and type of bleeding is not of any particular proven diagnostic value. Benign conditions represent the most frequent causes of postmenopausal bleeding and can cause considerable distress. The primary aim of initial investigations is to exclude endometrial carcinoma and atypical hyperplasia. It can be easier to demonstrate the presence of a malignant tumour if one exists in a given patient than it is to be certain there is no malignant lesion even though results of diagnostic procedures are all negative.

The risk of endometrial carcinoma in women with postmenopausal bleeding rises with age from approximately 1% at the age of 50 years to approximately 25% at the age of 80 years.[3] The risk is also increased significantly in obese women.[4] One population-based, case-control study conducted in Hawaii examining the

**Tom O'Gorman** MBChB BAO DCH MRCOG
Specialist Registrar in Obstetrics and Gynaecology, Whipps Cross University Hospital, Whipps Cross Road, Leytonstone, London, UK
E-mail: Thomas.OGorman@bartsandthelondon.nhs.uk

**Tony Hollingworth** MBChB MBA PhD FRCS(Ed) FRCOG
Consultant Obstetrician and Gynaecologist, Whipps Cross University Hospital, Whipps Cross Road, Leytonstone, London, UK
E-mail: tony.hollingworth@Whippsx.nhs.uk

**Table 1** Causes of postmenopausal bleeding

| | |
|---|---|
| • Normal/atrophic | 58.8% |
| • Endometrial carcinoma | 9.4% |
| • Endometrial polyp | 9.4% |
| • Carcinoma of the cervix | 6% |
| • Submucous fibroid | 4% |
| • Endometrial hyperplasia, pyometra, ovarian cancer and urethral caruncle | 12.4% |

Adapted from Weiderpass et al.[6]

association of diet, body size, and physical activity with the risk of endometrial cancer showed the odds ratio (OR) for endometrial cancer among women in the highest quartile of body mass index (BMI) was more than four times that among women in the lowest quartile.[5]

More than 90% of patients with endometrial carcinomas present with irregular or postmenopausal vaginal bleeding. However, only 20% of patients with postmenopausal bleeding will have any significant pathology as a cause for their bleeding (Table 1). The risk of endometrial cancer in non-hormone replacement therapy (HRT) users complaining of postmenopausal bleeding and in HRT users experiencing abnormal bleeding is sufficient to recommend referring all patients for investigation.[6,7]

## UROGENITAL ATROPHY AND VAGINAL MOISTURISERS

The histology of the vagina is a non-keratinised stratified squamous epithelium that changes extensively after the menopause. The epithelium often becomes quite thin and heavily infiltrated with neutrophils. Urogenital tissues are oestrogen sensitive and, following the menopause, they undergo changes, which include: (i) thinning of the epithelium; (ii) reduction in vascularity; and (iii) decreased muscle bulk and increased fat deposition.

Vaginal irritation, dryness, dyspareunia and itching are all symptoms associated with urogenital atrophy. The loss of elasticity and decreased thickness of the epithelium cause the vagina to be more easily traumatised and may result in vaginal bleeding. The extent of significant urogenital symptoms appears to be relatively low[8] and the majority of women are not significantly distressed. The hormonal changes associated with the menopause have also been shown to induce changes in the bacterial colonisation of the vagina.

An objective assessment of urogenital atrophy can be carried out by performing a vaginal smear for cytology. This will usually show a failure of epithelial maturation with a marked reduction in the proportion of superficial epithelial cells and a relative excess of parabasal epithelial cells. This pattern is reflected in indices such as the maturation index (percentage of superficial cells), which expresses the percentages of (para)basal, intermediate, and superficial cells in a predetermined number of cells in a smear.

The administration of exogenous oestrogens (either systemic or topical) is a common treatment for symptoms related to vaginal atrophy[9] and can restore vaginal epithelium maturation. However, the use of exogenous oestrogens has several adverse effects namely endometrial stimulation with an increased the risk

**Table 2** Probability of having endometrial cancer associated with postmenopausal bleeding in women with different risk factors: a meta-analysis

| Risk factor | Percentage (n/total) | References |
|---|---|---|
| Early menarche < 10 years | 80.0 (4/5) | 14 |
| Late menopause > 55 | 45.5 (5/11) | 14 |
| Nulliparity | 41.8 (28/67) | 14,15 |
| Unopposed oestrogen therapy | 40.0 (10/25) | 15,16 |
| Bleeding (moderate or severe) | 33.5 (77/230) | 14–16 |
| Obesity | 33.0 (30/91) | 14,15 |
| Diabetes | 31.0 (13/42) | 14,15 |
| Liver disease | 30.0 (9/30) | 14 |
| Persistent/recurrent bleeding | 27.0 (38/141) | 15 |
| Hypertension | 30.7 (42/137) | 14,15 |

Adapted from Ind.[13]

of endometrial hyperplasia and carcinoma and consequently needs to be used judiciously.[9,10]

Replens©, a polycarbophil-based vaginal moisturiser, is a non-hormonal alternative to oestrogen treatment. A characteristic of this bio-adhesive polymer is that it is water insoluble, but water swellable. When applied intravaginally, it binds to the vaginal epithelium, releasing purified water to hydrate the underlying cells. The gel produces a moist film over the vaginal tissue, which remains attached to the epithelial cell surface. The hydration of the epithelium lubricates the vaginal wall and reduces the incidence of vaginal itching, irritation, and dyspareunia.[10] Furthermore, Replens© restores the vaginal pH to premenopausal values[9] and has also been shown to increase maturation of vaginal epithelium.[11]

In a double-blind, placebo-controlled trial, phyto-oestrogens (these are naturally occurring compounds of plants, such as soybeans, or plant products, such as whole grain cereals, that act like oestrogen in the body) have not been shown to have a significant effect on vaginal maturation index scores.[12]

## INVESTIGATIONS

The principal aim of the investigation of postmenopausal bleeding is to identify or exclude endometrial pathology. A thorough history may reveal factors associated with increased risk of endometrial hyperplasia and cancer such as nulliparity, diabetes, obesity, hypertension and the use of unopposed oestrogens. The risk increases with age and the number of risk factors present.[3] Table 2 is a summary of a meta-analysis of three studies including 811 patients in all and gives the numbers of women with the various risks who presented with postmenopausal bleeding and the percentage of them within each category who were found to have invasive disease of the endometrium.

Examination may help in the diagnosis of vulval, vaginal, cervical or pelvic pathology. Vaginal and cervical pathology such as cervical polyps, atrophic vaginitis or ulceration from a ring pessary may be identified. Women presenting with postmenopausal bleeding should, therefore, receive a pelvic examination at some stage during the course of clinical assessment. A cervical smear test should be carried out to exclude cervical precancer, where appropriate (though this is usually asymptomatic), and invasive disease. Endometrial carcinoma has been detected on a cytology smear.[17] However, endometrial cytology has been found to be particularly unsuccessful due to difficulties in obtaining adequate numbers of endometrial cells and in making the diagnosis from such scanty specimens.

The mean endometrial thickness in postmenopausal women is much thinner than in premenopausal women. Thickening of the endometrium may indicate the presence of significant pathology. In general, the thicker the endometrium the higher the likelihood of significant pathology (*e.g.* endometrial cancer) being present.[18] Primary assessment in all cases should be with transvaginal ultrasound scanning (TVS), which can reliably assess endometrial thickness. Women with postmenopausal bleeding who have a thin endometrium are unlikely to have significant endometrial pathology. Further investigation may not be necessary unless there is recurrence of bleeding.[19] No endometrial thickness threshold completely excludes the possibility of an early endometrial carcinoma, which can be present in women who have no postmenopausal bleeding but have been scanned for other reasons and found to have a thickened endometrium as an incidental finding. Sensitivity depends on the cut off used for normal endometrial thickness (usually no more than 4 mm). The addition of colour Doppler imaging to transvaginal ultrasound scanning has not been found to be helpful in identifying pathological conditions of the endometrium.[20]

All postmenopausal women with an endometrial thickness greater than 4 mm or persistent bleeding despite a normal endometrial thickness should undergo an endometrial biopsy.[21] There appears to be no prognostic advantage for endometrial screening using transvaginal ultrasound on asymptomatic postmenopausal women compared with symptomatic patients who had bleeding of shorter than 8 weeks.[22] Moreover, patients who are at a high risk for endometrial cancer tend to avoid TVS screening. Endometrial screening often results in unnecessary operations, which are associated with increased morbidity and costs.[23]

Magnetic resonance imaging (MRI) will help identify the site and size of the primary tumour, any evident myometrial invasion and the presence of lymph node metastases. MRI is the optimum modality for assessing myometrial invasion and cervical involvement. Although MRI is superior to transvaginal sonography in evaluating myometrial invasion, it is expensive and time consuming, and is not suitable as a screening 'triage' test for postmenopausal bleeding or depth of invasion. On the other hand, transvaginal sonography is relatively low-cost technique, which can be easily performed and repeated though it does depends upon operator experience in order to achieve high accuracy.

Dilatation and curettage is a blind procedure that should no longer be used as the first-line method in investigating postmenopausal bleeding. Its sensitivity for detecting endometrial cancer is unknown. Less than half of the endometrium is sampled in 60% of patients and D&C prior to hysterectomy showed that endometrial lesions were missed in 10% of cases.[24] In postmenopausal women, specimens adequate for histological diagnosis were obtained in 74 of 88 (84.1%) by Pipelle and in only 22 of 48 (45.8%) by D&C.[25]

Various sampling devices are available to obtain an endometrial biopsy. They are usually tube-like devices, which are inserted into the uterine cavity, and a plunger is withdrawn. The negative pressure permits aspiration of tissue into the device. Randomised trials have shown that the Pipelle and Vabra aspirators give equal diagnostic accuracy although the Pipelle causes less discomfort and samples considerably less of the endometrial surface.[25,26] Both perform as well as diagnostic curettage in diagnostic accuracy and have lower complication rates. A meta-analysis carried out by Grimes[27] looking at endometrial sampling using the Vabra aspirator did not identify a single case where an unanticipated major operation was necessitated by complications.

Out-patient endometrial sampling has a procedure failure rate and a tissue yield failure rate approaching 10%.[28] In this study, the indications for sampling were abnormal menstrual bleeding (65 patients), intermenstrual or postcoital bleeding (7 patients), and postmenopausal bleeding (28 patients). Yield failure is much more likely with atrophic changes than when carcinoma is present. Out-patient sampling has been compared to in-patient hysteroscopy and curettage and found to be as effective in screening for endometrial hyperplasia but hysteroscopy prior to curettage was shown to be better at diagnosing polyps, uterine abnormalities and other benign lesions.[29] However, hysteroscopy without biopsy is unreliable in differentiating between premalignant and malignant endometrium.[30] Hysteroscopy is associated with more possible operative complications including uterine perforation, haemorrhage and anaesthetic complications. In one study, the pros and cons of different diagnostic strategies (*i.e.* expectant management after ultrasound or complete diagnostic work-up including invasive procedures) were offered. Most women wanted to be totally certain that carcinoma could be ruled out. Only 5% of the women were willing to accept more than 5% risk of false re-assurance. If the risk of recurrent bleeding due to benign disease exceeded 25%, the majority of women would prefer immediate diagnosis and treatment of benign lesions.[30] Women with postmenopausal bleeding are prepared to undergo hysteroscopy to rule out any malignancy which suggests that endometrial thickness measurement by initial transvaginal ultrasound may not be the patients' choice.[31]

A one-stop clinic is effective for early diagnosis of genital tract malignancy in a majority of patients with postmenopausal bleeding and significantly helps in reducing the hospital waiting list.[32] Asymptomatic postmenopausal women found to have a thickened endometrium on ultrasound have a low risk of endometrial cancer(0.002%) if the endometrium measures less than 11 mm. If the endometrium measures 11 mm or greater, the risk rises to 6.7% and biopsy should be considered.[33]

## UTERINE POLYPS

A polyp is defined as tumours projecting from the a mucosa into the lumen of a hollow viscus. Uterine polyps are a common cause of postmenopausal bleeding. They are usually inflammatory but may occasionally have hyperplastic or neoplastic changes of the covering endometrium. They can be of fibroid origin and much more common if other fibroids are present, though rarely display sarcomatous changes. Saline sonohysterography is a particularly useful diagnostic tool to identify intra-uterine polyps. The exact pathogenesis of endometrial polyps is not fully elucidated, but they are thought to originate as a localised hyperplasia of the basalis secondary to hormonal influences.[34] Since both endometrial polyps and endometrial hyperplasia are associated with hyperoestrogenism, they can co-exist and endometrial hyperplasia can be identified in 3% of polyps.[35] There are no standard recommendations for the follow-up of women with hyperplasia identified in a polyp in an endometrial biopsy or polypectomy specimen. Hysterectomy is the preferred treatment when a diagnosis of atypical hyperplasia occurs within a polyp. A retrospective study of 204 patients with endometrial carcinoma showed endometrial cancer arising in polyps in 27 patients (13.2%), which accounted for 1.8% of all polyps diagnosed during that period. The study conclusion was that postmenopausal women with endometrial polyps diagnosed by ultrasonography should undergo directed biopsies under hysteroscopic vision.[36]

## ENDOMETRIAL HYPERPLASIA

Endometrial hyperplasia is an oestrogen-dependent condition, and the same risk factors apply to it as endometrial carcinoma. The WHO classification of endometrial hyperplasia has four categories: (i) simple endometrial hyperplasia; (ii) complex endometrial hyperplasia; (iii) simple atypical endometrial hyperplasia, and (iv) complex atypical endometrial hyperplasia.

Predisposing factors to hyperplasia include: (i) obesity; (ii) anovulation; (iii) ovarian stromal hyperplasia; (iv) oestrogen tumours; (v) unopposed oestrogen HRT; and (vi) Tamoxifen therapy due to the unopposed oestrogen or oestrogen-like effect on the endometrium.

Endometrial hyperplasia may not always cause any symptoms and may remained undiagnosed; it is thought the condition may be self-limiting in a large number of women.[37] The incidence of progression to invasive carcinoma in untreated endometrial hyperplasia in the four categories is considered to be: (i) simple hyperplasia, 1%; (ii) complex hyperplasia, < 5%; (iii) simple hyperplasia with atypia, 5–10%; and (iv) complex atypical hyperplasia, 25–30%.

These risks appear to be over the short term as the data are derived from studies in which most women had their hysterectomy within 6 months of the diagnosis of endometrial hyperplasia being made.[38] Longer term follow-up of 170 patients with all grades of endometrial hyperplasia, who did not undergo a hysterectomy for at least 1 year (range, 1–26.7 years; mean, 13.4 years) revealed similar rates of progression in the four groups.[39]

### TREATMENT OF HYPERPLASIA

Endometrial hyperplasia without atypia is likely to respond to hormonal treatment.[40,41] The levonorgestrel IUS has been shown to be effective in the management of endometrial hyperplasia.[42] Women with atypical hyperplasia on histology should be offered total hysterectomy, especially if they are postmenopausal.[43]

## HORMONE REPLACEMENT THERAPY

Older HRT regimens that utilise unopposed oestrogen increase the relative risk of endometrial carcinoma around 6-fold after 5 years of use.[6] Progestogens are added to HRT regimens to prevent endometrial hyperplasia and cancer: their inclusion reduces the relative risk of endometrial cancer to around 1.5.[44] Protection is provided by either 10–12 days of cyclical progestogens or continuous combined regimens.

Sequential or cyclical combined regimens cause scheduled bleeding in most users. Continuous combined regimens are associated with a reduced relative risk of endometrial cancer but may cause unpredictable spotting or bleeding during initial use.[45,46]

The incidence of endometrial abnormalities in women receiving HRT may be higher in the general population than in clinical trial populations. In the latter population, any pre-existing condition may have been resolved before commencing HRT. Bleeding in HRT users is less likely to be associated with endometrial carcinoma than bleeding in non-HRT users although benign pathology, such as polyps, may be present.[47]

The use of sequential HRT causes endometrial thickening whereas tibolone and continuous combined HRT cause endometrial atrophy. Stopping HRT prior to investigation may result in an oestrogen withdrawal bleed and this may make acquiring tissue for histology less likely. There is a greater risk of false-positive results on transvaginal ultrasound screening of the endometrium in women who continue to use HRT during investigation.[48]

## TAMOXIFEN

Women receiving Tamoxifen in the treatment or prevention of breast cancer experience a 3–6-fold greater incidence of endometrial cancer than non-users.[49,50] An increasing number of women are now receiving this therapy, and the risk of endometrial cancer rises with both the use of higher doses and increasing duration of Tamoxifen use especially if treatment continues beyond 5 years.[51,52] Furthermore, there is evidence from one case control study that the endometrial cancers occurring in long-term users of Tamoxifen have a poorer prognosis (due to less favourable histology and higher stage).[53]

There has been some debate about how closely women on Tamoxifen should be monitored for the development of endometrial cancer irrespective of symptoms. However, evidence mainly from observational studies indicates that periodic investigations are unlikely to be cost effective.[54,55] Therefore, postmenopausal bleeding should remain as the primary trigger for the investigation of women on Tamoxifen. Tamoxifen has a sonotranslucent effect on both the endometrial stroma and myometrium. Some studies have suggested that a higher cut off of endometrial thickness of 9 mm should be used to prompt further investigation; however, the use of hysteroscopy and biopsy as first-line investigations may be more appropriate and provide less ambiguous results in this high-risk group of women as well as help allay their anxiety.[56] All women experiencing abnormal bleeding while taking Tamoxifen should be investigated to exclude malignancy.

Anastrozole has been shown to have superior efficacy and tolerability in comparison to Tamoxifen in the treatment of hormone receptor positive breast cancer in postmenopausal women and is associated with fewer episodes of postmenopausal bleeding (Anastrozole versus Tamoxifen, 1.0% versus 2.5%).[57] The ATAC (Arimidex, Tamoxifen, Alone or in Combination) trial showed only patients receiving Tamoxifen developed endometrial atypical hyperplasia.[58] Switching from Tamoxifen to Anastrozole treatment significantly reduced the need for a second hysteroscopy and D&C due to the decrease incidence of recurrent vaginal bleeding or thickening of the endometrium in postmenopausal breast cancer patients with Tamoxifen-induced endometrial abnormalities.[59]

## THE CERVIX AND CERVICAL SCREENING

Cervical lesions including cervicitis, cervical polyps or carcinoma may also result in postmenopausal bleeding, which can occur spontaneously, or following intercourse.

Cervical cancer has been shown to be twice as common as endometrial cancer in women presenting with postmenopausal bleeding who have a thin endometrium on ultrasound scan. During subsequent follow-up, the risk of endometrial cancer was as expected, whereas the risk of cervical cancer was higher than expected. At follow-up (3–15 years), cervical cancer was detected in 2 of 313 (0.6%) women; no additional case of endometrial cancer was found. The expected incidence of cervical and endometrial cancer during follow-up was 0.23 (standard incidence ratio [SIR], 8.7; 95% CI 1.1–31.4) and 1.34 (SIR, 0.0; 95% CI 0.0–2.7), respectively. Of the women, 13% (41 of 313) sought medical care because of re-bleeding. Endometrial pathology was found in 16% (4 of 25) and cervical pathology in 11% (3 of 28) of these women. The results support that the diagnostic focus should be directed at excluding cervical pathology and that repeated diagnostic procedures be performed in cases of re-bleeding.[60]

The aim of cervical screening is to prevent the development of cancer and relies on effective treatment of premalignant change plus the long latent interval between premalignant changes and development of occult cancer. The current UK screening programme changes the frequency of screening according to the woman's age and has been shown to be effective.[61] The majority of postmenopausal women eligible for screening will fall into the group offered screening every 5 years. The exit age of 65 years has been questioned particularly on reducing the age of screening to 50 years in women who have been well screened with a satisfactory negative history. Cervical screening is less efficient at detecting cervical intra-epithelial neoplasia 3 (CIN 3) in older women – more smears are required to detect a case of CIN 3 after the age of 50 years,[62] but it is more efficient at preventing invasive cancer.[61]

The prevalence of CIN 3 and invasive cancer in women over the age of 50 years is low – 11 in 100,000 in well-screened women compared with a prevalence rate of 59 in 100,000 women in the population as a whole.[63] Women who were diagnosed with invasive cancer after the age of 50 years had not participated adequately in the cervical screening programme.[64] Evidence from the US suggests that screening women over the age of 65 years, who have been poorly screened previously, still results in a reduction in the subsequent rate of cervical cancer.[65]

Women who are hypo-oestrogenic are at risk of genital tract atrophy. Cervical atrophy can reduce the accuracy of cervical cytology due to the difficulty in obtaining smears from the transformation zone as the squamocolumnar junction lies within the endocervical canal. Women presenting with postmenopausal bleeding do not require a cervical smear if they are up-to-date with their routine screening appointments. Speculum examination should be carried out and, if there are suspicious appearances on the cervix, a biopsy should be carried out. If the external cervix appears normal, the possibility of an endocervical glandular lesion needs to be excluded. A smear should be taken if routine screening has been missed.

Asymptomatic postmenopausal women with normal endometrial cells in their smear are at significant higher risk for (pre)cancerous endometrial lesion than women without these cells.[66,67] This increased risk has been reported in postmenopausal women taking HRT as well.[68] Nuclear enlargement in squamous cells is an expected normal reactive change present in postmenopausal atrophic cervical vaginal smears that resolves with the application of local oestrogen. Nuclear hyperchromasia and irregular nuclear contours remain the most reliable cellular characteristics for diagnosing SIL in atrophic CVS.[69]

## RISK OF RECURRENT BLEEDING

For women who present with postmenopausal bleeding and a benign tissue diagnosis, recurrent bleeding is a concern. Although the initial tissue diagnosis may be benign, the possibility of endometrial cancer or complex hyperplasia needs to be ruled out for women with recurrent postmenopausal bleeding. Diagnostic D&C or endometrial biopsy combined with other tools (vaginal ultrasound, hysteroscopy, transvaginal sonohysterography) is more reliable for evaluating women with recurrent postmenopausal bleeding than D&C or endometrial biopsy only. If these diagnostic results are negative, a total hysterectomy with bilateral salpingo-oophorectomy should be considered to reduce the risk of endometrial cancer in women who present with recurrent bleeding.[70] This study, with a 5-year follow-up, showed that postmenopausal women aged 65 years or over had a much greater chance (13 of 29; 44.8%) of having endometrial cancer or complex hyperplasia than women aged below 65 years (6 of 48; 12.5%) if they presented with recurrent postmenopausal bleeding and an initial benign tissue diagnosis ($P = 0.005$).

In patients presenting with postmenopausal bleeding, once an initial hysteroscopy and curettage has excluded uterine pathology there is no need to repeat the procedure unless there are very strong grounds for suspecting an occult carcinoma. By carefully tracking oestrogen levels subsequently, it can be possible to predict if and when recurrent episodes of bleeding will occur. A transvaginal ultrasound measured endometrial thickness of less than 5 mm provides additional re-assurance that there is no sinister underlying pathology.[71] However, other studies have looked at the histology associated with recurrent postmenopausal bleeding. The recurrence rate of uterine bleeding was shown to be very high in carcinoma of the endometrium, moderate in proliferative endometrium and low in secretory and atrophic endometrium.[72]

The cause and possible treatment of postmenopausal bleeding of 6 months' duration or longer has also been reviewed. A total of 110 women aged 40–90 years with persistent postmenopausal bleeding were evaluated by diagnostic hysteroscopy and managed by operative hysteroscopy. Only two patients had an early adenocarcinoma, the majority of the rest had benign causes for their symptoms with approximately 10% of the total having no significant pathology. Diagnostic and operative hysteroscopy was effective in controlling this prolonged postmenopausal bleeding in almost 90% of the patients as either polyps or submucous fibroids were the primary cause of the bleeding.[73]

## MISCELLANEOUS CAUSES OF BLEEDING FROM THE GENITAL TRACT

Adnexal tumours of ovarian and fallopian tube origin (benign or malignant) may also present with postmenopausal bleeding by virtue of functional ovarian tumours producing oestrogens or association of pelvic congestion and increased vascularity with non-functional tumours. Chronic endometritis of tuberculosis has also been known to cause postmenopausal spotting or bleeding. This is of particular relevance in countries with a high incidence of tuberculosis.[74]

Postmenopausal women may have a systemic cause of vaginal bleeding superimposed against a backdrop of severe atrophic endometritis. The common causes include: (i) thrombocytopenia; (ii) leukaemia; (iii) pancytopenia from immunosuppression, chemotherapy, bone marrow suppression; (iv) anticoagulation (iatrogenic) especially when a high INR is a therapeutic requirement; and (v) secondary coagulopathy from liver disease.

Non-vaginal bleeding can often be mistaken by women to be vaginal in origin. Surrounding structures and problems that need to be considered from the urogenital part of the perineum include a bleeding urethral caruncle, haematuria from acute or chronic cystitis, bladder polyp or even neoplasia. This bleeding is usually painless though may occasionally be associated with local perineal or pelvic pain. Likewise, rectal bleeding can also be mistaken for bleeding of vaginal origin. Anorectal piles, fissure *in ano* and malignancy may be other offending causes to be considered as the source of bleeding from the posterior part of the perineum.

---

### Key points for clinical practice

- Benign conditions represent the most frequent causes of postmeno-pausal bleeding though primary aim of initial investigations is to exclude endometrial carcinoma and atypical hyperplasia.

- The amount and type of bleeding is not of any particular proven diagnostic value as only 20% of patients with postmenopausal bleeding will have a significant pathology as a cause for their bleeding.

- In general, the thicker the endometrium in postmenopausal women, the higher the likelihood of significant pathology (*e.g.* endometrial cancer) being present; an endometrial thickness greater than 4 mm or persistent bleeding irrespective of thickness warrants an endometrial biopsy.

---

**Key points for clinical practice** *(continued)*

- The risk of endometrial carcinoma in women with postmenopausal bleeding rises with age from approximately 1% at the age of 50 years to approximately 25% at the age of 80 years

- Phyto-oestrogens have not been shown to have a significant effect on vaginal maturation index scores though Replens, a polycarbophil-based vaginal moisturiser, is a non-hormonal alternative to vaginal oestrogen treatment.

- There appears to be no prognostic advantage for endometrial screening using transvaginal ultrasound on asymptomatic postmenopausal women compared with symptomatic patients.

- Women receiving Tamoxifen therapy, particularly for longer than 5 years, are at increased risk of endometrial cancer; consequently, women experiencing abnormal bleeding while taking Tamoxifen should be investigated to exclude malignancy. Anastrazole (Arimidex) is an alternative to Tamoxifen and is associated with fewer episodes of postmenopausal bleeding.

- Women presenting with postmenopausal bleeding do not require a cervical smear if they are up-to-date with their routine screening appointments.

- Out-patient endometrial sampling has a procedure failure rate and a tissue yield failure rate approaching 10%; hysteroscopy with endometrial sampling is the diagnostic procedure of choice.

---

*References*

1. Report of a WHO Scientific Group. Research on the menopause in the 1990s. *World Health Organ Tech Rep Ser* 1996; **866**: 1–107.
2. Anon, Endometrial bleeding. *Hum Reprod Update* 2007; **13**: 421–431.
3. Gredmark T, Kvint S, Havel G, Mattsson LA. Histopathological findings in women with postmenopausal bleeding. *Br J Obstet Gynaecol* 1995; **102**: 133–136.
4. MacDonald PC, Edman CD, Hemsell DL, Porter JC, Siiteri PK. Effect of obesity on conversion of plasma androstenedione to estrone in postmenopausal women with and without endometrial cancer. *Am J Obstet Gynecol* 1978; **130**: 448–455.
5. Goodman MT, Hankin JH, Wilkens LR *et al.* Diet, body size, physical activity, and the risk of endometrial cancer. *Cancer Res* 1997; **57**: 5077–5085.
6. Weiderpass E, Adami HO, Baron JA *et al.* Risk of endometrial cancer following estrogen replacement with and without progestins. *J Natl Cancer Inst* 1999; **91**: 1131–1137.
7. Oehler MK, MacKenzie I, Kehoe S, Rees MC. Assessment of abnormal bleeding in menopausal women: an update. *J Br Menopause Soc* 2003; **9**: 117–121.
8. Barlow DH, Cardozo LD, Francis RM *et al.* Urogenital ageing and its effect on sexual health in older British women. *Br J Obstet Gynaecol* 1997; **104**: 87–91.
9. Nachtigall LE. Comparative study: Replens versus local estrogen in menopausal women. *Fertil Steril* 1994; **61**: 178–180.
10. Bygdeman M, Swahn ML. Replens versus dienoestrol cream in the symptomatic treatment of vaginal atrophy in postmenopausal women. *Maturitas* 1996; **23**: 259–263.
11. van der Laak JA, de Bie LM, de Leeuw H, de Wilde PC, Hanselaar AG. The effect of Replens on vaginal cytology in the treatment of postmenopausal atrophy: cytomorphology versus computerised cytometry. *J Clin Pathol* 2002; **55**: 446–451.

12. D'Anna R, Cannata ML, Atteritano M *et al*. Effects of the phytoestrogen genistein on hot flushes, endometrium, and vaginal epithelium in postmenopausal women: a 1-year randomized, double-blind, placebo-controlled study. *Menopause* 2007; **14**: 648–655.

13. Ind T. Management of post-menopausal bleeding. *Prog Obstet Gynaecol* 1998; **10**: 361–377.

14. Alberico S, Conoscenti G, Veglio P, Bogatti P, Di Bonito L, Mandruzzato G. A clinical and epidemiological study of 245 postmenopausal metrorrhagia patients. *Clin Exp Obstet Gynecol* 1989; **16**: 113–121.

15. Feldman S, Cook EF, Harlow BL, Berkowitz RS. Predicting endometrial cancer among older women who present with abnormal vaginal bleeding. *Gynecol Oncol* 1995; **56**: 376–381.

16. Miyazawa K. Clinical significance of an enlarged uterus in patients with postmenopausal bleeding. *Obstet Gynecol* 1983; **61**: 148–152.

17. Demirkiran F, Arvas M, Erkun E *et al*. The prognostic significance of cervico-vaginal cytology in endometrial cancer. *Eur J Gynaecol Oncol* 1995; **16**: 403–409.

18. Wolman I, Amster R, Hartoov J *et al*. Reproducibility of transvaginal ultrasonographic measurements of endometrial thickness in patients with postmenopausal bleeding. *Gynecol Obstet Invest* 1998; **46**: 191–194.

19. Garuti G, Sambruni I, Cellani F, Garzia D, Alleva P, Luerti M. Hysteroscopy and transvaginal ultrasonography in postmenopausal women with uterine bleeding. *Int J Gynaecol Obstet* 1999; **65**: 25–33.

20. Wilailak S, Jirapinyo M, Theppisai U. Transvaginal Doppler sonography: is there a role for this modality in the evaluation of women with postmenopausal bleeding? *Maturitas* 2005; **50**: 111–116.

21. Moodley M, Roberts C. Clinical pathway for the evaluation of postmenopausal bleeding with an emphasis on endometrial cancer detection. *J Obstet Gynaecol* 2004; **24**: 736–741.

22. Robertson G. Screening for endometrial cancer. *Med J Aust* 2003; **178**: 657–659.

23. Gerber B, Krause A, Muller H *et al*. Ultrasonographic detection of asymptomatic endometrial cancer in postmenopausal patients offers no prognostic advantage over symptomatic disease discovered by uterine bleeding. *Eur J Cancer* 2001; **37**: 64–71.

24. Stock RJ, Kanbour A. Prehysterectomy curettage. *Obstet Gynecol* 1975; **45**: 537–541.

25. Ben-Baruch G, Seidman DS, Schiff E, Moran O, Menczer J. Outpatient endometrial sampling with the Pipelle curette. *Gynecol Obstet Invest* 1994; **37**: 260–262.

26. Kaunitz AM, Masciello A, Ostrowski M, Rovira EZ. Comparison of endometrial biopsy with the endometrial Pipelle and Vabra aspirator. *J Reprod Med* 1988; **33**: 427–431.

27. Grimes DA. Diagnostic dilation and curettage: a reappraisal. *Am J Obstet Gynecol* 1982; **142**: 1–6.

28. Gordon SJ, Westgate J. The incidence and management of failed Pipelle sampling in a general outpatient clinic. *Aust NZ J Obstet Gynaecol* 1999; **39**: 115–118.

29. Etherington IJ HK, Read MD. A comparison of outpatient endometrial sampling with hysteroscopy, curettage and cystoscopyin the evaluation of postmenopausal bleeding. *J Obstet Gynaecol* 1995; **15**: 259–262.

30. Loverro G, Bettocchi S, Vicino M, Selvaggi L. Diagnosis of endometrial hyperplasia in women with abnormal uterine bleeding. *Acta Eur Fertil* 1994; **25**: 23–25.

31. Timmermans A, Opmeer BC, Veersema S, Mol BW. Patients' preferences in the evaluation of postmenopausal bleeding. *Br J Obstet Gynaecol* 2007; **114**: 1146–1149.

32. Panda JK. One-stop clinic for postmenopausal bleeding. *J Reprod Med* 2002; **47**: 761–766.

33. Smith-Bindman R, Weiss E, Feldstein V. How thick is too thick? When endometrial thickness should prompt biopsy in postmenopausal women without vaginal bleeding. *Ultrasound Obstet Gynecol* 2004; **24**: 558–565.

34. McGurgan P, Taylor LJ, Duffy SR, O'Donovan PJ. Are endometrial polyps from pre-menopausal women similar to post-menopausal women? An immunohistochemical comparison of endometrial polyps from pre- and post-menopausal women. *Maturitas* 2006; **54**: 277–284.

35. Kelly P, Dobbs SP, McCluggage WG. Endometrial hyperplasia involving endometrial polyps: report of a series and discussion of the significance in an endometrial biopsy specimen. *Br J Obstet Gynaecol* 2007; **114**: 944–950.

36. Martin-Ondarza C, Gil-Moreno A, Torres-Cuesta L *et al*. Endometrial cancer in polyps: a clinical study of 27 cases. *Eur J Gynaecol Oncol* 2005; **26**: 55–58.

37. Hammond R, Johnson J. Endometrial hyperplasia. *Curr Obstet Gynaecol* 2004; **14**: 99–103.
38. Hunter JE, Tritz DE, Howell MG *et al*. The prognostic and therapeutic implications of cytologic atypia in patients with endometrial hyperplasia. *Gynecol Oncol* 1994; **55**: 66–71.
39. Kurman RJ, Kaminski PF, Norris HJ. The behavior of endometrial hyperplasia. A long-term study of 'untreated' hyperplasia in 170 patients. *Cancer* 1985; **56**: 403–412.
40. Eichner E, Abellera M. Endometrial hyperplasia treated by progestins. *Obstet Gynecol* 1971; **38**: 739–742.
41. Wheeler DT, Bristow RE, Kurman RJ. Histologic alterations in endometrial hyperplasia and well-differentiated carcinoma treated with progestins. *Am J Surg Pathol* 2007; **31**: 988–998.
42. Wildemeersch D, Janssens D, Pylyser K *et al*. Management of patients with non-atypical and atypical endometrial hyperplasia with a levonorgestrel-releasing intrauterine system: long-term follow-up. *Maturitas* 2007; **57**: 210–213.
43. Horn LC, Schnurrbusch U, Bilek K, Hentschel B, Einenkel J. Risk of progression in complex and atypical endometrial hyperplasia: clinicopathologic analysis in cases with and without progestogen treatment. *Int J Gynecol Cancer* 2004; **14**: 348–353.
44. Lethaby A, Farquhar C, Sarkis A, Roberts H, Jepson R, Barlow D. Hormone replacement therapy in postmenopausal women: endometrial hyperplasia and irregular bleeding. Cochrane Database Syst Rev 2000; (2): CD000402.
45. Barrett-Connor E. Hormone replacement therapy. *BMJ* 1998; **317**: 457–461.
46. Archer DF, Pickar JH, Bottiglioni F. Bleeding patterns in postmenopausal women taking continuous combined or sequential regimens of conjugated estrogens with medroxyprogesterone acetate. Menopause Study Group. *Obstet Gynecol* 1994; **83**: 686–692.
47. Nagele F, O'Connor H, Baskett TF, Davies A, Mohammed H, Magos AL. Hysteroscopy in women with abnormal uterine bleeding on hormone replacement therapy: a comparison with postmenopausal bleeding. *Fertil Steril* 1996; **65**: 1145–1150.
48. Smith-Bindman R, Kerlikowske K, Feldstein VA *et al*. Endovaginal ultrasound to exclude endometrial cancer and other endometrial abnormalities. *JAMA* 1998; **280**: 1510–1517.
49. Rutqvist LE, Johansson H, Signomklao T, Johansson U, Fornander T, Wilking N. Adjuvant tamoxifen therapy for early stage breast cancer and second primary malignancies. Stockholm Breast Cancer Study Group. *J Natl Cancer Inst* 1995; **87**: 645–651.
50. Fisher B, Costantino JP, Wickerham DL *et al*. Tamoxifen for prevention of breast cancer: report of the National Surgical Adjuvant Breast and Bowel Project P-1 Study. *J Natl Cancer Inst* 1998; **90**: 1371–1388.
51. Bernstein L, Deapen D, Cerhan JR *et al*. Tamoxifen therapy for breast cancer and endometrial cancer risk. *J Natl Cancer Inst* 1999; **91**: 1654–1662.
52. van Leeuwen FE, Benraadt J, Coebergh JW *et al*. Risk of endometrial cancer after tamoxifen treatment of breast cancer. *Lancet* 1994; **343**: 448–452.
53. Bergman L, Beelen ML, Gallee MP, Hollema H, Benraadt J, van Leeuwen FE. Risk and prognosis of endometrial cancer after tamoxifen for breast cancer. Comprehensive Cancer Centres' ALERT Group. Assessment of Liver and Endometrial cancer Risk following Tamoxifen. *Lancet* 2000; **356**: 881–887.
54. Tepper R, Beyth Y, Altaras MM *et al*. Value of sonohysterography in asymptomatic postmenopausal tamoxifen-treated patients. *Gynecol Oncol* 1997; **64**: 386–391.
55. Love CD, Muir BB, Scrimgeour JB, Leonard RC, Dillon P, Dixon JM. Investigation of endometrial abnormalities in asymptomatic women treated with tamoxifen and an evaluation of the role of endometrial screening. *J Clin Oncol* 1999; **17**: 2050–2054.
56. Franchi M, Ghezzi F, Donadello N, Zanaboni F, Beretta P, Bolis P. Endometrial thickness in tamoxifen-treated patients: an independent predictor of endometrial disease. *Obstet Gynecol* 1999; **93**: 1004–1008.
57. Nabholtz JM, Bonneterre J, Buzdar A, Robertson JF, Thurlimann B. Anastrozole (Arimidex) versus tamoxifen as first-line therapy for advanced breast cancer in postmenopausal women: survival analysis and updated safety results. *Eur J Cancer* 2003; **39**: 1684–1689.
58. Buzdar AU. The ATAC (Arimidex, Tamoxifen, Alone or in Combination) trial: an update. *Clin Breast Cancer* 2004; **5 (Suppl 1)**: S6–S12.

59. Gerber B, Krause A, Reimer T *et al*. Anastrozole versus tamoxifen treatment in postmenopausal women with endocrine-responsive breast cancer and tamoxifen-induced endometrial pathology. *Clin Cancer Res* 2006; **12**: 1245–1250.

60. Epstein E, Jamei B, Lindqvist PG. High risk of cervical pathology among women with postmenopausal bleeding and endometrium < or = 4.4 mm: long-term follow-up results. *Acta Obstet Gynecol Scand* 2006; **85**: 1368–1374.

61. Sasieni P, Adams J, Cuzick J. Benefit of cervical screening at different ages: evidence from the UK audit of screening histories. *Br J Cancer* 2003; **89**: 88–93.

62. Gustafsson L, Sparen P, Gustafsson M *et al*. Low efficiency of cytologic screening for cancer *in situ* of the cervix in older women. *Int J Cancer* 1995; **63**: 804–809.

63. Cruickshank ME, Angus V, Kelly M, McPhee S, Kitchener HC. The case for stopping cervical screening at age 50. *Br J Obstet Gynaecol* 1997; **104**: 586–589.

64. Van Wijngaarden WJ, Duncan ID. Rationale for stopping cervical screening in women over 50. *BMJ* 1993; **306**: 967–971.

65. Cornelison TL, Montz FJ, Bristow RE, Chou B, Bovicelli A, Zeger SL. Decreased incidence of cervical cancer in Medicare-eligible California women. *Obstet Gynecol* 2002; **100**: 79–86.

66. Siebers AG, Verbeek AL, Massuger LF, Grefte JM, Bulten J. Normal appearing endometrial cells in cervical smears of asymptomatic postmenopausal women have predictive value for significant endometrial pathology. *Int J Gynecol Cancer* 2006; **16**: 1069–1074.

67. Geier CS, Wilson M, Creasman W. Clinical evaluation of atypical glandular cells of undetermined significance. *Am J Obstet Gynecol* 2001; **184**: 64–69.

68. Montz FJ. Significance of 'normal' endometrial cells in cervical cytology from asymptomatic postmenopausal women receiving hormone replacement therapy. *Gynecol Oncol* 2001; **81**: 33–39.

69. Abati A, Jaffurs W, Wilder AM. Squamous atypia in the atrophic cervical vaginal smear: a new look at an old problem. *Cancer* 1998; **84**: 218–225.

70. Twu NF, Chen SS. Five-year follow-up of patients with recurrent postmenopausal bleeding. *Zhonghua Yi Xue Za Zhi (Taipei)* 2000; **63**: 628–633.

71. Fliegner JR. The use of hormone assays and transvaginal ultrasound measurement of endometrial thickness in the management of recurrent postmenopausal bleeding. *J Obstet Gynaecol* 1998; **18**: 76–77.

72. Iatrakis G, Diakakis I, Kourounis G *et al*. Postmenopausal uterine bleeding. *Clin Exp Obstet Gynecol* 1997; **24**: 157.

73. Townsend DE, Fields G, McCausland A, Kauffman K. Diagnostic and operative hysteroscopy in the management of persistent postmenopausal bleeding. *Obstet Gynecol* 1993; **82**: 419–421.

74. Gungorduk K, Ulker V, Sahbaz A, Ark C, Tekirdag AI. Postmenopausal tuberculosis endometritis. *Infect Dis Obstet Gynecol* 2007; **2007**: 27028 E-pub.

*Thozhukat Sathyapalan   Stephen L. Atkin*

**18**

# Insulin resistance and polycystic ovary syndrome

Polycystic ovary syndrome (PCOS) is an common disorder of premenopausal women with a prevalence of 5–10% in women of reproductive age.[1,2] Since it was first shown that PCOS was associated with hyperinsulinaemia in 1980,[3] it has become clear that the syndrome has major metabolic as well as reproductive morbidities. The recognition of this association has also stimulated extensive investigation of the relationship between insulin and gonadal function.[4–6] This article will summarise the current understanding of the role of insulin resistance in PCOS.

The association between a disorder of carbohydrate metabolism and hyperandrogenism was first described in 1921 by Achard and Thiers[7] and was called 'the diabetes of bearded women (diabete des femmes a barbe)'. Polycystic ovaries were subsequently described in 1935 by Stein and Leventhal.[8] In 1980, it was reported that women with PCOS, had basal and glucose-stimulated hyperinsulinaemia compared with weight-matched control women, suggesting the presence of insulin resistance.[3] There were significant positive linear correlations between insulin and androgen levels which suggested that this might have aetiological significance. In the mid-1980s, several groups noted that acanthosis nigricans occurred frequently in obese hyperandrogenic women.[9–12] These women had hyperinsulinaemia basally and during an oral glucose tolerance test, compared with appropriately age- and weight-matched control women. The presence of hyperinsulinaemia in PCOS women, independent of obesity, was confirmed by a number of further studies.[13–15]

**Thozhukat Sathyapalan** MRCP
The Michael White Centre for Diabetes and Endocrinology, University of Hull, 220–236 Anlaby Road, Hull HU3 2JX, UK

**Stephen L. Atkin** PhD FRCP (for correspondence)
Professor in Diabetes and Endocrinology, The Michael White Centre for Diabetes and Endocrinology, University of Hull, 220–236 Anlaby Road, Hull HU3 2JX, UK
E-mail: s.l.atkin@hull.ac.uk

Insulin resistance is a metabolic state in which physiological concentrations of insulin produce subnormal effects on glucose homeostasis and utilisation.[16] Although insulin resistance is not a disease, its presence in both obese and non-obese subjects is associated with an increased risk of cardiovascular morbidity and mortality as well as type 2 diabetes mellitus.[17] Obesity, body fat location and muscle mass all have important independent effects on insulin sensitivity.[18-21] Alterations in any of these parameters could potentially contribute to insulin resistance in PCOS. PCOS women have an increased prevalence of obesity,[22] and women with upper, as opposed to lower, body obesity have an increased frequency of hyperandrogenism.[21] Studies in which body composition, assessed by hydrostatic weighing, have been matched to normal control women, and in which lean PCOS women, who had body composition and waist-to-hip girth ratios similar to controls, have confirmed that PCOS women are insulin resistant.[23,24] Women with PCOS are more insulin resistant than are unaffected counterparts matched for body mass index, fat-free body mass, and body fat distribution.[1,25,26]

Obese women with PCOS, particularly those with the abdominal obesity phenotype, are usually more insulin resistance and more hyperinsulinaemic than their normal-weight counterparts.[1,27] Both fasting and glucose-stimulated insulin concentrations are, in fact, significantly higher in obese than in non-obese PCOS subgroups. Accordingly, studies examining insulin sensitivity by using different methods, such as the euglycaemic hyperinsulinaemic clamp technique, the frequent-sample intravenous glucose test and the insulin test have further demonstrated that obese PCOS women have significantly lower insulin sensitivity than their non-obese PCOS counterparts and, therefore, a more severe insulin resistance state.[1,27,28]

## METABOLIC SYNDROME AND PCOS

The consequences of PCOS extend beyond the reproductive axis; women with the disorder are at substantial risk for the development of metabolic and cardiovascular abnormalities similar to those that make up metabolic syndrome.[29] This finding is not surprising, since both PCOS and metabolic syndrome share insulin resistance as a central pathogenetic feature.[30] The PCOS might thus be viewed as a sex-specific form of metabolic syndrome, and the term 'syndrome XX' has been suggested as an apt term to underscore this association.[31]

Metabolic syndrome is a consistent feature of the majority of obese women with PCOS, although it can also be detected in many normal-weight affected women.[1,32] Studies using ATPIII criteria to assess the prevalence of the metabolic syndrome in PCOS women has found prevalence rate ranging from 43% to 46%.[29,33] It has also been described that there is higher free testosterone and lower sex-hormone-binding globulin (SHBG) levels in those women with the metabolic syndrome with respect to those without it, as well as a higher prevalence of acanthosis nigricans and a greater tendency to have a family history of PCOS.[33] These results were in accordance with a cross-sectional, population-based study which reported a different concentration of some sex hormones between premenopausal women with and without the ATPIII defined metabolic syndrome.[34] Therefore, collectively, 82% of PCOS women had at least one feature of metabolic syndrome, a finding consistent with a very large presence of single or grouped metabolic abnormalities in this disorder. Compared to those without any criteria, the other two groups were progressively more obese and had a higher prevalence of the abdominal pattern of fat distribution.

In addition, women presenting with metabolic syndrome were characterised by higher systolic and diastolic blood pressure, higher pulse rate, greater frequency of liver enzyme abnormalities, worsened insulin resistance, higher glycosylated haemoglobin and a more severe hyperandrogenaemia with respect to those without the metabolic syndrome. Taken together, these findings demonstrate that the prevalence of the metabolic syndrome in women with PCOS is higher than that of the general population, regardless of ethnicity and geographical area. They also indicate a strong association between the metabolic syndrome and the hyperandrogenic state.[35]

The cause of obesity in PCOS remains unknown, but obesity is present in at least 30% of cases; in some series, as high as 75%.[36] Women in the US with PCOS generally have a higher body weight than their European counterparts.[2,36–38] This fact has been cited as an explanation for the increase in the incidence of PCOS in the US population – an increase that parallels the increase in obesity.[39] Increased adiposity, particularly visceral adiposity that is reflected by an elevated waist circumference (> 88 cm [35 inches]) or waist-to-hip ratio, has been associated with hyperandrogenaemia, insulin resistance, glucose intolerance, and dyslipidaemia. Attenuation of insulin resistance, whether accomplished by weight loss or with medication, ameliorates (but not necessarily normalises) many of the metabolic aberrations in women with PCOS.[30]

Hypertension develops in some women with PCOS during their reproductive years,[29,40] and sustained hypertension may develop in later life in women with the disorder.[41,42] Reduced vascular compliance[43] and vascular endothelial dysfunction were noted in most,[43–46] but not all,[47] studies of women with PCOS.

Furthermore, the degree of impairment in vascular reactivity is significantly greater than can be explained by obesity alone.[43] Insulin-lowering therapies appear to improve the vascular endothelial dysfunction in patients with PCOS.[45]

A predisposition to macrovascular disease and thrombosis[48,49] in women with PCOS has also been described. A recent study of premenopausal women showed that those with PCOS had a higher prevalence of coronary-artery calcification as detected by electron-beam computed tomography.[50] Increased levels of plasminogen-activator inhibitor type 1 may contribute to this risk.[51–53] Levels of plasminogen-activator inhibitor type 1 in patients with PCOS may exceed those typically seen in type 2 diabetes mellitus.[53] A reduction in insulin levels decreases levels and activity of plasminogen-activator inhibitor type 1.[53]

Hypertriglyceridaemia, increased levels of very low-density lipoprotein and low-density lipoprotein cholesterol, and decreased levels of high-density lipoprotein cholesterol[54] also predispose patients to vascular disease in PCOS. Both insulin resistance and hyperandrogenaemia contribute to this atherogenic lipid profile. Testosterone decreases lipoprotein lipase activity in abdominal fat cells, and insulin resistance impairs the ability of insulin to exert its antilipolytic effects. Although these abnormalities would be expected to increase the morbidity and mortality from coronary artery disease and other vascular disorders in women with PCOS, this has been difficult to establish.[55–57]

# IMPAIRED GLUCOSE TOLERANCE AND PCOS

Studies in American,[58,59] Asian[60] and Italian[61] subjects have also shown that women with PCOS have an increased risk for the selective development of impaired glucose tolerance and type 2 diabetes mellitus, with a tendency to early development of glucose intolerance states,[62] when compared to the general population. The close connection between PCOS and glucose intolerance is further emphasised by the finding of a high prevalence of polycystic ovarian morphology on ultrasound scans in both premenopausal women with type 2 diabetes mellitus[63] and in those with previous gestational diabetes.[64] Similar to the general population,[65] there is evidence that insulin resistance may play a major pathophysiological role in the development of glucose intolerance in PCOS women also. The decrease of insulin sensitivity in PCOS appears, in fact, to be quite similar to that found in patients with type 2 diabetes mellitus and to be relatively independent of obesity, fat distribution and lean body mass.[1,32] However, there is strong evidence that obesity, particularly the abdominal phenotype, *per se* represents an important independent risk factor for glucose intolerance in PCOS women.[28]

Moreover, an impaired early-phase, insulin secretion appears to play a role in the development of glucose intolerance in obese PCOS, at least in Hispanic-American subgroups,[1,66]) particularly when they have a positive family history for diabetes.[66,67] The prevalence of impaired glucose tolerance and type 2 diabetes mellitus in PCOS women living in various cities in Italy[61] was significantly higher than that described in the general population of a similar age,[68] but somewhat lower with respect to that reported in previous studies performed on US or Asian PCOS women.[58–60]

This suggests that environmental factors may play a dominant role in determining individual susceptibility to metabolic disorders, which is probably more important than genetic background, as supported by recent long-term epidemiological studies demonstrating that the appearance of type 2 diabetes mellitus can be prevented by adequate life-style intervention, focusing on dietary habits and increased physical activity.[69,70]

Obese PCOS women had significantly increased glucose levels during an oral glucose tolerance test compared with age- and weight-matched ovulatory hyperandrogenic and control women.[71] There were no significant differences, however, in glucose levels during the oral glucose tolerance test in the non-obese PCOS women compared with age- and weight-matched control women. Interestingly, anovulatory women with PCOS display insulin resistance whereas those with a regular menstrual cycle with symptoms of hyperandrogenism do not demonstrate insulin resistance.[25,72]

The prevalence of glucose intolerance is significantly higher in obese PCOS women of around 30% than in concurrently studied age-, ethnicity-, and weight-matched ovulatory control women which is around 10%.[73] In contrast, it was found that non-obese PCOS women have impaired glucose tolerance only occasionally, consistent with the synergistic negative effect of obesity and PCOS on glucose tolerance.[23,25]

Based on the prevalence of glucose intolerance in women,[68] the prevalence of glucose intolerance in PCOS,[71] and on a conservative estimate of the prevalence of PCOS of around 5%, it can be extrapolated that PCOS-related insulin resistance contributes to approximately 10% of cases of glucose intolerance in premenopausal women.[1]

Although obesity and age substantially increase the risk, impaired glucose tolerance and diabetes are frequent even among non-obese PCOS women (10% and 1.5%, respectively).[58] Other factors found be associated with glucose intolerance are waist-to-hip ratio[58] and family history of type 2 diabetes mellitus.[59,61] The risk of glucose intolerance among PCOS women appears to be equally increased in mixed ethnicities of the US population and Asian PCOS groups.[58–60]

Glucose intolerance is present in as many as 30–40% of obese PCOS women in the US[1] and probably to a lower extent in those living in Europe,[61] whilst it is uncommon in their normal-weight counterparts.[1,74] In any case, the prevalence rate for impaired glucose tolerance in the population of obese PCOS subjects appears to be higher than that reported in population-based studies on the incidence of glucose intolerance in women of similar ages,[68] although epidemiological studies are lacking. These findings indicate that obesity may contribute to determining the insulin-resistant state and may impair glucose tolerance in PCOS.

Although insulin resistance seems to play a determining role in the development of diabetes, the presence of insulin resistance does not immediately imply a concomitant alteration of glucose tolerance. In fact, most obese, insulin-resistant PCOS women still have normal glucose tolerance. However, it has recently been found that PCOS women with impaired glucose tolerance or type 2 diabetes mellitus are significantly more insulin resistant and hyperinsulinaemic than those with normal glucose tolerance, regardless of the presence of obesity.[61]

It has also been reported that the development of states of glucose intolerance can be predicted to a certain extent, since there are early markers such as low birth weight and early menarche age in PCOS, as in the general population.[75,76] Prospective studies in which PCOS women were followed for approximately 10 years have also found that insulin resistance tends to worsen over time, together with an increment of insulin and C-peptide response to an oral glucose challenge, and that, in several cases, glucose intolerance appears.[62] Taken together, these findings strongly support the role of insulin resistance in the development of altered glucose tolerance states in PCOS women.

## TYPE 2 DIABETES MELLITUS AND PCOS

The overall risk of developing type 2 diabetes mellitus was found to be increased 3–7-fold in patients with PCOS.[42,55,58,71] The study in postmenopausal women with a history of PCOS found a 15% prevalence of type 2 diabetes mellitus.[42] Oligomenorrhoea was found to be a risk factor for the development of type 2 diabetes mellitus and this risk was accentuated, but not totally explained, by obesity.[77] Thus PCOS poses a major risk factor for type 2 diabetes mellitus in women, regardless of age.

Of women with PCOS, 30–40% have impaired glucose tolerance, and as many as 10% have type 2 diabetes mellitus by their fourth decade.[58,59,78] These prevalence rates are among the highest known among women of similar age.[79] An enhanced rate of deterioration in glucose tolerance is also evident in PCOS.[59,80]

Insulin resistance alone cannot fully account for the predisposition to, and development of, type 2 diabetes mellitus among patients with PCOS. In patients with normal glucose tolerance, insulin secretion is (by definition) sufficient for the degree of insulin resistance; when the pancreatic β-cell is no longer able to compensate sufficiently, glucose tolerance begins to deteriorate.[81,82] Most women with PCOS are able to compensate fully for their insulin resistance, but a substantial proportion (particularly those with a first-degree relative with type 2 diabetes mellitus[66]) have a disordered and insufficient β-cell response to meals or a glucose challenge.[66,83–86] Before the development of frank glucose intolerance, defects in insulin secretion may be latent and revealed only in circumstances that augment insulin resistance, as with the development of gestational diabetes in pregnancy[87] or glucose intolerance associated with glucocorticoid administration.[85]

## GESTATIONAL DIABETES AND PCOS

An association between gestational diabetes and PCOS has also been observed. The prevalence of polycystic ovarian morphology in women with previous gestational diabetes is significantly higher than control women (41–52%).[64,87,88] These observations reinforce the increased risk of developing type 2 diabetes mellitus in later life.

## BIOLOGICAL VARIATION OF INSULIN RESISTANCE IN PATIENTS WITH PCOS

It was found that the intra-individual variation of insulin resistance using HOMA is higher in patients with PCOS compared to normal controls. In PCOS subjects, there was a wide degree of variation of the value of insulin resistance both as a group and between each individual within the group; that is, the inter-individual as well as intra-individual variations were high.

As a consequence, at any level of insulin resistance, a subsequent sample must rise by more than 322% or fall by more than 31% to be considered significantly different from the first. insulin resistance, measured using the homeostasis model assessment model, is significantly greater and more variable for overweight patients with PCOS.[89] It has been also shown that, for patients with PCOS, SHBG is an integrated marker of insulin resistance that may be of use to identify insulin-resistant individuals for targeted treatment with insulin-sensitising agents.[90]

## INSULIN RESISTANCE IN PATIENTS WITH POLYCYSTIC OVARIES

The polycystic ovary morphology (detected by ultrasonography) has been reported to be inherited as an autosomal dominant, if premature balding is used as the male phenotype.[91] It was found that Caribbean Hispanic women have twice the prevalence of PCOS compared with other ethnic groups.[92] Brothers, as well as sisters, of PCOS women can be insulin resistant.[93] The insulin resistant sisters usually also have PCOS.[132] Finally, in 50% of PCOS women, defects in insulin receptor phosphorylation persist in cultured cells.[94] All of these observations support the hypothesis that there is a genetic component to PCOS and the insulin resistance associated with it. Caribbean Hispanic women are also significantly more insulin resistant than non-Hispanic White women by euglycaemic clamp determination of insulin-mediated glucose disposal.[92] PCOS independently further decreases insulin action. Non-Hispanic White PCOS women have similar degrees of insulin resistance to Caribbean Hispanic normal ovulatory women.[92] These findings suggest that the increased prevalence of PCOS in this ethnic group may be secondary to an increased prevalence of insulin resistance.

Hyperinsulinaemia resulting from a spectrum of defects in insulin action, at least some of which are genetic, may play a permissive role in the development of PCOS in genetically susceptible women. Polycystic ovaries may secrete excessive androgens when hyperinsulinaemia and/or insulin resistance are also present. This hypothesis is supported by the finding of the full-blown PCOS (hyperandrogenism and anovulation) primarily in women with polycystic ovaries who are also hyperinsulinaemic.[72,95]

## DEFECTS OF INSULIN SECRETION, ACTION AND CLEARANCE IN PCOS

### BETA-CELL DYSFUNCTION IN PCOS

In the presence of peripheral insulin resistance, pancreatic β-cell insulin secretion increases in a compensatory fashion. Type 2 diabetes mellitus develops when the compensatory increase in insulin levels is no longer sufficient to maintain euglycaemia.[96,97] Under normal circumstances, the relationship of β-cell function and peripheral insulin sensitivity is constant.[81,96] This relationship can be quantified as the product of insulin sensitivity and first-phase insulin release known as the disposition index.[96]

Fasting hyperinsulinaemia is present in obese PCOS women and this is, in part, secondary to increased basal insulin secretion rates. Insulin responses to an oral glucose load are increased in lean and obese PCOS women, but acute insulin responses to an intravenous glucose load, first-phase insulin secretion, are similar to weight-matched control women.[71,86]

When the relationship between insulin secretion and sensitivity is examined, lean and obese PCOS women fall below the relationship in weight-matched control women, and the disposition index is significantly decreased by PCOS as well as by obesity.[92] It has been shown that there are defects in β-cell entrainment to an oscillatory glucose infusion and decreased meal-related insulin secretory responses in PCOS further confirming β-cell dysfunction.[66,83]

These defects are much more pronounced in PCOS women who have a first-degree relative with type 2 diabetes mellitus, suggesting that such women may be at particularly high risk to develop glucose intolerance.[66] There are reports of increased insulin secretion in PCOS, but these studies have not examined insulin secretion in the context of insulin sensitivity and/or have included women in whom the diagnosis was made on the basis of ovarian morphological changes rather than endocrine criteria.[98,99] In summary, the most compelling evidence suggests that β-cell dysfunction, in addition to insulin resistance, is a feature of PCOS.

Studies examining the extent of insulin secretion in relation to insulin sensitivity have demonstrated that a β-cell dysfunction may co-exist with insulin resistance in obese PCOS women. In particular, a defective early phase β-cell insulin secretion and a reduced insulin secretory response to boluses or graded intravenous infusion of glucose, when expressed in relation to the degree of insulin resistance, have been reported in these women.[62,86] Notably, these findings have been described in Hispanic-American insulin-resistant obese PCOS women, but not in PCOS women living in Europe or in Mediterranean areas.[61,100]). It is, therefore, possible that several environmental factors, such as habitual diet or other life-style behaviour, may be involved in this difference.

## DEFECTS OF INSULIN ACTION IN PCOS

Euglycaemic glucose clamp studies have demonstrated significant and substantial decreases in insulin-mediated glucose disposal in PCOS.[23,25] This decrease of around 35–40% is of a similar magnitude to that seen in type 2 diabetes mellitus.

Studies in cultured cells have confirmed the impression from *in vivo* studies that an intrinsic defect in insulin action is present in PCOS.[94] Basal hepatic glucose production and the $ED_{50}$ value of insulin for suppression of hepatic glucose production are significantly increased only in obese PCOS women.[23,25] This synergistic negative effect of obesity and PCOS on hepatic glucose production is an important factor in the pathogenesis of glucose intolerance.[23,25,71,101] This is analogous to type 2 diabetes mellitus in general, where defects in insulin action, presumably genetic, synergise with environmentally induced insulin resistance, primarily obesity-related, to produce glucose intolerance.[102,103]

Sequential multiple-insulin-dose euglycaemic clamp studies have indicated that the $ED_{50}$ insulin for glucose uptake is significantly increased, and that maximal rates of glucose disposal are significantly decreased in lean and in obese PCOS women.[23] It appears, however, that body fat has a more pronounced negative effect on insulin sensitivity in women with PCOS.[24,98]

There were significant decreases in insulin-mediated glucose disposal in both lean and obese PCOS women.[23,25,92] Similarly, it was found that there is significant decreases in insulin sensitivity determined by modified frequently sampled intravenous glucose tolerance test with minimal model analysis in such PCOS women.[24,86] Insulin resistance has been found in PCOS women of many racial and ethnic groups including Japanese, Caribbean and Mexican Hispanics, non-Hispanic Whites, and African Americans.[23,92,104,105]

## DEFECTS OF INSULIN CLEARANCE IN PCOS

Hyperinsulinaemia can result from decreases in insulin clearance as well as from increased insulin secretion. Decreased insulin clearance is usually present in insulin-resistant states since insulin clearance is receptor-mediated, and acquired decreases in receptor number and/or function are often present in insulin resistance secondary to hyperinsulinaemia and/or hyperglycaemia.[106,107] Thus, PCOS would be expected to be associated with decreases in insulin clearance.

Direct measurement of post-hepatic insulin clearance during euglycaemic clamp studies has not been abnormal in PCOS.[25,92] Circulating insulin to C-peptide molar ratios are increased in PCOS, suggesting decreased hepatic extraction of insulin, but such ratios also reflect insulin secretion.[13,108] Direct measurement of hepatic insulin clearance in non-PCOS hyperandrogenic women has found it to be decreased.[109]

In PCOS women, it was found that there is decreased hepatic insulin extraction by model analysis of C-peptide levels.[83] Therefore, in PCOS, hyperinsulinaemia is probably the result of a combination of increased basal insulin secretion and decreased hepatic insulin clearance.

## DEFECTS IN CELLULAR MECHANISMS OF INSULIN ACTION

Insulin acts on cells by binding to its cell surface receptor.[102,110,111] The insulin receptor belongs to a family of protein tyrosine kinase receptors that includes the insulin-like growth factor-I (IGF-I) receptor, with which it shares substantial sequence and structural homology, as well as epidermal growth factor (EGF), fibroblast growth factor, platelet-derived growth factor, and colony-stimulating factor-1 receptors.[112] A variety of phosphorylation–dephosphorylation signalling cascades are then activated, leading to the pleiotropic actions of insulin.

Insulin has numerous target tissue actions, such as stimulation of glucose uptake, gene regulation, DNA synthesis, and amino acid uptake.[102,110] Insulin receptor numbers and affinities of receptors for insulin have been shown to be normal in women with PCOS.[113,114] Therefore, abnormalities in sub-cellular signalling of insulin are a more probable mechanism for insulin resistance. Several investigators have found that adipocytes from women with PCOS have down-regulated insulin-stimulated glucose transport early in the insulin signalling pathway.[94,115,116] These cells also have decreased insulin-stimulated lipolysis.[115]

It was also found that fibroblasts isolated from women with PCOS displayed decreased serine autophosphorylation of the insulin receptor.[94] These data suggest that there is a defect in the serine kinase regulating this activity in women with PCOS. Other studies support the concept that increased free fatty acids in women with PCOS at least contribute to the insulin resistance of muscle, liver and adipose tissue.

There is evidence that women with PCOS have abnormalities in processing a non-classical mediator of insulin action called D-chiro-inositolphosphoglycan (DCI-IPG); this is an inositolphosphoglycan known to be present in the muscle and adipose tissue of primates and humans.[117] Insulin stimulates the intracellular transport of this mediator via G-protein activation[118] and, once intracellular, DCI-IPG can directly increase pyruvate dehydrogenase activity and increase glucose utilisation.[119,120] Type 2 diabetic men have been shown to be deficient in DCI-IPG as compared to normal men.[117] In one study, it was found that women with PCOS treated with D-chiro-inositol (DCI), a synthetic mediator of DCI-IPG, can reduce insulin resistance and androgen production and increase ovulatory rates in women with PCOS.[121] It was also found that metformin increases insulin-stimulated DCI-IPG activity in women with PCOS.[122] These data support the concept that more than one pathway may lead to insulin resistance in PCOS, including a non-classical mechanism of insulin action.

Insulin may directly increase theca-cell production of testosterone by affecting sub-cellular substrates of androgen production. For instance, metformin given to women with PCOS decreases the activity of the rate-limiting enzyme in testosterone synthesis, cytochrome P450-17-alpha (gene CYP17). In line with this hypothesis, it is demonstrated that decreased insulin-stimulated phosphorylation of mitogen-activated protein kinase (MEK) 1/2 and extracellular regulated kinase (ERK) 1/2 in the MAP kinase pathway from theca cells of women in PCOS as compared to normal resulting in increased expression of CYP17.[123] Other *in vitro* studies have also confirmed up-regulation of CYP17 activity in theca cells of women with PCOS, although a mutation in CYP17 itself has not been identified.[124]

In addition to insulin resistance *per se*, there are a number of epiphenomena that occur in response to improving insulin resistance in women with PCOS that seem to suggest that insulin's action on the ovary may not be the only mechanism by which insulin acts to induce hyperandrogenism in these women. For example, insulin-like growth factor 1 (IGF-1) can also stimulate ovarian androgen production.[125–127] It has been suggested that insulin-sensitising drugs reduce ovarian androgen production by decreasing free IGF-1 levels.[128–132] Insulin itself has also been shown to decrease sex hormone binding globulin (SHBG) production from liver and can, in turn, increase free testosterone concentrations in women with PCOS.[133–137] Indeed, insulin-sensitising therapy has been shown to increase SHBG and decrease free testosterone in women with PCOS.[136,138–144]

Although the mechanisms of insulin resistance in PCOS have not been specifically elucidated, it is clear that insulin resistance plays a significant role in the pathogenesis of this disease. Unfortunately, there are really no reliable out-patient tests of insulin resistance to quantify this in any one individual, as random insulin levels and fasting glucose-to-insulin ratios have notoriously poor correlation to the gold standard, the euglycaemic clamp. Since it seems clear that insulin resistance is present in many women with PCOS, it is of questionable value to measure insulin resistance *per se* in PCOS. Given the risk for metabolic syndrome and diabetes in these women, it is prudent to screen patients for abnormal glucose tolerance particularly in obese patients with a body mass index greater than 30 kg/m$^2$, or others with a family history of type 2 diabetes mellitus, which may help prevent atherosclerosis and type 2 diabetes mellitus. However, even with dyslipidaemia, these subjects have a low cardiovascular risk; unless there is a family history for premature cardiovascular disease, screening of fasting lipids is unnecessary as treatment with prophylactic statin therapy likely in these patients is unproven.

## HYPERINSULINAEMIA AND HYPERANDROGENISM IN PCOS

IGF-I is produced by human ovarian tissue, and IGF-I receptors are present in the ovary.[145,146] Insulin in high concentrations can mimic IGF-I actions by occupancy of the IGF-I receptor.[147,148] and this has been a proposed mechanism for insulin-mediated hyperandrogenism.[4,5] However, it has recently been shown that insulin has specific actions on steroidogenesis acting through its own receptor.[149] Moreover, these actions appear to be preserved in insulin-resistant states,[149,150] presumably because of differences in receptor sensitivity to this insulin action or because of differential regulation of the receptor in this tissue.

Studies in which insulin levels have been lowered for prolonged periods have been much more informative. This has been accomplished for 7 days to 3 months with agents that either decrease insulin secretion (diazoxide[151] or somatostatin[152]) or that improve insulin sensitivity (metformin[153] or troglitazone[154]). Circulating androgen levels have decreased significantly in women with PCOS in these studies. Sex hormone binding globulin (SHBG) levels have increased,[151,154] compatible with a major role for insulin in regulating hepatic production of this protein.[155,156] However, oestrogen levels also decreased significantly, suggesting that insulin has diffuse effects on steroidogenesis.[154]

In summary, studies in which insulin levels have been lowered by a variety of modalities indicate that hyperinsulinaemia augments androgen production in PCOS. Moreover, this action appears to be directly mediated by insulin acting through its cognate receptor rather than by spill-over occupancy of the IGF-I receptor. Intrinsic abnormalities in steroidogenesis appear to be necessary for this insulin action to be manifested, since lowering insulin levels does not affect circulating androgen levels in normal women. Further, in many PCOS women, lowering insulin levels ameliorates. but does not abolish. hyperandrogenism.

On the other hand, modest hyperandrogenism characteristic of PCOS may contribute to the associated insulin resistance. Additional factors are necessary to explain the insulin resistance, since suppressing androgen levels does not completely restore normal insulin sensitivity.[157,158] Further, androgen administration does not produce insulin resistance of the same magnitude as that seen in PCOS.[23,25,159] Finally, there are clearly defects in insulin action that persist in cultured PCOS skin fibroblasts removed from the hormonal milieu for generations.[94]

## LEPTIN IN PCOS

Leptin, the recently identified product of the *ob* gene,[160] has been investigated in PCOS. Since leptin is a fat cell product that acts on the hypothalamus,[160] it could link the metabolic and neuro-endocrine derangements characteristic of PCOS. Leptin production is regulated by insulin and could be modulated in insulin-resistant PCOS women via this mechanism. An initial report suggested that leptin levels were elevated in some PCOS women.[161] However, in this study the confounding effects of differences in body weight were not adjusted for appropriately. Subsequent studies in PCOS that have contained appropriately weight- or fat mass-matched control women have not found significant differences in leptin levels in PCOS women.[162,163]

## WEIGHT LOSS AND IMPROVEMENT OF INSULIN RESISTANCE IN PCOS

Since a high percentage of PCOS patients are obese, the role of weight loss in the management of this syndrome may be significant. The literature is encouraging on this point, although most studies have not included a control group;[164,165] statistical samples have also been small[100,166,167] and heterogeneous[164] but all studies agree that weight loss has a positive effect on hyperinsulinaemia in women with PCOS. The effect did not seem to require great weight loss, but became evident with losses of 2–5%.[168] In addition to a reduction in insulin resistance, weight loss also involves a parallel improvement in endocrine status of PCOS patients. Significant improvements in hirsutism and ovulation, with restoration of regular cycles and an increased incidence of spontaneous pregnancies in 30% of patients, have also been reported.[100,164–167]

A significant reduction in total T and A, with increased SHBG and reduced free T, are also reported. Some authors found a reduction in basal levels of LH,[164] which, together with the increase in SHBG and reduced levels of insulin, could explain the improvement in hyperandrogenism in obese women with PCOS.

The selective cannabinoid type-1 (CB1) receptor blocker, rimonabant, has been shown to reduce weight, insulin resistance and other features of metabolic syndrome[169,170] and might prove useful for treatment for PCOS.

## THE ROLE OF INSULIN SENSITISERS IN PCOS

A reduction in insulin levels pharmacologically ameliorates sequelae of both hyperinsulinaemia and hyperandrogenaemia. The place of insulin-reduction therapies in treating PCOS is evolving. These therapies can effectively manage the established metabolic derangements in PCOS, but whether they can prevent them is not yet established.

Both metformin and thiazolidinediones have been used to reduce insulin resistance. Although metformin appears to influence ovarian steroidogenesis directly,[171,172] this effect does not appear to be primarily responsible for the attenuation of ovarian androgen production in women with PCOS. Rather, metformin inhibits the output of hepatic glucose, necessitating a lower insulin concentration and, thereby, probably reducing the androgen production of theca cells. Subject characteristics and control measures for effects of weight change, dose of metformin, and outcome vary widely among published studies of metformin in PCOS.

Metformin also improved fasting insulin levels, blood pressure, and levels of low-density lipoprotein cholesterol.[173] These effects were judged to be independent of any changes in weight that were associated with metformin, but controversy persists as to whether the beneficial effects of metformin are entirely independent of the weight loss[174] that is typically seen early in the course of therapy. Finally, the rates of spontaneous miscarriage and gestational diabetes are reportedly lower among women with PCOS who conceive while taking metformin.[175–178] However, the long-term effects of metformin in pregnancy are unknown.

In one recent randomised trial involving 626 infertile women with PCOS with metformin, clomiphene or a combination, clomiphene was superior to metformin in achieving live birth although metformin significantly reduced body weight, insulin resistance and hyperandrogenaemia compared to clomiphene[179] suggesting that reduction of insulin resistance alone does not improve fertility.

The thiazolidinediones improve the action of insulin in the liver, skeletal muscle, and adipose tissue and have only a modest effect on hepatic glucose output. As with metformin, the thiazolidinediones are reported to affect ovarian steroid synthesis directly, although most evidence indicates that the reduction in insulin levels is responsible for decreased concentrations of circulating androgen.[180] Obese women with PCOS who took troglitazone had consistent improvements in insulin resistance, hyperandrogenaemia, and glucose tolerance.[51,154]

In addition, troglitazone treatment was associated with a relative improvement in pancreatic β-cell function and a reduction in levels of the prothrombotic factor plasminogen-activator inhibitor type 1.[51] These findings led to a double-blind, randomised, placebo-controlled study of troglitazone in PCOS.[36] Ovulation was significantly greater for women who received troglitazone than for those who received placebo; free testosterone levels decreased, and levels of sex hormone-binding globulin increased in a dose-dependent fashion. Nearly all glycaemic measures showed dose-related decreases with troglitazone treatment. Although troglitazone is no longer available, subsequent studies using rosiglitazone[181,182] and pioglitazone[183] have had similar results. Because of concern about using thiazolidinediones in pregnancy, the drugs have been less readily adopted for routine clinical use.

Somatostatin is a 14-amino acid endogenous hypothalamic peptide with a short half-life that, besides blunting the LH response to gonadotropin-releasing hormone (GnRH) and decreasing growth hormone (GH) pituitary secretion,[111] inhibits pancreatic insulin release.[184] Somatostatin analogues should, therefore, be potential drugs for the treatment of PCOS. A few prospective, non-controlled, short-term studies using octreotide[185–190] confirmed these findings and definitively demonstrated the ability of octreotide to reduce insulin levels in PCOS patients. These studies also showed that administration of octreotide in PCOS improved pulsatile gonadotropin patterns, reduced LH, androgen and IGF-I levels,[114–121] and increased spontaneous and stimulated ovulation.[191]

Unfortunately, the daily multiple s.c. injections required by the short life of octreotide makes this procedure inappropriate for long-term treatment. In a placebo-controlled study to evaluate the effect of prolonged therapy with a long-acting somatostatin analogue formulation release (octreotide-LAR), injected i.m. every 28 days, in a selected group of anovulatory PCOS women with abdominal obesity.[192] The addition of octreotide-LAR significantly amplified the effects of a low-calorie diet in decreasing fasting and glucose-stimulated insulin levels and the insulin-resistant state. Moreover, androgen, GH and IGF-1 concentrations were reduced, while the circulating levels of IGF binding proteins 1–3 were increased by octreotide-LAR. This treatment also significantly improved hirsutism and acanthosis nigricans, and, interestingly, presented particularly strong efficacy in improving the ovulatory rate, as all women treated with octreotide-LAR ovulated, compared to only one of those receiving placebo. An additional advantage of this formulation is a lowering in the occurrence of side-effects, such as gallstone formation.

## References

1. Dunaif A. Insulin resistance and the polycystic ovary syndrome: mechanism and implications for pathogenesis. *Endocr Rev* 1997; **18**: 774–800.
2. Franks S. Polycystic ovary syndrome: a changing perspective. *Clin Endocrinol (Oxf)* 1989; **31**: 87–120.
3. Burghen GA, Givens JR, Kitabchi AE. Correlation of hyperandrogenism with

hyperinsulinism in polycystic ovarian disease. *J Clin Endocrinol Metab* 1980; **50**: 113–116.

4.  Barbieri RL, Ryan KJ. Hyperandrogenism, insulin resistance, and acanthosis nigricans syndrome: a common endocrinopathy with distinct pathophysiologic features. *Am J Obstet Gynecol* 1983; **147**: 90–101.

5.  Poretsky L, Kalin MF. The gonadotropic function of insulin. *Endocr Rev* 1987; **8**: 132–141.

6.  Poretsky L. On the paradox of insulin-induced hyperandrogenism in insulin-resistant states. *Endocr Rev* 1991; **12**: 3–13.

7.  Achard C Thiers J. Le virilisme pilaire et son association a l'insuffisance glycolytique (diabete des femmes abarb). *Bull Acad Natl Med* 1921; **86**: 51–64.

8.  Stein IF. Amenorrhea associated with bilateral polycystic ovaries. *Am J Obstet Gynecol* 1935; **29**: 181–191.

9.  Flier JS, Eastman RC, Minaker KL, Matteson D, Rowe JW. Acanthosis nigricans in obese women with hyperandrogenism. Characterization of an insulin-resistant state distinct from the type A and B syndromes. *Diabetes* 1985; **34**: 101–107.

10. Dunaif A, Hoffman AR, Scully RE *et al*. Clinical, biochemical, and ovarian morphologic features in women with acanthosis nigricans and masculinization. *Obstet Gynecol* 1985; **66**: 545–552.

11. Stuart CA, Peters EJ, Prince MJ, Richards G, Cavallo A, Meyer 3rd WJ. Insulin resistance with acanthosis nigricans: the roles of obesity and androgen excess. *Metabolism* 1986; **35**: 197–205.

12. Peters EJ, Stuart CA, Prince MJ. Acanthosis nigricans and obesity: acquired and intrinsic defects in insulin action. *Metabolism* 1986; **35**: 807–813.

13. Pasquali R, Venturoli S, Paradisi R, Capelli M, Parenti M, Melchionda N. Insulin and C-peptide levels in obese patients with polycystic ovaries. *Horm Metab Res* 1982; **14**: 284–287.

14. Shoupe D, Kumar DD, Lobo RA. Insulin resistance in polycystic ovary syndrome. *Am J Obstet Gynecol* 1983; **147**: 588–592.

15. Chang RJ, Nakamura RM, Judd HL, Kaplan SA. Insulin resistance in nonobese patients with polycystic ovarian disease. *J Clin Endocrinol Metab* 1983; **57**: 356–359.

16. Reaven GM. Banting Lecture 1988. Role of insulin resistance in human disease. *Diabetes* 1988; **37**: 1595–1607.

17. Reaven G. Metabolic syndrome: pathophysiology and implications for management of cardiovascular disease. *Circulation* 2002; **106**: 286–288.

18. Yki-Jarvinen H, Koivisto VA. Effects of body composition on insulin sensitivity. *Diabetes* 1983; **32**: 965–969.

19. Bogardus C, Lillioja S, Mott DM, Hollenbeck C, Reaven G. Relationship between degree of obesity and in vivo insulin action in man. *Am J Physiol* 1985; **248**: E286–E291.

20. Caro JF, Dohm LG, Pories WJ, Sinha MK. Cellular alterations in liver, skeletal muscle, and adipose tissue responsible for insulin resistance in obesity and type II diabetes. *Diabetes Metab Rev* 1989; **5**: 665–689.

21. Kissebah AH, Peiris AN. Biology of regional body fat distribution: relationship to non-insulin-dependent diabetes mellitus. *Diabetes Metab Rev* 1989; **5**: 83–109.

22. Goldzieher JW, Green JA. The polycystic ovary. I. Clinical and histologic features. *J Clin Endocrinol Metab* 1962; **22**: 325–338.

23. Dunaif A, Segal KR, Shelley DR, Green G, Dobrjansky A, Licholai T. Evidence for distinctive and intrinsic defects in insulin action in polycystic ovary syndrome. *Diabetes* 1992; **41**: 1257–1266.

24. Morales AJ, Laughlin GA, Butzow T, Maheshwari H, Baumann G, Yen SS. Insulin, somatotropic, and luteinizing hormone axes in lean and obese women with polycystic ovary syndrome: common and distinct features. *J Clin Endocrinol Metab* 1996; **81**: 2854–2864.

25. Dunaif A, Segal KR, Futterweit W, Dobrjansky A. Profound peripheral insulin resistance, independent of obesity, in polycystic ovary syndrome. *Diabetes* 1989; **38**: 1165–1174.

26. Dunaif A, Wu X, Lee A, Diamanti-Kandarakis E. Defects in insulin receptor signaling *in vivo* in the polycystic ovary syndrome (PCOS). *Am J Physiol* 2001; **281**: E392–E399.

27. Pasquali R, Casimirri F. The impact of obesity on hyperandrogenism and polycystic ovary syndrome in premenopausal women. *Clin Endocrinol (Oxf)* 1993; **39**: 1–16.

28. Gambineri A, Pelusi C, Vicennati V, Pagotto U, Pasquali R. Obesity and the polycystic ovary syndrome. *Int J Obes Relat Metab Disord* 2002; **26**: 883–896.

29. Glueck CJ, Papanna R, Wang P, Goldenberg N, Sieve-Smith L. Incidence and treatment of metabolic syndrome in newly referred women with confirmed polycystic ovarian syndrome. *Metabolism* 2003; **52**: 908–915.

30. Ehrmann DA. Polycystic ovary syndrome. *N Engl J Med* 2005; **352**: 1223–1236.

31. Sam S, Dunaif A. Polycystic ovary syndrome: syndrome XX? *Trends Endocrinol Metab* 2003; **14**: 365–370.

32. Poretsky L, Cataldo NA, Rosenwaks Z, Giudice LC. The insulin-related ovarian regulatory system in health and disease. *Endocr Rev* 1999; **20**: 535–582.

33. Apridonidze T, Essah PA, Iuorno MJ, Nestler JE. Prevalence and characteristics of the metabolic syndrome in women with polycystic ovary syndrome. *J Clin Endocrinol Metab* 2005; **90**: 1929–1935.

34. Korhonen S, Hippelainen M, Vanhala M, Heinonen S, Niskanen L. The androgenic sex hormone profile is an essential feature of metabolic syndrome in premenopausal women: a controlled community-based study. *Fertil Steril* 2003; **79**: 1327–1334.

35. Pasquali R, Gambineri A. Insulin-sensitizing agents in polycystic ovary syndrome. *Eur J Endocrinol* 2006; **154**: 763–775.

36. Azziz R, Ehrmann D, Legro RS *et al.* Troglitazone improves ovulation and hirsutism in the polycystic ovary syndrome: a multicenter, double blind, placebo-controlled trial. *J Clin Endocrinol Metab* 2001; **86**: 1626–1632.

37. Conway GS, Honour JW, Jacobs HS. Heterogeneity of the polycystic ovary syndrome: clinical, endocrine and ultrasound features in 556 patients. *Clin Endocrinol (Oxf)* 1989; **30**: 459–470.

38. Carmina E, Legro RS, Stamets K, Lowell J, Lobo RA Difference in body weight between American and Italian women with polycystic ovary syndrome: influence of the diet. *Hum Reprod* 2003; **18**: 2289–2293.

39. Mokdad AH, Ford ES, Bowman BA *et al.* Prevalence of obesity, diabetes, and obesity-related health risk factors, 2001. *JAMA* 2003; **289**: 76–79.

40. Zimmermann S, Phillips RA, Dunaif A *et al.* Polycystic ovary syndrome: lack of hypertension despite profound insulin resistance. *J Clin Endocrinol Metab* 1992; **75**: 508–513.

41. Dahlgren E, Janson PO, Johansson S, Lapidus L, Oden A. Polycystic ovary syndrome and risk for myocardial infarction. Evaluated from a risk factor model based on a prospective population study of women. *Acta Obstet Gynecol Scand* 1992; **71**: 599–604.

42. Dahlgren E, Johansson S, Lindstedt G *et al.* Women with polycystic ovary syndrome wedge resected in 1956 to 1965: a long-term follow-up focusing on natural history and circulating hormones. *Fertil Steril* 1992; **57**: 505–513.

43. Kelly CJ, Speirs A, Gould GW, Petrie JR, Lyall H, Connell JM. Altered vascular function in young women with polycystic ovary syndrome. *J Clin Endocrinol Metab* 2002; **87**: 742–746.

44. Paradisi G, Steinberg HO, Hempfling A *et al.* Polycystic ovary syndrome is associated with endothelial dysfunction. *Circulation* 2001; **103**: 1410–1415.

45. Paradisi G, Steinberg HO, Shepard MK, Hook G, Baron AD. Troglitazone therapy improves endothelial function to near normal levels in women with polycystic ovary syndrome. *J Clin Endocrinol Metab* 2003; **88**: 576–580.

46. Orio Jr F, Palomba S, Cascella T *et al.* Early impairment of endothelial structure and function in young normal-weight women with polycystic ovary syndrome. *J Clin Endocrinol Metab* 2004; **89**: 4588–4593.

47. Mather KJ, Verma S, Corenblum B, Anderson TJ. Normal endothelial function despite insulin resistance in healthy women with the polycystic ovary syndrome. *J Clin Endocrinol Metab* 2000; **85**: 1851–1856.

48. Yildiz BO, Haznedaroglu IC, Kirazli S, Bayraktar M. Global fibrinolytic capacity is decreased in polycystic ovary syndrome, suggesting a prothrombotic state. *J Clin Endocrinol Metab* 2002; **87**: 3871–3875.

49. Orio Jr F, Palomba S, Spinelli L *et al.* The cardiovascular risk of young women with polycystic ovary syndrome: an observational, analytical, prospective case-control study. *J Clin Endocrinol Metab* 2004; **89**: 3696–3701.

50. Christian RC, Dumesic DA, Behrenbeck T, Oberg AL, Sheedy 2nd PF, Fitzpatrick LA. Prevalence and predictors of coronary artery calcification in women with polycystic ovary syndrome. *J Clin Endocrinol Metab* 2003; **88**: 2562–2568.

51. Ehrmann DA, Schneider DJ, Sobel BE *et al.* Troglitazone improves defects in insulin action,

insulin secretion, ovarian steroidogenesis, and fibrinolysis in women with polycystic ovary syndrome. *J Clin Endocrinol Metab* 1997; **82**: 2108–2116.

52. Dahlgren E, Janson PO, Johansson S, Lapidus L, Lindstedt G, Tengborn L. Hemostatic and metabolic variables in women with polycystic ovary syndrome. *Fertil Steril* 1994; **61**: 455–460.

53. Atiomo WU, Bates SA, Condon JE, Shaw S, West JH, Prentice AG. The plasminogen activator system in women with polycystic ovary syndrome. *Fertil Steril* 1998; **69**: 236–241.

54. Talbott E, Guzick D, Clerici A *et al.* Coronary heart disease risk factors in women with polycystic ovary syndrome. *Arterioscler Thromb Vasc Biol* 1995; **15**: 821–826.

55. Wild S, Pierpoint T, Jacobs H, McKeigue P. Long-term consequences of polycystic ovary syndrome: results of a 31 year follow-up study. *Hum Fertil (Camb)* 2000; **3**: 101–105.

56. Talbott EO, Zborowskii JV, Boudraux MY. Do women with polycystic ovary syndrome have an increased risk of cardiovascular disease? Review of the evidence. *Minerva Ginecol* 2004; **56**: 27–39.

57. Legro RS. Polycystic ovary syndrome and cardiovascular disease: a premature association? *Endocr Rev* 2003; **24**: 302–312.

58. Legro RS, Kunselman AR, Dodson WC, Dunaif A. Prevalence and predictors of risk for type 2 diabetes mellitus and impaired glucose tolerance in polycystic ovary syndrome: a prospective, controlled study in 254 affected women. *J Clin Endocrinol Metab* 1999; **84**: 165–169.

59. Ehrmann DA, Barnes RB, Rosenfield RL, Cavaghan MK, Imperial J. Prevalence of impaired glucose tolerance and diabetes in women with polycystic ovary syndrome. *Diabetes Care* 1999; **22**: 141–146.

60. Weerakiet S, Srisombut C, Bunnag P, Sangtong S, Chuangsoongnoen N, Rojanasakul A. Prevalence of type 2 diabetes mellitus and impaired glucose tolerance in Asian women with polycystic ovary syndrome. *Int J Gynaecol Obstet* 2001; **75**: 177–184.

61. Gambineri A, Pelusi C, Manicardi E *et al.* Glucose intolerance in a large cohort of Mediterranean women with polycystic ovary syndrome: phenotype and associated factors. *Diabetes* 2004; **53**: 2353–2358.

62. Pasquali R, Gambineri A, Anconetani B *et al.* The natural history of the metabolic syndrome in young women with the polycystic ovary syndrome and the effect of long-term oestrogen-progestagen treatment. *Clin Endocrinol (Oxf)* 1999; **50**: 517–527.

63. Conn JJ, Jacobs HS, Conway GS. The prevalence of polycystic ovaries in women with type 2 diabetes mellitus. *Clin Endocrinol (Oxf)* 2000; **52**: 81–86.

64. Holte J, Gennarelli G, Wide L, Lithell H, Berne C. High prevalence of polycystic ovaries and associated clinical, endocrine, and metabolic features in women with previous gestational diabetes mellitus. *J Clin Endocrinol Metab* 1998; **83**: 1143–1150.

65. DeFronzo RA, Ferrannini E. Insulin resistance. A multifaceted syndrome responsible for NIDDM, obesity, hypertension, dyslipidemia, and atherosclerotic cardiovascular disease. *Diabetes Care* 1991; **14**: 173–194.

66. Ehrmann DA, Sturis J, Byrne MM, Karrison T, Rosenfield RL, Polonsky KS. Insulin secretory defects in polycystic ovary syndrome. Relationship to insulin sensitivity and family history of non-insulin-dependent diabetes mellitus. *J Clin Invest* 1995; **96**: 520–527.

67. Colilla S, Cox NJ, Ehrmann DA. Heritability of insulin secretion and insulin action in women with polycystic ovary syndrome and their first degree relatives. *J Clin Endocrinol Metab* 2001; **86**: 2027–2031.

68. Harris MI, Hadden WC, Knowler WC, Bennett PH. Prevalence of diabetes and impaired glucose tolerance and plasma glucose levels in U.S. population aged 20–74 yr. *Diabetes* 1987; **36**: 523–534.

69. Norris SL, Zhang X, Avenell A *et al.* Long-term effectiveness of lifestyle and behavioral weight loss interventions in adults with type 2 diabetes: a meta-analysis. *Am J Med* 2004; **117**: 762–774.

70. Kanaya AM, Narayan KM. Prevention of type 2 diabetes: data from recent trials. *Prim Care* 2003; **30**: 511–526.

71. Dunaif A, Graf M, Mandeli J, Laumas V, Dobrjansky A. Characterization of groups of hyperandrogenic women with acanthosis nigricans, impaired glucose tolerance, and/or hyperinsulinemia. *J Clin Endocrinol Metab* 1987; **65**: 499–507.

72. Robinson S, Kiddy D, Gelding SV *et al.* The relationship of insulin insensitivity to

menstrual pattern in women with hyperandrogenism and polycystic ovaries. *Clin Endocrinol (Oxf)* 1993; **39**: 351–355.

73. Quintana B CV, Sieber J, Fultz P, George N, Dunaif A. High risk glucose intolerance (GI) in women with oligomenorrhea (oligo) or with polycystic ovary syndrome (PCOS). Program of the 77th Annual Meeting of The Endocrine Society, Washington DC. 1995; Abstract OR3-5:50.

74. Pasquali R, Patton L, Pagotto U, Gambineri A. Metabolic alterations and cardiovascular risk factors in the polycystic ovary syndrome. *Minerva Ginecol* 2005; **57**: 79–85.

75. Hofman PL, Cutfield WS, Robinson EM *et al.* Insulin resistance in short children with intrauterine growth retardation. *J Clin Endocrinol Metab* 1997; **82**: 402–406.

76. Phillips DI. Insulin resistance as a programmed response to fetal undernutrition. *Diabetologia* 1996; **39**: 1119–1122.

77. Solomon CG, Hu FB, Dunaif A *et al.* Long or highly irregular menstrual cycles as a marker for risk of type 2 diabetes mellitus. *JAMA* 2001; **286**: 2421–2426.

78. Nelson VL, Qin Kn KN, Rosenfield RL *et al.* The biochemical basis for increased testosterone production in theca cells propagated from patients with polycystic ovary syndrome. *J Clin Endocrinol Metab* 2001; **86**: 5925–5933.

79. Krosnick A. The diabetes and obesity epidemic among the Pima Indians. *N Engl J Med* 2000; **97**: 31–37.

80. Norman RJ, Masters L, Milner CR, Wang JX, Davies MJ. Relative risk of conversion from normoglycaemia to impaired glucose tolerance or non-insulin dependent diabetes mellitus in polycystic ovarian syndrome. *Hum Reprod* 2001; **16**: 1995–1998.

81. Kahn SE, Prigeon RL, McCulloch DK *et al.* Quantification of the relationship between insulin sensitivity and beta-cell function in human subjects. Evidence for a hyperbolic function. *Diabetes* 1993; **42**: 1663–1672.

82. Polonsky KS, Sturis J, Bell GI. Seminars in Medicine of the Beth Israel Hospital, Boston. Non-insulin-dependent diabetes mellitus – a genetically programmed failure of the beta cell to compensate for insulin resistance. *N Engl J Med* 1996; **334**: 777–783.

83. O'Meara NM, Blackman JD, Ehrmann DA *et al.* Defects in beta-cell function in functional ovarian hyperandrogenism. *J Clin Endocrinol Metab* 1993; **76**: 1241–1247.

84. Ehrmann DA, Breda E, Cavaghan MK *et al.* Insulin secretory responses to rising and falling glucose concentrations are delayed in subjects with impaired glucose tolerance. *Diabetologia* 2002; **45**: 509–517.

85. Ehrmann DA, Breda E, Corcoran MC *et al.* Impaired beta-cell compensation to dexamethasone-induced hyperglycemia in women with polycystic ovary syndrome. *Am J Physiol* 2004; **287**: E241–E246.

86. Dunaif A, Finegood DT. Beta-cell dysfunction independent of obesity and glucose intolerance in the polycystic ovary syndrome. *J Clin Endocrinol Metab* 1996; **81**: 942–947.

87. Kousta E, Cela E, Lawrence N *et al.* The prevalence of polycystic ovaries in women with a history of gestational diabetes. *Clin Endocrinol (Oxf)* 2000; **53**: 501–507.

88. Anttila L, Karjala K, Penttila RA, Ruutiainen K, Ekblad U. Polycystic ovaries in women with gestational diabetes. *Obstet Gynecol* 1998; **92**: 13–16.

89. Jayagopal V, Kilpatrick ES, Holding S, Jennings PE, Atkin SL. The biological variation of insulin resistance in polycystic ovarian syndrome. *J Clin Endocrinol Metab* 2002; **87**: 1560–1562.

90. Jayagopal V, Kilpatrick ES, Jennings PE, Hepburn DA, Atkin SL. The biological variation of testosterone and sex hormone-binding globulin (SHBG) in polycystic ovarian syndrome: implications for SHBG as a surrogate marker of insulin resistance. *J Clin Endocrinol Metab* 2003; **88**: 1528–1533.

91. Carey AH, Chan KL, Short F, White D, Williamson R, Franks S. Evidence for a single gene effect causing polycystic ovaries and male pattern baldness. *Clin Endocrinol (Oxf)* 1993; **38**: 653–658.

92. Dunaif A, Sorbara L, Delson R, Green G. Ethnicity and polycystic ovary syndrome are associated with independent and additive decreases in insulin action in Caribbean-Hispanic women. *Diabetes* 1993; **42**: 1462–1468.

93. Norman RJ, Masters S, Hague W. Hyperinsulinemia is common in family members of women with polycystic ovary syndrome. *Fertil Steril* 1996; **66**: 942–947.

94. Dunaif A, Xia J, Book CB, Schenker E, Tang Z. Excessive insulin receptor serine phosphorylation in cultured fibroblasts and in skeletal muscle. A potential mechanism for insulin resistance in the polycystic ovary syndrome. *J Clin Invest* 1995; **96**: 801–810.

95. Sampson M, Kong C, Patel A, Unwin R, Jacobs HS. Ambulatory blood pressure profiles and plasminogen activator inhibitor (PAI-1) activity in lean women with and without the polycystic ovary syndrome. *Clin Endocrinol (Oxf)* 1996; **45**: 623–629.

96. Bergman RN, Phillips LS, Cobelli C. Physiologic evaluation of factors controlling glucose tolerance in man: measurement of insulin sensitivity and beta-cell glucose sensitivity from the response to intravenous glucose. *J Clin Invest* 1981; **68**: 1456–1467.

97. Bergman RN. Lilly lecture 1989. Toward physiological understanding of glucose tolerance. Minimal-model approach. *Diabetes* 1989; **38**: 1512–1527.

98. Holte J, Bergh T, Berne C, Berglund L, Lithell H. Enhanced early insulin response to glucose in relation to insulin resistance in women with polycystic ovary syndrome and normal glucose tolerance. *J Clin Endocrinol Metab* 1994; **78**: 1052–1058.

99. Weber RF, Pache TD, Jacobs ML *et al.* The relation between clinical manifestations of polycystic ovary syndrome and beta-cell function. *Clin Endocrinol (Oxf)* 1993; **38**: 295–300.

100. Holte J, Bergh T, Berne C, Wide L, Lithell H. Restored insulin sensitivity but persistently increased early insulin secretion after weight loss in obese women with polycystic ovary syndrome. *J Clin Endocrinol Metab* 1995; **80**: 2586–2593.

101. Dunaif A. Hyperandrogenic anovulation (PCOS): a unique disorder of insulin action associated with an increased risk of non-insulin-dependent diabetes mellitus. *Am J Med* 1995; **98**: 33S–39S.

102. Kahn CR. Banting Lecture. Insulin action, diabetogenes, and the cause of type II diabetes. *Diabetes* 1994; **43**: 1066–1084.

103. DeFronzo RA. Lilly lecture 1987. The triumvirate: beta-cell, muscle, liver. A collusion responsible for NIDDM. *Diabetes* 1988; **37**: 667–687.

104. Carmina E, Koyama T, Chang L, Stanczyk FZ, Lobo RA. Does ethnicity influence the prevalence of adrenal hyperandrogenism and insulin resistance in polycystic ovary syndrome? *Am J Obstet Gynecol* 1992; **167**: 1807–1812.

105. Norman RJ, Mahabeer S, Masters S. Ethnic differences in insulin and glucose response to glucose between white and Indian women with polycystic ovary syndrome. *Fertil Steril* 1995; **63**: 58–62.

106. Flier JS, Minaker KL, Landsberg L, Young JB, Pallotta J, Rowe JW. Impaired *in vivo* insulin clearance in patients with severe target-cell resistance to insulin. *Diabetes* 1982; **31**: 132–135.

107. Marshall S. Kinetics of insulin receptor internalization and recycling in adipocytes. Shunting of receptors to a degradative pathway by inhibitors of recycling. *J Biol Chem* 1985; **260**: 4136–4144.

108. Mahabeer S, Jialal I, Norman RJ, Naidoo C, Reddi K, Joubert SM. Insulin and C-peptide secretion in non-obese patients with polycystic ovarian disease. *Horm Metab Res* 1989; **21**: 502–506.

109. Peiris AN, Mueller RA, Struve MF, Smith GA, Kissebah AH. Relationship of androgenic activity to splanchnic insulin metabolism and peripheral glucose utilization in premenopausal women. *J Clin Endocrinol Metab* 1987; **64**: 162–169.

110. Cheatham B, Kahn CR. Insulin action and the insulin signaling network. *Endocr Rev* 1995; **16**: 117–142.

111. Kahn CR. The molecular mechanism of insulin action. *Annu Rev Med* 1985; **36**: 429–451.

112. Ullrich A, Schlessinger J. Signal transduction by receptors with tyrosine kinase activity. *Cell* 1990; **61**: 203–212.

113. Conway GS, Avey C, Rumsby G. The tyrosine kinase domain of the insulin receptor gene is normal in women with hyperinsulinaemia and polycystic ovary syndrome. *Hum Reprod* 1994; **9**: 1681–1683.

114. Tarkun I, Arslan BC, Canturk Z, Turemen E, Sahin T, Duman C. Endothelial dysfunction in young women with polycystic ovary syndrome: relationship with insulin resistance and low-grade chronic inflammation. *J Clin Endocrinol Metab* 2004; **89**: 5592–5596.

115. Rosenbaum D, Haber RS, Dunaif A. Insulin resistance in polycystic ovary syndrome:

decreased expression of GLUT-4 glucose transporters in adipocytes. *Am J Physiol* 1993; **264**: E197–E202.

116. Ciaraldi TP, Morales AJ, Hickman MG, Odom-Ford R, Olefsky JM, Yen SS. Cellular insulin resistance in adipocytes from obese polycystic ovary syndrome subjects involves adenosine modulation of insulin sensitivity. *J Clin Endocrinol Metab* 1997; **82**: 1421–1425.

117. Asplin I, Galasko G, Larner J. Chiro-inositol deficiency and insulin resistance: a comparison of the chiro-inositol- and the myo-inositol-containing insulin mediators isolated from urine, hemodialysate, and muscle of control and type II diabetic subjects. *Proc Natl Acad Sci USA* 1993; **90**: 5924–5928.

118. Sleight S, Wilson BA, Heimark DB, Larner J. G(q/11) is involved in insulin-stimulated inositol phosphoglycan putative mediator generation in rat liver membranes: co-localization of G(q/11) with the insulin receptor in membrane vesicles. *Biochem Biophys Res Commun* 2002; **295**: 561–569.

119. Ortmeyer HK, Huang LC, Zhang L, Hansen BC, Larner J. Chiroinositol deficiency and insulin resistance. II. Acute effects of D-chiroinositol administration in streptozotocin-diabetic rats, normal rats given a glucose load, and spontaneously insulin-resistant rhesus monkeys. *Endocrinology* 1993; **132**: 646–651.

120. Ortmeyer HK, Larner J, Hansen BC. Effects of D-chiroinositol added to a meal on plasma glucose and insulin in hyperinsulinemic rhesus monkeys. *Obes Res* 1995; **3 (Suppl 4)**: 605S–608S.

121. Nestler JE, Jakubowicz DJ, Reamer P, Gunn R, Allan G. Effects of D-chiroinositol (INS-1) on insulin, glucose and spontaneous ovulation in obese women with polycystic ovary syndrome (PCOS). 58th Scientific Sessions of the American Diabetes Association, A91, 1988; abstract 0353.

122. Baillargeon JP, Iuorno MJ, Jakubowicz DJ, Apridonidze T, He N, Nestler JE. Metformin therapy increases insulin-stimulated release of D-chiro-inositol-containing inositolphosphoglycan mediator in women with polycystic ovary syndrome. *J Clin Endocrinol Metab* 2004; **89**: 242–249.

123. Nelson-Degrave VL, Wickenheisser JK, Hendricks KL *et al*. Alterations in mitogen-activated protein kinase kinase and extracellular regulated kinase signaling in theca cells contribute to excessive androgen production in polycystic ovary syndrome. *Mol Endocrinol* 2005; **19**: 379–390.

124. Daneshmand S, Weitsman SR, Navab A, Jakimiuk AJ, Magoffin DA. Overexpression of theca-cell messenger RNA in polycystic ovary syndrome does not correlate with polymorphisms in the cholesterol side-chain cleavage and 17alpha-hydroxylase/C(17-20) lyase promoters. *Fertil Steril* 2002; **77**: 274–280.

125. Homburg R, Pariente C, Lunenfeld B, Jacobs HS. The role of insulin-like growth factor-1 (IGF-1) and IGF binding protein-1 (IGFBP-1) in the pathogenesis of polycystic ovary syndrome. *Hum Reprod* 1992; **7**: 1379–1383.

126. Mason HD, Margara R, Winston RM, Seppala M, Koistinen R, Franks S. Insulin-like growth factor-I (IGF-I) inhibits production of IGF-binding protein-1 while stimulating estradiol secretion in granulosa cells from normal and polycystic human ovaries. *J Clin Endocrinol Metab* 1993; **76**: 1275–1279.

127. Nahum R, Thong KJ, Hillier SG. Metabolic regulation of androgen production by human thecal cells *in vitro*. *Hum Reprod* 1995; **10**: 75–81.

128. De Leo V, La Marca A, Orvieto R, Morgante G. Effect of metformin on insulin-like growth factor (IGF) I and IGF-binding protein I in polycystic ovary syndrome. *J Clin Endocrinol Metab* 2000; **85**: 1598–1600.

129. Kowalska I, Kinalski M, Straczkowski M, Wolczyski S, Kinalska I. Insulin, leptin, IGF-I and insulin-dependent protein concentrations after insulin-sensitizing therapy in obese women with polycystic ovary syndrome. *Eur J Endocrinol* 2001; **144**: 509–515.

130. Stadtmauer LA, Toma SK, Riehl RM, Talbert LM. Metformin treatment of patients with polycystic ovary syndrome undergoing *in vitro* fertilization improves outcomes and is associated with modulation of the insulin-like growth factors. *Fertil Steril* 2001; **75**: 505–509.

131. Ibanez L, Aulesa C, Potau N, Ong K, Dunger DB, de Zegher F. Plasminogen activator inhibitor-1 in girls with precocious pubarche: a premenarcheal marker for polycystic ovary syndrome? *Pediatr Res* 2002; **51**: 244–248.

132. Pawelczyk L, Spaczynski RZ, Banaszewska B, Duleba AJ. Metformin therapy increases insulin-like growth factor binding protein-1 in hyperinsulinemic women with polycystic ovary syndrome. *Eur J Obstet Gynecol Reprod Biol* 2004; **113**: 209–213.

133. Buyalos RP, Geffner ME, Watanabe RM, Bergman RN, Gornbein JA, Judd HL. The influence of luteinizing hormone and insulin on sex steroids and sex hormone-binding globulin in the polycystic ovarian syndrome. *Fertil Steril* 1993; **60**: 626–633.

134. Fendri S, Arlot S, Marcelli JM, Dubreuil A, Lalau JD. Relationship between insulin sensitivity and circulating sex hormone-binding globulin levels in hyperandrogenic obese women. *Int J Obes Relat Metab Disord* 1994; **18**: 755–759.

135. Ebeling P, Stenman UH, Seppala M, Koivisto VA. Acute hyperinsulinemia, androgen homeostasis and insulin sensitivity in healthy man. *J Endocrinol* 1995; **146**: 63–69.

136. Pasquali R, Macor C, Vicennati V *et al.* Effects of acute hyperinsulinemia on testosterone serum concentrations in adult obese and normal-weight men. *Metabolism* 1997; **46**: 526–529.

137. Ciampelli M, Fulghesu AM, Cucinelli F *et al.* Impact of insulin and body mass index on metabolic and endocrine variables in polycystic ovary syndrome. *Metabolism* 1999; **48**: 167–172.

138. Crave JC, Fimbel S, Lejeune H, Cugnardey N, Dechaud H, Pugeat M. Effects of diet and metformin administration on sex hormone-binding globulin, androgens, and insulin in hirsute and obese women. *J Clin Endocrinol Metab* 1995; **80**: 2057–2062.

139. Nestler JE, Jakubowicz DJ. Decreases in ovarian cytochrome P450c17 alpha activity and serum free testosterone after reduction of insulin secretion in polycystic ovary syndrome. *N Engl J Med* 1996; **335**: 617–623.

140. Nestler JE, Jakubowicz DJ. Lean women with polycystic ovary syndrome respond to insulin reduction with decreases in ovarian P450c17 alpha activity and serum androgens. *J Clin Endocrinol Metab* 1997; **82**: 4075–4079.

141. Nestler JE, Jakubowicz DJ, Evans WS, Pasquali R. Effects of metformin on spontaneous and clomiphene-induced ovulation in the polycystic ovary syndrome. *N Engl J Med* 1998; **338**: 1876–1880.

142. Diamanti-Kandarakis E, Kouli CR, Bergiele AT *et al.* A survey of the polycystic ovary syndrome in the Greek island of Lesbos: hormonal and metabolic profile. *J Clin Endocrinol Metab* 1999; **84**: 4006–4011.

143. Chou KH, von Eye Corleta H, Capp E, Spritzer PM. Clinical, metabolic and endocrine parameters in response to metformin in obese women with polycystic ovary syndrome: a randomized, double-blind and placebo-controlled trial. *Horm Metab Res* 2003; **35**: 86–91.

144. Glueck CJ, Moreira A, Goldenberg N, Sieve L, Wang P. Pioglitazone and metformin in obese women with polycystic ovary syndrome not optimally responsive to metformin. *Hum Reprod* 2003; **18**: 1618 1625.

145. el-Roeiy A, Chen X, Roberts VJ, LeRoith D, Roberts Jr CT, Yen SS. Expression of insulin-like growth factor-I (IGF-I) and IGF-II and the IGF-I, IGF-II, and insulin receptor genes and localization of the gene products in the human ovary. *J Clin Endocrinol Metab* 1993; **77**: 1411–1418.

146. el-Roeiy A, Chen X, Roberts VJ *et al.* Expression of the genes encoding the insulin-like growth factors (IGF-I and II), the IGF and insulin receptors, and IGF-binding proteins-1-6 and the localization of their gene products in normal and polycystic ovary syndrome ovaries. *J Clin Endocrinol Metab* 1994; **78**: 1488–1496.

147. Froesch ER, Zapf J. Insulin-like growth factors and insulin: comparative aspects. *Diabetologia* 1985; **28**: 485–493.

148. LeRoith D, Werner H, Beitner-Johnson D, Roberts Jr CT. Molecular and cellular aspects of the insulin-like growth factor I receptor. *Endocr Rev* 1995; **16**: 143–163.

149. Willis D, Franks S. Insulin action in human granulosa cells from normal and polycystic ovaries is mediated by the insulin receptor and not the type-I insulin-like growth factor receptor. *J Clin Endocrinol Metab* 1995; **80**: 3788–3790.

150. Willis D, Mason H, Gilling-Smith C, Franks S. Modulation by insulin of follicle-stimulating hormone and luteinizing hormone actions in human granulosa cells of normal and polycystic ovaries. *J Clin Endocrinol Metab* 1996; **81**: 302–309.

151. Nestler JE, Barlascini CO, Matt DW *et al.* Suppression of serum insulin by diazoxide reduces serum testosterone levels in obese women with polycystic ovary syndrome. *J Clin Endocrinol Metab* 1989; **68**: 1027–1032.

152. Prelevic GM, Wurzburger MI, Balint-Peric L, Nesic JS. Inhibitory effect of sandostatin on

secretion of luteinising hormone and ovarian steroids in polycystic ovary syndrome. *Lancet* 1990; **336**: 900–903.

153. Velazquez EM, Mendoza S, Hamer T, Sosa F, Glueck CJ. Metformin therapy in polycystic ovary syndrome reduces hyperinsulinemia, insulin resistance, hyperandrogenemia, and systolic blood pressure, while facilitating normal menses and pregnancy. *Metabolism* 1994; **43**: 647–654.

154. Dunaif A, Scott D, Finegood D, Quintana B, Whitcomb R. The insulin-sensitizing agent troglitazone improves metabolic and reproductive abnormalities in the polycystic ovary syndrome. *J Clin Endocrinol Metab* 1996; **81**: 3299–3306.

155. Plymate SR, Matej LA, Jones RE, Friedl KE. Inhibition of sex hormone-binding globulin production in the human hepatoma (Hep G2) cell line by insulin and prolactin. *J Clin Endocrinol Metab* 1988; **67**: 460–464.

156. Nestler JE. Sex hormone-binding globulin: a marker for hyperinsulinemia and/or insulin resistance? *J Clin Endocrinol Metab* 1993; **76**: 273–274.

157. Dunaif A, Green G, Futterweit W, Dobrjansky A. Suppression of hyperandrogenism does not improve peripheral or hepatic insulin resistance in the polycystic ovary syndrome. *J Clin Endocrinol Metab* 1990; **70**: 699–704.

158. Moghetti P, Tosi F, Castello R *et al*. The insulin resistance in women with hyperandrogenism is partially reversed by antiandrogen treatment: evidence that androgens impair insulin action in women. *J Clin Endocrinol Metab* 1996; **81**: 952–960.

159. Polderman KH, Gooren LJ, Asscheman H, Bakker A, Heine RJ. Induction of insulin resistance by androgens and estrogens. *J Clin Endocrinol Metab* 1994; **79**: 265–271.

160. Caro JF, Sinha MK, Kolaczynski JW, Zhang PL, Considine RV. Leptin: the tale of an obesity gene. *Diabetes* 1996; **45**: 1455–1462.

161. Brzechffa PR, Jakimiuk AJ, Agarwal SK, Weitsman SR, Buyalos RP, Magoffin DA. Serum immunoreactive leptin concentrations in women with polycystic ovary syndrome. *J Clin Endocrinol Metab* 1996; **81**: 4166–4169.

162. Mantzoros CS, Dunaif A, Flier JS. Leptin concentrations in the polycystic ovary syndrome. *J Clin Endocrinol Metab* 1997; **82**: 1687–1691.

163. Laughlin GA, Morales AJ, Yen SS. Serum leptin levels in women with polycystic ovary syndrome: the role of insulin resistance/hyperinsulinemia. *J Clin Endocrinol Metab* 1997; **82**: 1692–1696.

164. Pasquali R, Antenucci D, Casimirri F *et al*. Clinical and hormonal characteristics of obese amenorrheic hyperandrogenic women before and after weight loss. *J Clin Endocrinol Metab* 1989; **68**: 173–179.

165. Kiddy DS, Hamilton-Fairley D, Bush A *et al*. Improvement in endocrine and ovarian function during dietary treatment of obese women with polycystic ovary syndrome. *Clin Endocrinol (Oxf)* 1992; **36**: 105–111.

166. Harlass FE, Plymate SR, Fariss BL, Belts RP. Weight loss is associated with correction of gonadotropin and sex steroid abnormalities in the obese anovulatory female. *Fertil Steril* 1984; **42**: 649–652.

167. Guzick DS, Wing R, Smith D, Berga SL, Winters SJ. Endocrine consequences of weight loss in obese, hyperandrogenic, anovulatory women. *Fertil Steril* 1994; **61**: 598–604.

168. Huber-Buchholz MM, Carey DG, Norman RJ. Restoration of reproductive potential by lifestyle modification in obese polycystic ovary syndrome: role of insulin sensitivity and luteinizing hormone. *J Clin Endocrinol Metab* 1999; **84**: 1470–1474.

169. Pi-Sunyer FX, Aronne LJ, Heshmati HM, Devin J, Rosenstock J, for the RIONASG. Effect of rimonabant, a cannabinoid-1 receptor blocker, on weight and cardiometabolic risk factors in overweight or obese patients: RIO-North America: a randomized controlled trial. *JAMA* 2006; **295**: 761–775.

170. Van Gaal LF, Rissanen AM, Scheen AJ, Ziegler O, Rossner S. Effects of the cannabinoid-1 receptor blocker rimonabant on weight reduction and cardiovascular risk factors in overweight patients: 1-year experience from the RIO-Europe study. *Lancet* 2005; **365**: 1389–1397.

171. Mansfield R, Galea R, Brincat M, Hole D, Mason H. Metformin has direct effects on human ovarian steroidogenesis. *Fertil Steril* 2003; **79**: 956–962.

172. Attia GR, Rainey WE, Carr BR. Metformin directly inhibits androgen production in human thecal cells. *Fertil Steril* 2001; **76**: 517–524.

173. Lord JM, Flight IH, Norman RJ. Insulin-sensitising drugs (metformin, troglitazone, rosiglitazone, pioglitazone, D-chiro-inositol) for polycystic ovary syndrome. Cochrane Database Syst Rev 2003; CD003053

174. Crave JC, Lejeune H, Brebant C, Baret C, Pugeat M. Differential effects of insulin and insulin-like growth factor I on the production of plasma steroid-binding globulins by human hepatoblastoma-derived (Hep G2) cells. *J Clin Endocrinol Metab* 1995; **80**: 1283–1289.

175. Glueck CJ, Phillips H, Cameron D, Sieve-Smith L, Wang P. Continuing metformin throughout pregnancy in women with polycystic ovary syndrome appears to safely reduce first-trimester spontaneous abortion: a pilot study. *Fertil Steril* 2001; **75**: 46–52.

176. Glueck CJ, Goldenberg N, Pranikoff J, Loftspring M, Sieve L, Wang P. Height, weight, and motor-social development during the first 18 months of life in 126 infants born to 109 mothers with polycystic ovary syndrome who conceived on and continued metformin through pregnancy. *Hum Reprod* 2004; **19**: 1323–1330.

177. Glueck CJ, Wang P, Kobayashi S, Phillips H, Sieve-Smith L. Metformin therapy throughout pregnancy reduces the development of gestational diabetes in women with polycystic ovary syndrome. *Fertil Steril* 2002; **77**: 520–525.

178. Glueck CJ, Wang P, Goldenberg N, Sieve-Smith L. Pregnancy outcomes among women with polycystic ovary syndrome treated with metformin. *Hum Reprod* 2002; **17**: 2858–2864.

179. Legro RS, Barnhart HX, Schlaff WD *et al*. Clomiphene, metformin, or both for infertility in the polycystic ovary syndrome. *N Engl J Med* 2007; **356**: 551–566.

180. Mitwally MF, Witchel SF, Casper RF. Troglitazone: a possible modulator of ovarian steroidogenesis. *J Soc Gynecol Invest* 2002; **9**: 163–167.

181. Ghazeeri G, Kutteh WH, Bryer-Ash M, Haas D, Ke RW. Effect of rosiglitazone on spontaneous and clomiphene citrate-induced ovulation in women with polycystic ovary syndrome. *Fertil Steril* 2003; **79**: 562–566.

182. Belli SH, Graffigna MN, Oneto A, Otero P, Schurman L, Levalle OA. Effect of rosiglitazone on insulin resistance, growth factors, and reproductive disturbances in women with polycystic ovary syndrome. *Fertil Steril* 2004; **81**: 624–629.

183. Romualdi D, Guido M, Ciampelli M *et al*. Selective effects of pioglitazone on insulin and androgen abnormalities in normo- and hyperinsulinaemic obese patients with polycystic ovary syndrome. *Hum Reprod* 2003; **18**: 1210–1218.

184. Hsu WH, Xiang HD, Rajan AS, Kunze DL, Boyd 3rd AE. Somatostatin inhibits insulin secretion by a G-protein-mediated decrease in $Ca^{2+}$ entry through voltage-dependent $Ca^{2+}$ channels in the beta cell. *J Biol Chem* 1991; **266**: 837–843.

185. Wurzburger MI, Prelevic GM, Sonksen PH, Balint-Peric LA. The effect of the somatostatin analogue octreotide on growth hormone secretion in insulin-dependent diabetics without residual insulin secretion. *Horm Metab Res* 1992; **24**: 329–332.

186. Prelevic GM, Ginsburg J, Maletic D *et al*. The effects of the somatostatin analogue octreotide on ovulatory performance in women with polycystic ovaries. *Hum Reprod* 1995; **10**: 28–32.

187. Morris RS, Carmina E, Vijod MA, Stanczyk FZ, Lobo RA. Alterations in the sensitivity of serum insulin-like growth factor 1 and insulin-like growth factor binding protein-3 to octreotide in polycystic ovary syndrome. *Fertil Steril* 1995; **63**: 742–746.

188. Fulghesu AM, Lanzone A, Andreani CL, Pierro E, Caruso A, Mancuso S. Effectiveness of a somatostatin analogue in lowering luteinizing hormone and insulin-stimulated secretion in hyperinsulinemic women with polycystic ovary disease. *Fertil Steril* 1995; **64**: 703–708.

189. Morris RS, Karande VC, Dudkiewicz A, Morris JL, Gleicher N. Octreotide is not useful for clomiphene citrate resistance in patients with polycystic ovary syndrome but may reduce the likelihood of ovarian hyperstimulation syndrome. *Fertil Steril* 1999; **71**: 452–456.

190. Ciotta L, De Leo V, Galvani F, La Marca A, Cianci A. Endocrine and metabolic effects of octreotide, a somatostatin analogue, in lean PCOS patients with either hyperinsulinaemia or lean normoinsulinaemia. *Hum Reprod* 1999; **14**: 2951–2958.

191. Wenzl R, Lehner R, Schurz B, Karas H, Huber JC. Successful ovulation induction by sandostatin-therapy of polycystic ovarian disease. *Acta Obstet Gynecol Scand* 1996; **75**: 298–299.

192. Gambineri A, Patton L, De Iasio R *et al*. Efficacy of octreotide-LAR in dieting women with abdominal obesity and polycystic ovary syndrome. *J Clin Endocrinol Metab* 2005; **90**: 3854–3862.

# Index